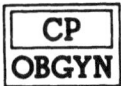 Clinical Perspectives in Obstetrics and Gynecology

Series Editor:

Herbert J. Buchsbaum, M.D.

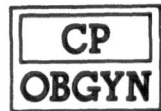 Clinical Perspectives in Obstetrics and Gynecology

perspective *noun:* . . . the capacity to view subjects in their true relations or relative importance.

*Each volume in Clinical Perspectives in Obstetrics and
Gynecology will cover in depth a major clinical area in the
health care of women. The objective is to present to the reader
the pathophysiologic and biochemical basis of the condition
under discussion, and to provide a scientific basis for clinical
management. These volumes are not intended as "how to"
books, but as a ready reference by authorities in the field.*

*Though the obstetrician and gynecologist may be the primary
provider of health care for the female, this role is shared with
family practitioners, pediatricians, medical and surgical
specialists, and geriatricians. It is to all these physicians that
the series is addressed.*

Series Editor: Herbert J. Buchsbaum, M.D.

Buchsbaum (ed.):   *The Menopause*
Aiman (ed.):   *Infertility*

Forthcoming Volumes:

Galask (ed.):   *Infectious Disease in the Female Patient*
Lavery and Sanfilippo (eds.):   *Pediatric and Adolescent Gynecology*

Walter Futterweit, M.D.

Polycystic Ovarian Disease

With 49 Illustrations

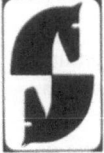

Springer-Verlag
New York Berlin Heidelberg Tokyo

Walter Futterweit, M.D., Associate Clinical Professor of
Medicine, Division of Endocrinology, Department of Medicine,
Mount Sinai School of Medicine of the City University of New
York, 1 Gustave L. Levy Place, New York, New York 10029

Series Editor: Herbert J. Buchsbaum, M.D., Department of Obstetrics and
Gynecology, University of Pittsburgh—Magee Women's Hospital,
Pittsburgh, Pennsylvania 15213

Library of Congress Cataloging in Publication Data
Futterweit, Walter.
    Polycystic ovarian disease.
    (Clinical perspectives in obstetrics and gynecology)
    Bibliography: p.
    1. Stein-Leventhal syndrome. I. Title. II. Series.
[DNLM: 1. Stein-Leventhal syndrome   WP 320 F996p]
RG480.S7F88   1984   618.1'1   84–5324

Typeset by Progressive Typographers, York, Pennsylvania.

9 8 7 6 5 4 3 2 1

ISBN-13: 978-1-4613-8291-1   e-ISBN-13: 978-1-4613-8289-8
DOI: 10.1007/978-1-4613-8289-8

*To Gloria—Lorelle, Stephen, and Debra;
my Grandmother Frieda and my parents*

Contents

Foreword

Polycystic ovarian disease, or polyfollicular ovarian disease, as Dr. Futterweit prefers to call it, is a disease of uncertain etiology and for which numerous modes of therapy have been advanced. Understanding of its pathophysiology should shed light on factors regulating normal ovarian function; the converse is also true.

Recent years have brought about great understanding of the neuroendocrine regulation of gonadal function, as well as of factors in the microenvironment of the ovary which affect its function. It is also appreciated that cases classified as polycystic ovarian disease actually represent a clinical and pathological spectrum which may reflect the effects of diverse etiological factors. In the present volume, Dr. Futterweit presents the fruits of his long interest in and extensive experience with this disease. He thoroughly and thoughtfully reviews the vast amount of basic and clinical information that has been garnered with regard to this condition over the past decade. The numerous theories that have been advanced to explain its etiology are presented in balanced fashion, in addition to a hypothesis, which is well formulated and amenable to clinical testing. His clinical interests and judgment are well represented by his presentation of the diverse manifestations of this condition, the approach to proper diagnosis, and the available therapeutic options.

Patients with this disease represent diagnostic and therapeutic problems in a situation where manifestations of disease may lead to major emotional stress. The availability in this volume of a well-reasoned, balanced review of the problems encountered, and a thorough summary of existing knowledge, should provide a much-needed reference point for focusing on the current state of the art and to foresee the significance of future developments.

Dorothy T. Krieger, M.D., D.Sc.
Director, Division of Endocrinology
Mount Sinai Medical Center
New York

Preface

Galen first described the ovary around 200 A.D. as a "female testis." In 1844, Chereau described a patient with sclerocystic disease of the ovaries. He observed a thick, pearly white sclerotic capsule in ovaries that were removed in the belief that they were diseased or damaged. Partial resection of such ovaries was practiced in Europe by a number of surgeons. This was the beginning of an enthusiastic increase of gynecologic surgery for a variety of disease states. In 1872, Robert Battey, of Georgia, suggested ovarian extirpation "for severe dysmenorrhea, for sufferers of pelvic engorgement and nervous exaltation, excessive menorrhagia, hysteroneurosis, and for those who had a tendency to epilepsy at the time of menstruation." This procedure was to be appropriately known as the "Battey operation." Removal of both ovaries became a popular procedure particularly in cystic degeneration or sclerocystic disease. Fortunately, less radical surgery was later advocated by Pozzi in 1894 and Waldo in 1895 using wedge resection. Although Findley, in America, in 1904 performed bilateral ovariectomy in many cases, he also utilized wedge resection for the treatment of cystic degeneration of the ovaries. Microcystic degeneration was described by Forgue and Massabuau in 1910 as a condition with many pea-sized follicular cysts occupying the cortex of the ovary. Between the years 1929 and 1935, two gynecologists from the Michael Reese Hospital in Chicago, Irving F. Stein and Michael L. Leventhal, noted the presence of polycystic ovaries in some of their patients with amenorrhea. It appears that prior to 1935 instances of amenorrhea usually had been associated with ovarian deficiency and, by inference, with small atrophic ovaries. As a consequence, diagnostic studies of wedge biopsies were performed by Stein and Leventhal and "from an ovarian biopsy, a syndrome was born." In 1935, Stein and Leventhal described a syndrome which consisted of amenorrhea, infertility, and hirsutism associated with bilaterally enlarged cystic ovaries (880). Biopsies of ovaries performed for histologic study revealed that patients incidentally menstruated regularly following this procedure. Observing this interesting phenomenon, Stein advocated wedge resection of the ovaries as the treatment of choice for this syndrome (875,877). It became increasingly clear that the criteria used by Stein and Leventhal were restrictive and that many patients were observed with typical polycystic, albeit not necessarily enlarged, ovaries, who were not hirsute or amenorrheic. Thus the eponym "Stein-Leventhal syndrome" has now only been variably applied to those patients presenting with their previously described criteria. Most prefer to categorize these patients into a wider clinical spectrum of disease called polycystic ovarian disease (PCOD). The delineation of PCOD together with initial medical treatment has yielded good results following ovarian wedge resection and subsequently has made PCOD no less enigmatic 49 years after the initial description of this "syndrome."

The term PCOD is applied to clinically poorly defined heterogeneous entities that are characterized by ovaries that are actually polyfollicular rather than polycystic, and which is usually associated with luteinizing-hormone (LH)-dependent increased androgen secretion. It may also be seen in a variety of disorders including congenital adrenocortical hyperfunction, virilizing tumors of the adrenals, and pituitary tumors. The common thread that binds these diverse syndromes together is a multifollicular ovary in various stages of growth and atresia, usually associated with some thickening of the tunica albuginea. Masculinizing syndromes mimicking ovarian or adrenal virilizing tumors may also be associated with gross features of PCOD with a moderate to severe degree of stromal thecal cell luteinization (ovarian "hyperthecosis"). Although the latter findings may be minimal in most instances of PCOD, extensive stromal luteinization may be associated with virilization, hypertension, massive obesity or diabetes mellitus. Hyperthecosis appears to be at one end of the spectrum of PCOD, the other being asymptomatic fertile women with minimal or no hirsutism who on exploratory laparotomy for a related or unrelated condition are found to have polycystic ovaries. In view of the absence of any absolute clinical or laboratory criteria for the disease, the author has found it useful to reconsider the term PCOD and redefine it as *polyfollicular ovarian disease* (PFOD). This is in keeping with the observation of others who frequently find no pathological difference between the ovaries of normal women and those with polycystic ovarian disease, other than the presence of numerous atretic follicles and a thickened capsule in the latter. The pathogenesis of this spectrum of diseases is elusive, but more evidence is accumulating that it may possibly be genetic with variable expression. In addition, a hypothalamic disturbance may be a factor in its pathogenesis, although the role of increased estrogens produced by peripheral conversion of ovarian and/or adrenal androgens may modulate hypothalamic-pituitary function. In essence, PFOD (or PCOD) is the human model of a "continuous estrus syndrome," with chronic anovulation and/or inappropriate gonadotropin secretion being a hallmark of the disease.

The complexity of polycystic ovarian disease has been well recognized by numerous investigators since it is a multi-faceted entity with no specific clinical signs nor specific histopathological features. In the last 5 to 10 years a number of important developments in the understanding of the control of luteinizing hormone-releasing hormone (LHRH) release, and pituitary modulation of LH and follicle-stimulating hormone (FSH), as well as a more detailed understanding of the microenvironment of the ovary, has led to a better appreciation of the control of ovarian function. The present volume is an attempt to review the many factors involved in the delicate interplay between the hypothalamic-pituitary unit, the adrenal cortex, and the ovary. Research must be oriented so that different subgroups of PCOD may be identified, each with a possible distinct pathogenetic mechanism and treatment. A comprehensive review of the hypothalamic-pituitary-gonadal axis, the clinical and laboratory features, as well as the use of more sophisticated laboratory tools in the diagnosis of polycystic ovarian disease, has been attempted. The various theories of possible pathogenesis of PCOD are critically reviewed and hopefully may direct further research to a better understanding and appropriate treatment of this disease complex. An exhaustive literature review has purposely been prepared to this end.

It is at times difficult to reconcile the various conclusions drawn by many eminent investigators who have contributed so much to our knowledge of PCOD. The fact that PCOD is indeed multi-faceted makes the diversity of proposed etiologic mechanisms an understandable consequence. Perhaps the dictum of Francis Bacon may be worth remembering:

If a man will begin with certainties,
He shall end in doubts,
But if he is content to begin with doubts,
He shall end in certainties.

(Advancement in Learning, Book I; 1605)

My sincerest thanks to Dr. Dorothy Krieger, Chief of the Division of Endocrinology of the Mount Sinai School of Medicine, for her encouragement, helpful comments and criticisms. I am also grateful to Dr. Arthur R. Sohval, Emeritus Clinical Professor of Medicine, Mount Sinai School of Medicine of the City University of New York, for his expert comments on the pathologic anatomy of PCOD, and to Dr. J. Lester Gabrilove, Baumritter Professor of Medicine of the Mount Sinai School of Medicine, for his helpful review of the section on virilizing adrenal and ovarian tumors. I am indebted to Dr. Mamoru Kaneko, Professor of Clinical Pathology of the Mount Sinai School of Medicine for his kind assistance, and to Mr. Richard A. Weiss for his expertise on the word-processor. My thanks to Dr. Christopher Longcope, Professor of Obstetrics and Gynecology and Medicine of the University of Massachusetts Medical School, and Dr. Erlio Gurpide, Professor of Obstetrics and Gynecology of the Mount Sinai School of Medicine, for their helpful data on the sources, metabolic clearance rates, and production rates of sex hormones. I would also like to acknowledge the association of Jeffrey I. Mechanick, third-year student at the Mount Sinai School of Medicine of the City University of New York, in the formulation of the hypothesis of PCOD. My thanks also to Marva Williams for her secretarial assistance.

Finally it is only fitting that I owe a deep sense of gratitude to my many patients who have been afflicted with PCOD and who have contributed in their way to much of what I have learned.

Walter Futterweit

Neuroendocrine Regulation of Gonadal Function

Production and Transport of Hypophysiotropic Hormones

The central nervous system (CNS) has an essential role in regulation of gonadal function. Electric stimulation or anatomic lesions of the hypothalamus can provoke or prevent ovulation. Furthermore, extrahypothalamic structures, such as those in the limbic system are connected functionally and anatomically with the hypothalamus. The hypothalamus controls the function of the anterior pituitary gland by a series of chemical messengers (hypophysiotropic hormones) that are synthesized in specific areas of the hypothalamus. Although many use the term *releasing hormones* for these messengers, they may either inhibit or stimulate the release of anterior pituitary hormones. Hypothalamic and extrahypothalamic neurosecretory neurons are involved in the elaboration of gonadotropin-releasing hormone (GnRH), also called luteinizing hormone-releasing hormone (LHRH), from the hypothalamus (603). This substance with apparent LH- as well as FSH-releasing activity was chemically identified as a decapeptide whose neurons have been located by immunologic and biologic techniques mainly in the arcuate-ventromedial region of the medial basal hypothalamus (MBH) (Fig. 1-1) (495), also in the preoptic suprachiasmatic area (Fig. 1-2) (494), and to some extent in neuronal terminals within the organum vasculosum located at the rostral tip of the third ventricle (99). The LHRH neurons located over the optic chiasm in the preoptic anterior hypothalamic region appear to be stimulated by estrogens to evoke the preovulatory surge of LHRH (positive feedback) (603). Those LHRH neurons located in a more caudal location in the arcuate regions have short axons that project to the median eminence (a specialized portion of the ventral hypothalamus), and may be inhibited by estrogens to bring about the negative feedback. The hypothalamic neurons that secrete and synthesize LHRH integrate neuronal input from higher centers with feedback signals from the developing follicle (see later section of this chapter). Most of the LHRH is stored in secretory granules in the axon terminals. LHRH is transported by a process of axonal flow to its terminals in the region of the median eminence. LHRH and other hypophysiotropic hormones are released there in response to certain stimuli, passing into the portal venous system down the pituitary stalk to the anterior lobe, where they affect the synthesis and release of pituitary hormones.

The anterior pituitary gland is under neural control via release of neurohormones into the primary capillary plexus of the hypophyseal portal system of veins. The primary capillary plexus is located in the median eminence of the tuber cinereum. The capillaries in the median eminence join into portal vessels which run parallel down the hypophyseal stalk and then break up into the adenohypophyseal sinusoids. The sinusoids give rise to the hypophyseal veins which exit from the gland and drain into the cavernous sinus. An area within the organum vasculosum of the lamina terminalis has LHRH present in the neuronal terminals of this structure. Special ependymal cells called tanycytes are in direct contact with the third ventricle.

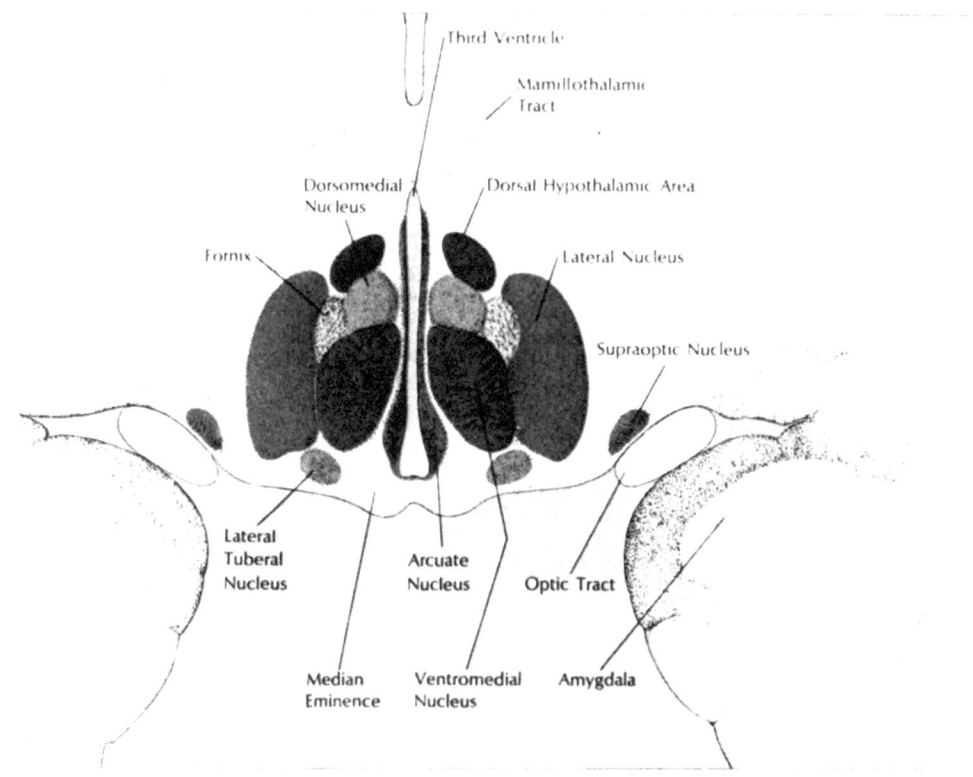

Fig. 1-1. Major nuclear centers of the hypothalamus. (Reprinted by permission from Krieger DT. The hypothalamus and neuroendocrinology. In: Krieger DT, Hughes JC, eds. Neuroendocrinology. Sunderland, Mass: Sinauer Associates, 1980.3–12.) (495).

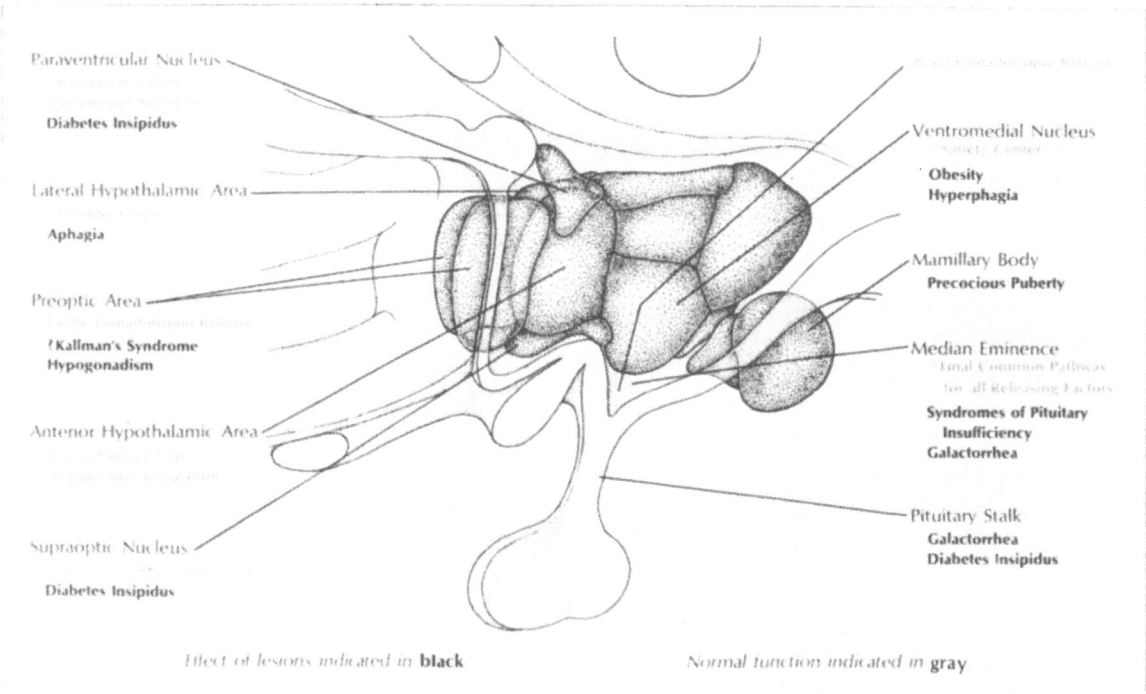

Fig. 1-2. Frontal section of major nuclear centers of the hypothalamus. Lesions in afferent projections to this area as well as in specific hypothalamic sites may result in disturbances of endocrine function. (Reprinted by permission from Krieger DT. The hypothalamus and neuroendocrine pathology. In: Krieger DT, Hughes JC, eds. Neuroendocrinology. Sunderland, Mass: Sinauer Associates, 1980:13–22.) (494).

Thus an alternative delivery system for LHRH may exist to allow it to be released into the cerebrospinal fluid of the third ventricle and to be picked up by tanycytes and transported to external layers of the median eminence and portal vessels. The proposed alternative tanycyte LHRH delivery system is, however, open to question since no major evidence has been presented that LHRH is present in the cerebrospinal fluid (CSF), tanycytes do not contain immunoreactive LHRH, and estrous cyclicity in rats proceeds normally after destruction of the median eminence tanycytes (56).

Activation of LHRH-containing neurons depends upon neurotransmitters such as the biogenic amines, peptides and sex steroids. Neurotransmitters alter gonadotropin release from the anterior pituitary directly or indirectly by affecting release of LHRH from the hypothalamus. The neurotransmitters which may control LHRH release in women include catecholamines, endorphins (endogenous opiate-like peptides) and—probably to a lesser degree—indoleamines (such as melatonin and serotonin), acetylcholine, histamine, neuroactive amino acids (e.g., gamma-aminobutyric acid), and neurogenic peptides such as thyrotropin-releasing hormone (TRH). There appear to be many neural connections to the hypothalamus both excitatory and inhibitory from the midbrain, the limbic system and the rhinencephalic nuclei of the forebrain. Altered activity of these systems profoundly influences hypothalamic neurosecretion. Thus the hypothalamic neurosecretory cell may be considered to be a "final common pathway" representing the terminus of a multisynaptic pathway involved in the regulation of a neurohormone release. "Aminergic" (noradrenergic, serotoninergic and dopaminergic) pathways to the hypothalamus have been identified by histochemical fluorescence techniques.

So far, four distinct hypothalamic releasing (or regulatory) hormones have been fully characterized:

1. thyrotropin-releasing hormone (TRH)
2. luteinizing hormone-releasing hormone (LHRH) (795)
3. growth hormone-release inhibiting hormone (somatostatin)
4. corticotropin releasing factor (CRF) (936)

Hypothalamic extracts and synthetic LHRH have FSH-releasing activity. Although some have reported partial purification of a separate FSH-releasing factor, it is clear that the major FSH-releasing activity in hypothalamic extracts is accounted for by LHRH. Resolution of the question whether a separate releasing hormone for FSH is present will require specific isolation of a factor for FSH.

Luteinizing Hormone-Releasing Hormone (LHRH)

MECHANISM OF ACTION OF LHRH. The decapeptide LHRH produces a brief but prompt release of LH from the pituitary gland within a minute after an injection of a 150 μg bolus intravenously. A peak serum LH usually occurs in 30 minutes. A prolonged effect can be produced by a continuous infusion or by subcutaneous injection. Specific plasma membrane receptors exist on the gonadotropes (pituitary cells specialized to secrete LH or FSH), and the combination of LHRH molecules with these receptors is essential for its action (Fig. 1-3) (603). The increase in LH release is brought about by activation of adenylate cyclase, which results in an increase in intracellular cyclic adenosine monophosphate (cyclic AMP, or cAMP). The cyclic AMP then activates a protein kinase which dephosphorylates membrane proteins, altering the permeability of the cell membrane. An alteration in membrane permeability brings about extrusion of secretory granules that contain stored LH (Fig. 1-4) (603). This process of exocytosis involves fusion of the granule with the cell membrane before the transfer into the extracellular space. As with other pituitary cells, calcium is necessary for the secretory process (156,603). In addition to stimulating release of LH, LHRH also increases its synthesis on the rough endoplasmic reticulum which is packaged into secretory granules by the Golgi apparatus. During exocytosis the mature secretory granule migrates to the cell membrane, with expulsion of the contents into the extracellular space (156).

There is no known specific gonadotropin-binding protein in the blood. Thus all of the circulating LH and FSH is available to clearance. The half-life of LH averages 30 minutes, while that of FSH is about ten times that of LH.

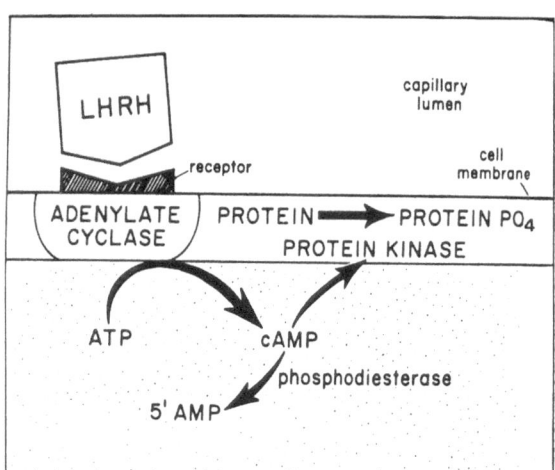

Fig. 1-3. Schematic representation of the mechanism of action of LHRH on the cell membrane of the gonadotropes. ATP = adenosine triphosphate, cAMP = cyclic adenosine monophosphate, AMP = adenosine monophosphate (Reprinted by permission from McCann SM. Luteinizing-Hormone-Releasing-Hormone. N Eng J Med. 1977; 296 797–802.) (603)

3. Intermediate frequency changes of gonadotropins also occur every 24 hours, and are called "diurnal" (circadian). These occur during puberty and are characterized by sleep-related peaks of LH and FSH.

The medial basal hypothalamus (MBH) in the region of the arcuate nucleus (778) is probably the major area of the CNS that controls gonadotropin secretion, the adequacy of negative and positive feedback and the continuation of circhoral pulses of LHRH, LH and FSH. The suprachiasmatic nucleus may perhaps also be involved for adequacy of positive feedback (653).

Studies of collection of hypothalamic-pituitary portal venous blood demonstrates that LHRH is secreted in a pulsatile manner. Knobil and his associates (479) have demonstrated that the pulsatile pattern of LHRH is fundamental

PULSATILE RELEASE OF GONADOTROPINS AND LHRH. Gonadotropins are released in rapid, rhythmic pulses, superimposed on a low level tonic secretion (789) reflecting intermittent hypothalamic stimulation (65). In the castrate individual with removal of the negative feedback of gonadal hormones, release of LH is augmented and occurs in bursts at relatively constant intervals, depending on the species (*ultradian* rhythm of LH release). Three types of gonadotropin secretions may be distinguished based on their frequency of fluctuations in the blood:

1. Low-frequency changes occurring approximately every 30 days; these are called "trigintan," "circatrigintan" or "infradian."
2. High frequency changes superimposed on these low-frequency changes, with pulses repeating themselves every 70–100 minutes; these are called "circhoral." This reflects the fact that they repeat themselves approximately every hour.

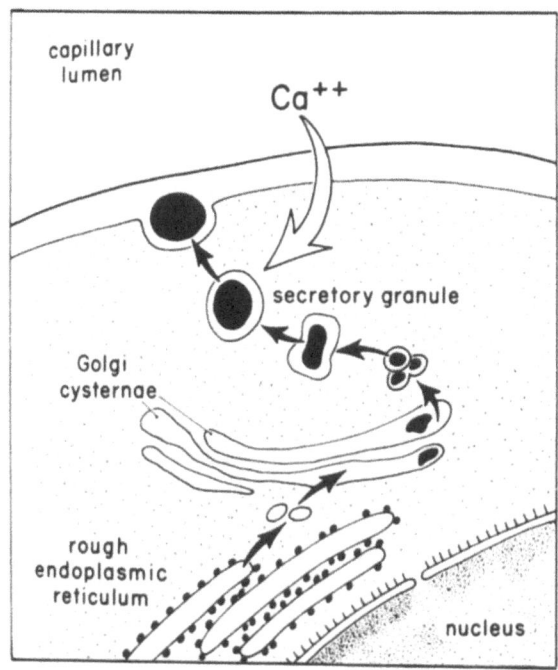

Fig. 1-4. Schematic representation of the pathway of LH biosynthesis and release from the cell by exocytosis. LHRH increases cell permeability to calcium. Uptake of calcium ions is involved in inducing exocytosis (Reprinted by permission from McCann SM. Luteinizing-Hormone-Releasing-Hormone. N Eng J Med. 1977; 296 797–802) (603)

for the control of gonadotropin secretion. Following destruction of the arcuate nucleus or stalk section, pituitary FSH and LH secretion is only activated by administering LHRH in a pulsatile manner (6 minutes on and 54 minutes off). A continuous infusion of LHRH is incapable of stimulating FSH and LH, nor does it allow for the restoration of estrogen induced negative and positive feedback (480).

The dynamic term "pulsatile" is used rather than "episodic" in that incremental changes in LH may occur within five minutes, while the rate of decay for the downside of LH pulses is linear with a mean half-life of 60 minutes. In view of this relatively slow decay, it is probable that the pulsatile component for LH release is superimposed on continuous secretion (743, 1023). A periodicity of approximately 90 minutes is observed in all phases of the menstrual cycle except during the mid and late luteal phases, when the frequency of the pulses is decreased to 3–4 hours intervals. The magnitude of the LH pulses is greatest during the midcycle LH surge and least during the early follicular phase. Since infusions of exogenous estradiol (E_2) rapidly dampen the pulsatile pattern of LH release (1023), it is likely that the change observed between the early and late follicular phase (day 14) is related to feedback modulation of the circulating E_2 from the preovulatory follicle. Progesterone also may have a dampening effect on the central neuronal mechanisms of LH release and thus account for the diminished pulse frequency seen during the mid to late luteal phase.

Unlike LH, pulsatile fluctuations in circulating FSH are poorly defined. However, some minor oscillations are seen during the early follicular phase (with low circulating E_2 levels) and during the midcycle FSH surge.

Direct measurement of LHRH in portal plasma of the pituitary stalk of sectioned rhesus monkeys demonstrates its episodic fluctuation (846). Measurements of immunoreactive LHRH in normal cycling women have recently demonstrated these hourly pulses in plasma (229). A specific and sensitive radioimmunoassay for LHRH has made it possible to measure small amounts of LHRH in human plasma (Table 1-1).

The pulses of LHRH are of a greater magnitude during the periovulatory period than during the follicular and luteal phases of the menstrual cycle, but no difference in the frequency of pulses is noted. These bursts are inhibited by estradiol leading to a fall in plasma LH. Similarly, LHRH release increases at the time of the preovulatory discharge of LH secondary to a rapid rise in estradiol. The latter provides a dramatic example of positive feedback whereby the preovulatory estrogen augments both the release of LHRH and the response of the anterior pituitary to the released LHRH.

TABLE 1-1. Plasma LHRH Levels (pg/ml).

	Mean ± SEM	Range
Normal male	1 6 ± 0 4	<0 3 – 4 0
Normal cycling women		
Follicular phase	1.4 ± 0.1	<0.3 – 4.7
Luteal phase	2 0 ± 0 2	<0 3 – 10 7
Periovulatory phase	10.0 ± 3.5	<0.64 – 34 7

From Elkind-Hirsch K, Ravnikar V, Schiff I, et al Determinations of endogenous immunoreactive luteinizing hormone-releasing hormone in human plasma J Clin Endocrinol Metab 1982, 54 602–607 (229)

INVOLVEMENT OF NEUROTRANSMITTERS IN GONADOTROPIN RELEASE. Many neural inputs converge on the medial basal hypothalamus and operate through synaptic neurotransmitters to effect release of LHRH from neurosecretory neurons present there. The structure of some of these neurotransmitters is indicated in Fig. 1-5. (587). Morphologic evidence indicates that LHRH-secreting neurons are in close contact with axons of noradrenergic neurons whose cell bodies lie in the brainstem tuberoinfundibular dopaminergic tract and terminals of serotoninergic, and histaminergic neurons that exist in the hypothalamus (296,627). In hypogonadal (ovariectomized) women, the increased release and synthesis of LH and FSH occurs with an increased magnitude of the pulsatile pituitary discharge of LH as well as FSH (789,1024). This suggests that the pulsatile pattern of gonadotropin release from the anterior pituitary is related to pulsatile increase in LHRH (117). The pulsatile LHRH discharge may be mediated by catecholamines (602), and animal experiments suggest that the pulsatile LH release may be abolished by α-adrenergic blocking agents such as phentolamine (481). Experiments in the rat have demonstrated that norepinephrine (NE) has a stimulatory role on LHRH release (145), while the dopaminergic system has an inhibitory effect (216,431). This has not been confirmed in experiments in rhesus monkeys (481). The site of the hypothesized noradrenergic synapse has been localized by electrical stimulation in the preoptic and in the arcuate-median-eminence regions. Preoptic stimulation induces a release of LH that can be blocked by inhibitors of NE synthesis (603). The release of LH by stimulation of the arcuate-median-eminence region cannot be blocked by these inhibitors. This site probably activates axons of LHRH neurons so that the inhibitors of norepinephrine synthesis are ineffective. The preovulatory discharge of LH may be due to increased impulse traffic across a noradrenergic synapse in the preoptic or anterior hypothalamic area, or both, which would result in an increased release of LHRH from the LHRH neurons. The LHRH acts on the primed pituitary to allow a massive discharge of LH. These pharmacologic studies are consistent with the concept that the stimulatory

feedback of LHRH may be exerted on the preoptic-anterior hypothalamic area where there is a faciliatory noradrenergic synapse. Negative feedback of gonadal hormones which inhibit LH release may be exerted on more basal structures where a noradrenergic synapse may be located (603). This is of potential clinical value since receptor-blocking drugs may be useful as antifertility agents. An extensive review of the role of catecholamines in the regulation of LHRH has been published by Barraclough and Wise (56).

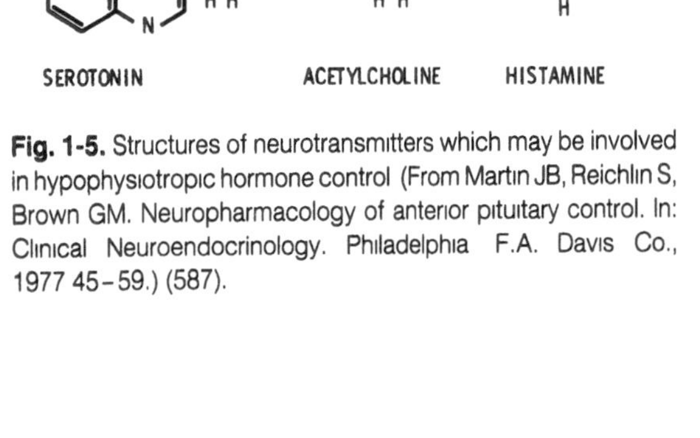

It has been stated previously that NE clearly exerts a stimulatory effect on LHRH release (145) while dopamine (DA), the immediate precursor of NE in catecholamine synthesis (587), has an inhibitory role on LHRH release (431), as well as a direct inhibitory effect on the pituitary lactotrope (Fig. 1-6). It appears that an intricate balance of noradrenergic stimulation and dopaminergic inhibition is involved in LHRH secretion. The central estrogen feedback control of LHRH may be exerted at least in part at the hypothalamic level by modulating or reducing the inhibitory influence of tuberoinfundibular dopaminergic neurons on LHRH release (511). Estrogen receptors are present in the cell bodies of arcuate dopaminergic neurons (355), as well as in the preoptic area, the hypothalamus and the pituitary gland (190). These intracellular cytosol receptors appear to be similar to those found outside the brain (668). Injections of E_2 increase dopamine neuronal activity while decreasing noradrenergic activity in the median eminence (295).

Prolactin stimulates dopaminergic neuronal activity in the median eminence (295). Dopamine infusion reduces serum LH, but not FSH in normal and hyperprolactinemic women (1012). Dopamine infusion studies by Judd et al. (431) suggest that there is a mid-cycle decrease in endogenous DA activity by tuberoinfundibular neurons which facilitates LHRH release for an LH surge. During the follicular phase, the increased dopaminergic tone suppresses endogenous LHRH.

Hyperprolactinemic states may stimulate DA through a short loop mechanism resulting in an altered LHRH release pattern which may lead to anovulation and amenorrhea. Both estrogens and progesterone exert a direct feedback action on catecholamine hormonal activities. Seroto-

Fig. 1-5. Structures of neurotransmitters which may be involved in hypophysiotropic hormone control (From Martin JB, Reichlin S, Brown GM. Neuropharmacology of anterior pituitary control. In: Clinical Neuroendocrinology. Philadelphia F.A. Davis Co., 1977 45–59.) (587).

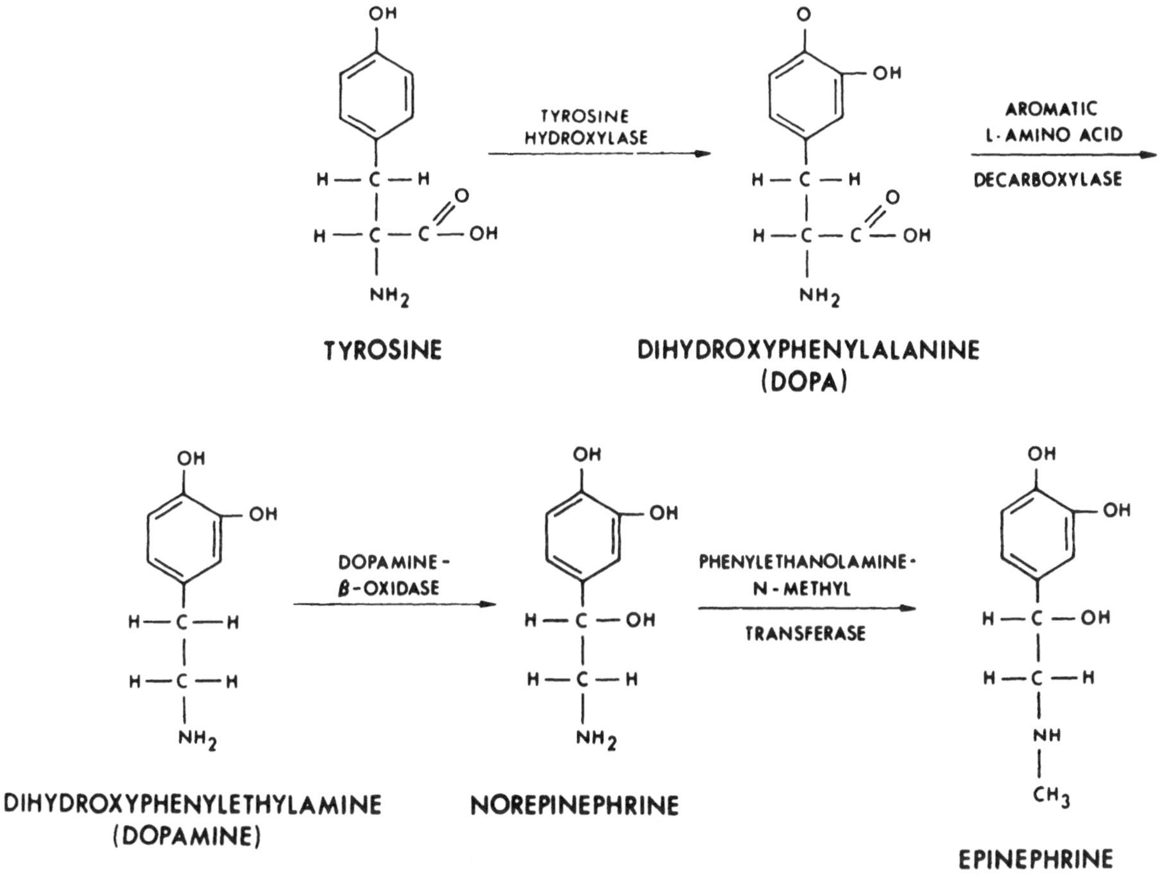

Fig. 1-6. Metabolic pathway for synthesis of dopamine, norepinephrine and epinephrine (From Martin JB, Reichlin S, Brown GM. Neuropharmacology of anterior pituitary control. In Clinical Neuroendocrinology. Philadelphia. F.A. Davis Co , 1977.45–59) (587).

nin and melatonin inhibit the release of LHRH from the median eminence. Gamma-aminobutyric acid (GABA) and acetylcholine have been shown experimentally to stimulate the release of LHRH from the median eminence (602).

The Endorphins. The endorphins are endogenous opiate peptides derived from a common ACTH b-lipotropin precursor, called pro-opiomelanocortin or POMC (Fig. 1-7). The highest concentrations of beta-endorphin (β-endorphin) in the human hypothalamus are found in the arcuate nucleus and median eminence. β-endorphin concentrations in the pituitary are a thousand-fold higher than in the hypothalamic

region (1010). Endorphins appear to have an effect on gonadotropin release as well as regulation of prolactin secretion (779). A hypothalamic site of action of β-endorphin has been suggested for its stimulatory effect on prolactin (PRL) release. The presence of opiate receptors on dopaminergic neurons, and the fact that endorphins inhibit release of dopamine into the portal blood, suggests that the hyperprolactinemic effect of endorphins may be due to decreasing tonic inhibition of PRL release (369). Elevated PRL levels follow injection of β-endorphin during the early follicular phase, and this is associated with a decline in LH concentration (746). β-endorphin may reduce dopaminergic

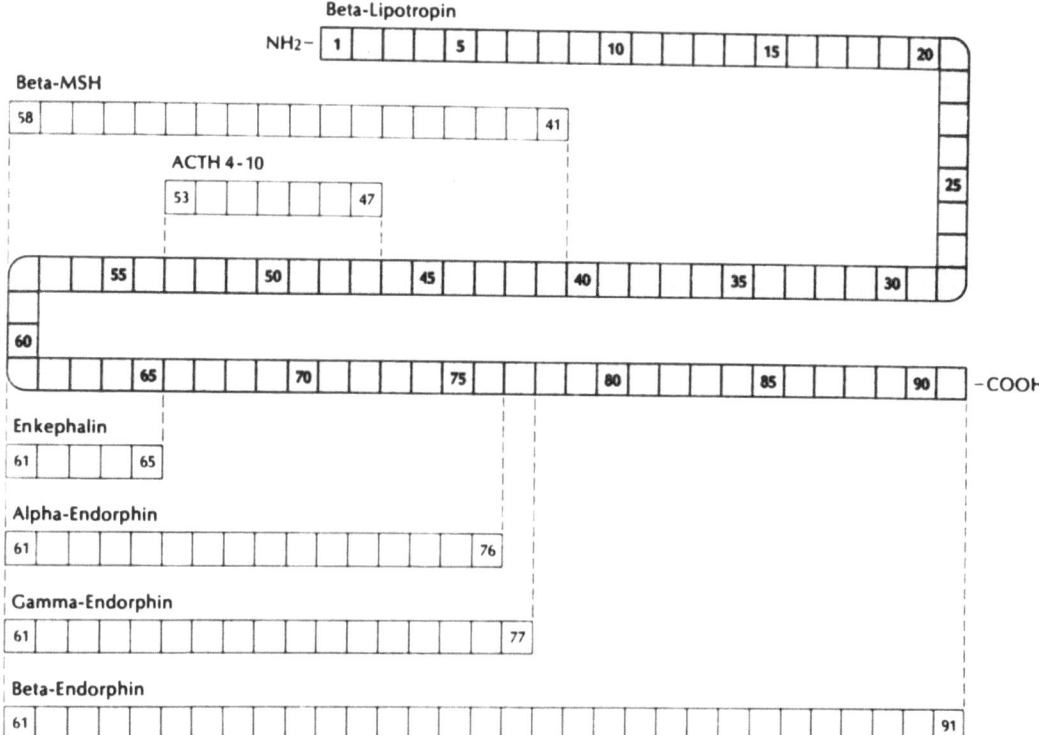

Fig. 1-7. The large 91-amino-acid beta-lipotropin molecule contains the amino-acid sequences of several smaller biologically active peptide molecules, as illustrated in the schematic above. These include beta-melanocyte-stimulating hormone (beta-MSH), the ACTH fragment 4–10, the enkephalins, and alpha-, gamma-, and β-endorphin. (Reprinted by permission from Guillemin R. Beta-lipotropin and endorphins: implications of current knowledge. In: Krieger DT, Hughes JC, eds. Neuroendocrinology. Sunderland, Mass: Sinauer Associates, 1980:67–74.) (370)

activity, leading to PRL stimulation which prompts an increase in dopamine release, resulting in suppression of LHRH. The hypothesized neuroanatomic relationships of noradrenergic, dopaminergic, β-endorphin and LHRH neurons may be seen in Fig. 1-8 (1010). Stress, exercise and other causes of hypothalamic amenorrhea may be associated with increased endogenous opiate activity and suppressed gonadotropins and perhaps elevated PRL levels (735,868). The endorphins also inhibit LHRH neuronal activity or do so indirectly by suppression of noradrenergic neurons.

The low frequency high amplitude pulsatile secretion of LH during the normal luteal cycle differs from that of the high frequency, low amplitude pulses seen during the follicular phase of the human menstrual cycle (Fig. 1-9) (1021). Short term infusion of a specific opiate receptor antagonist, naloxone (1.6 mg/hr × 4 hrs), causes an increase in LH release during the late-follicular phase, a marked increase during the mid-luteal phase, and no increase in the early follicular phase of the human menstrual cycle (734). A similar study using 2.8 mg naloxone/hr × 8 hrs, however, yielded a minimal but significant rise of LH in the early follicular phase as well (661). In another report by Ropert et al. (766), six normal subjects in the mid-luteal phase were given naloxone infusion. An increased frequency and magnitude of LH (> FSH) pulses occurred with naloxone. This suggests that an increased opiate inhibition of LHRH neuronal activity may, in part, participate in the attenuated pulsatile pattern of LH release, particularly during mid-luteal phase of the menstrual cycle (766). The inhibition appears to be a hypothalamic one and not via a pituitary mechanism, since the highest concentration of endogenous opiates in the brain is in the arcuate-median eminence region. Parenthetically, naloxone and opiate peptides fail to alter LH secretion by cultured pituitaries (631). The exact mechanism by which endogenous opiates modulate LHRH pulsatile release is still unknown, but may involve a dopaminergic mechanism as well as the nature of the gonadal steroid environment.

The Catecholestrogens. The hypothalamus has a great potential for 2-hydroxylation of E_2 and E_1. The addition of a hydroxyl (-OH) group at the 2-position gives estrogens a structural similarity to the neurotransmitters NE and dopamine. The enzyme that degrades catecholamines has a greater affinity for the catecholestrogens. Thus by competing for the enzyme, catechol-O-methyl-transferase (COMT), the catechol-estrogens have the capacity to alter the synthesis and concentrations of neurotransmitters. The catecholestrogens may play a role in the feedback modulation of gonadotropins and PRL by gonadal steroids (761,762).

The Role of Prostaglandins. The brain can synthesize and release prostaglandins, and as in many other organs of the body, they may in-crease or decrease cAMP levels. Although prostaglandins are not neurotransmitters, PGE_2 enhances LHRH release in vivo and has no direct effect on pituitary gonadotropes (232). Brain prostaglandin (PG) production may be decreased and modified by estrogen, thus allowing estrogen to act directly on LHRH neurons (757).

Factors Affecting of the Pituitary Response to LHRH

A multiplicity of factors must be considered in the evaluation of the adequacy or inadequacy of the anterior pituitary gonadotrope response to LHRH. Table 1-2 lists some of the factors involved in pituitary responsiveness to LHRH stimulation.

The signals which initiate the circhoral pulsatile discharges of gonadotropins originate from

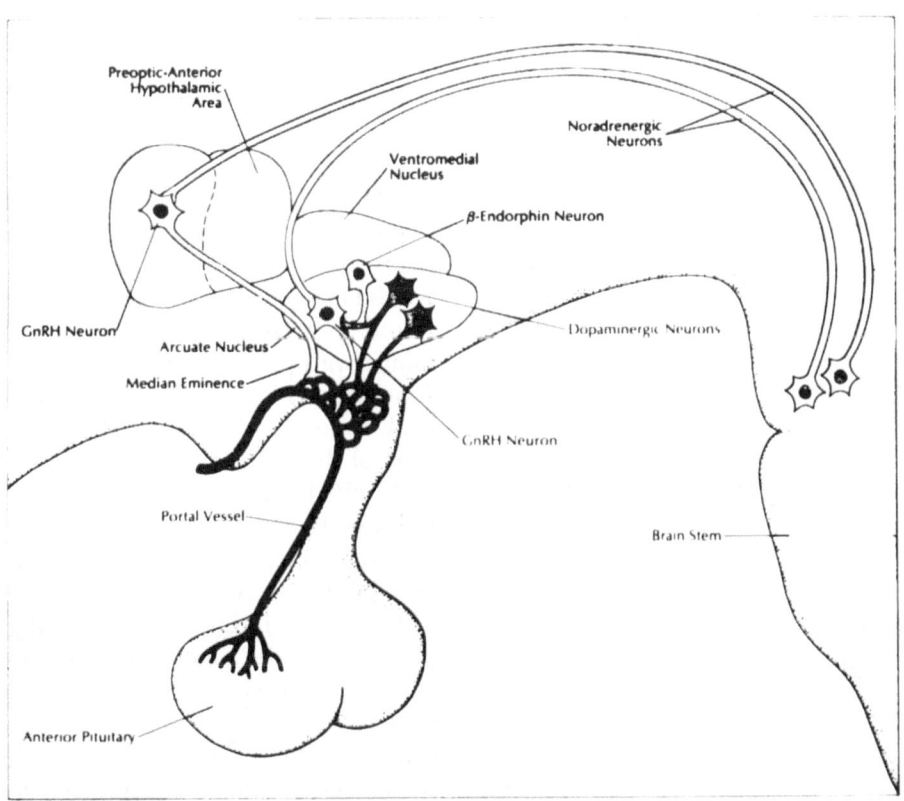

Fig. 1-8. Neuroanatomic relationships of noradrenergic, dopaminergic, β-endorphin, and GnRH (LHRH) neurons are hypothesized. Activation of noradrenergic neurons is believed to stimulate GnRH release, while dopaminergic neurons may inhibit or stimulate GnRH release, depending on the steroid milieu and degree of activation. β-endorphin may modulate these catecholaminergic functions GnRH neurons project to the median eminence where they release GnRH in close proximity to the primary capillary plexus of the portal vessels. (Reprinted by permission from Yen SSC. Neuroendocrine regulation of the menstrual cycle. In. Krieger DT, Hughes JC, eds Neuroendocrinology Sunderland, Mass Sinauer Associates, 1980 259–272.) (1010)

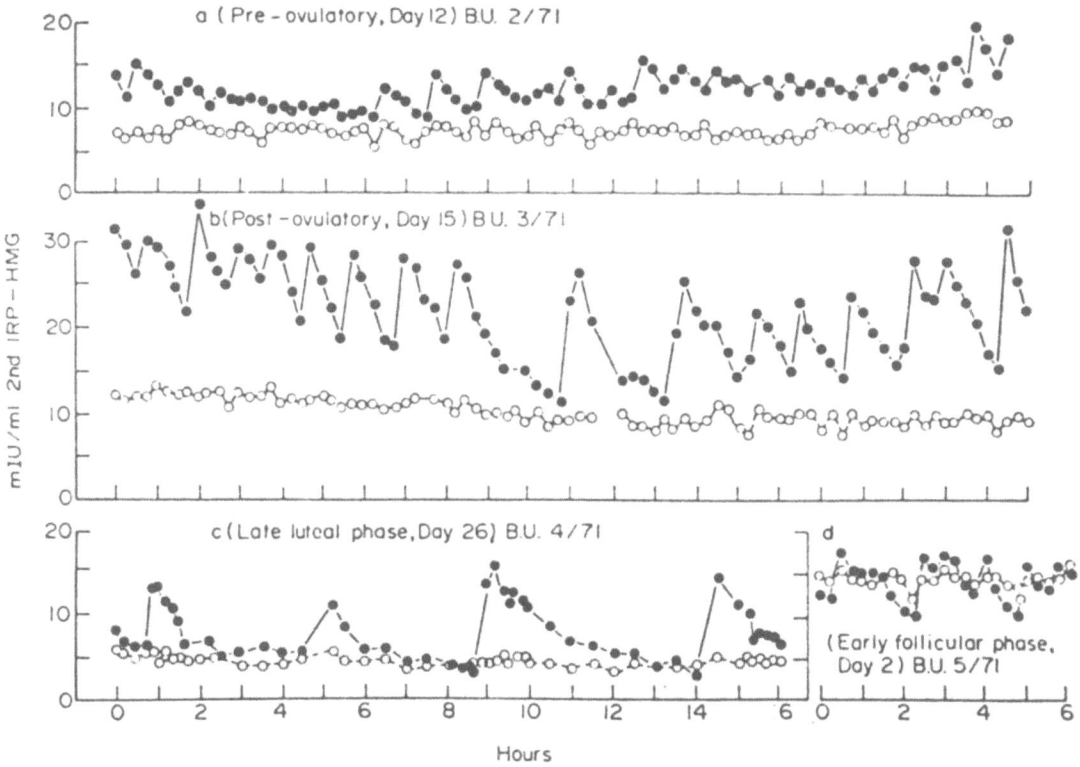

Fig. 1-9. Variations in the frequency and magnitude of the pulsatile pattern of circulating gonadotropins in a representative subject during different phases of the menstrual cycle (From Yen SSC, Rebar R, Vandenberg G, Ehara Y, Siler T Pituitary gonadotrophin responsiveness to synthetic LRF in subjects with normal and abnormal hypothalamic–pituitary–gonadal axis J Reprod Fertil (Suppl) 1973, 20 137–161) (1021).

the CNS. Experiments with specific antiserum to LHRH produce inhibition of gonadotropin secretion (606). In contrast to the rat, surgical disconnection of the medial basal hypothalamus which contains the arcuate nucleus in monkeys does not interfere with initiation of estrogen-induced gonadotropin surges (480).

The major feedback actions of estradiol on gonadotropin secretion may occur at the level of the arcuate region of the MBH controlling

TABLE 1-2. Factors Involved in the Anteror Pituitary Gonadotrope Response to LHRH.

1 Pulse amplitude and frequency of LHRH stimulus
2 Quality, quantity and exposure to the estrogen stimulus (or its absence)
3 Gonadotrope plasma membrane LHRH receptor content
4 Integrity or adequacy of the gonadotrope response to LHRH and/or estrogen stimulus
5 Role of other sex hormones (e.g., progesterone, testosterone)
6 Role of inhibin (See Chapter 6)
7 Role of endorphins
8 Role of dopamine and/or hyperprolactinemia (See Chapter 8)

LHRH release and/or at the level of the adeno-hypophysis modulating the response of the gonadotropes to hypophysiotropic stimulation. Knobil (481) demonstrated that in the ovariectomized arcuate-enucleated monkey maintained with pulsatile administration of LHRH, E_2 may exert both a positive and negative feedback action on LH and FSH secretion at the level of the pituitary gland. A biphasic pattern with initial suppression of gonadotropins was followed by a discharge of LH and FSH (481). Passive immunization with antiserum to LHRH or administration of neuroactive drugs (481) does not interfere with E_2-induced gonadotropin surges in the rhesus monkey. This is consonant with the view of some investigators that LHRH may be a permissive hormone whose principal role is to maintain the functional integrity of the gonadotropes while the "control" of gonadotropin secretion is exerted by E_2 primarily at the pituitary level (277). It appears that pituitary responsiveness to LHRH is a combination of the relative inputs of LHRH and E_2, and to a lesser extent progesterone (P).

Gonadal steroids affect not only the release of LHRH from the hypothalamus but also the response of the pituitary to the LHRH that is being discharged. Changes in gonadotrope responsiveness to LHRH (frequency and amplitude) occur during the human menstrual cycle (963,1022), reflecting changes in ovarian steroid titers in the blood. Thus responsiveness to LHRH increases during the late follicular phase as estradiol is secreted from the preovulatory follicle into the plasma, and becomes maximal 24 hours prior to the preovulatory discharge of LH (484). At this time when plasma LH is elevated approximately fifty-fold, responsiveness to sustained LHRH stimulation is also increased approximately fifty-fold and appears to be due to a "self-priming action of LHRH" (963)—a potentiating effect of the first dose of LHRH on the subsequent release of LH by a second dose of LHRH given soon thereafter. The degree of the gonadotrope's prior exposure to LHRH determines its response to an acute bolus of LHRH. Since there is increased LHRH release at the time of preovulatory discharge, self-priming action could be responsible in causing the observed increased gonadotrope responsiveness and episodic fluctuations of LH and FSH to LHRH (659). Decreased responsiveness to LHRH is present during the mid-luteal to late luteal phase of the menstrual cycle (832), with least responsivenes noted during the early follicular phase of the menstrual cycle (1022).

The two component concept of releasable LH in the anterior pituitary implies an acutely readily releasable LH pool (gonadotrope sensitivity to LHRH) and a larger releasable reserve LH pool (gonadotrope reserve) which requires sustained LHRH stimulation (963). The latter reserve pool of gonadotropin is activated and becomes more readily available with increased exposure or priming to LHRH—an event which depends largely on the endogenous steroid environment. The priming effect may also be noted clinically in the brisk and sustained response of the pituitary gland to LHRH in patients with hypergonadotropic hypogonadism (780,845). An absence of negative feedback by estrogens results in increased serum gonadotropins in primary ovarian failure. The enhanced response to LHRH may be a reflection of an increase of the readily releasable pool of pituitary gonadotropins, and/or increased sensitivity of the pituitary gonadotrope to LHRH (845).

The sum of activity of the acutely releasable pool and the releasable reserve pool of LH is referred to as pituitary gonadotropin capacity (1010).

As already indicated, during the early follicular phase a minimum of pituitary sensitivity and reserve is noted (Fig. 1-10) (1010). With increasing E_2 levels during the late follicular phase, there is a preferential increase of pituitary reserve over sensitivity in response to LHRH, which implies increased synthesis of LH rather than release (963). The latter appears to be a prerequisite for the mid-cycle gonadotropin surge. From the late follicular phase to the mid-cycle a self-priming effect of LHRH occurs with an increased pituitary activation of the reserve pool and its transfer to the more readily releasable pool. A dramatic increased pituitary sensitivity occurs on the day before and during the mid-cycle surge (963). This may be further enhanced by progesterone acting on a fully estrogen-primed gland (827). A gradual reduction of pituitary sensitivity and reserve occurs from the mid-luteal to late-luteal phase of the cycle. Although FSH responses to LHRH are less obvious, they parallel the pattern of LH response (963). It appears that the gonadotropes are target cells which react in sensitivity and capacity to the variables of controlling inputs, namely, LHRH, E_2 and P (1016).

Augmentation by estrogen treatment results in a near doubling of the LH response and a minimal rise of FSH following LHRH stimulation. A direct action of estradiol on pituitary gonadotropes may induce an increase in both sensitivity and reserve of the gonadotropes, and the quantitative release following LHRH stimulation may reflect the size of the acute releasable gonadotropin and the stored gonadotropin pools (508).

A constant infusion of 0.2 μg/min of LHRH demonstrates a biphasic pituitary release pattern of LH (early and late). This finding also supports the hypothesis of two pools of LH in the human pituitary (940,1018). A small bolus of LHRH induces LH increments, which is a measure of the size of the acute releasable pool of pituitary gonadotropins. On the other hand, an evaluation of pituitary reserve requires a longer duration of LHRH stimulation (508). Gonadotropin release was assessed by repeated administration of 10 μg LHRH every 2 hours for 5 doses during the early follicular phase of

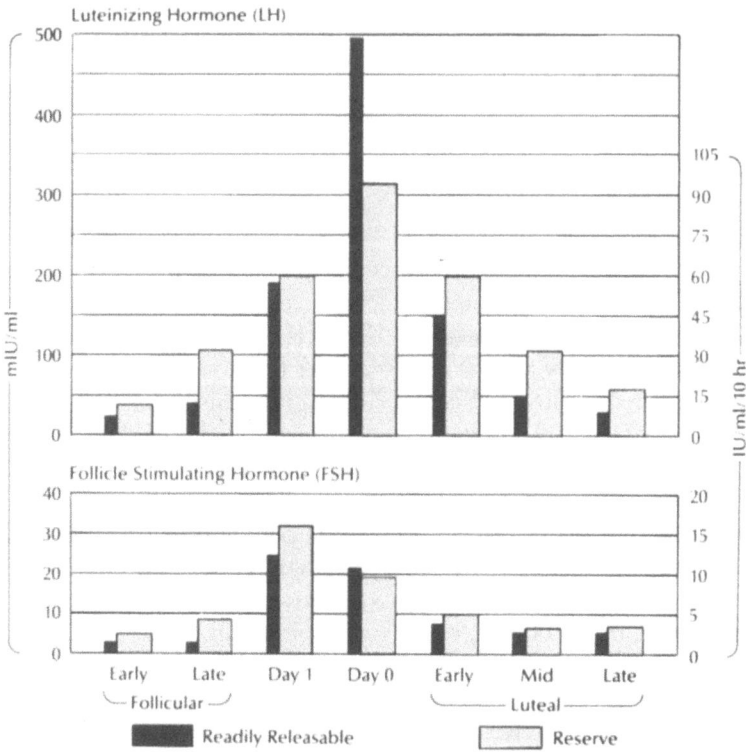

Fig. 1-10. The dynamics of pituitary gonadotropin capacity during the menstrual cycle provide evidence for the existence of two pools of gonadotropin. The first is readily releasable in response to GnRH (LHRH) stimulation. The second, or reserve pool, requires sustained GnRH stimulation. In the early follicular phase, both pools are at a minimum. From the midfollicular phase, reserve pool increases preferentially, but a shift occurs just prior to ovulation (day 0) and the readily releasable pool exceeds the reserve pool. Capacity, high during early luteal phase, then declines. (Reprinted by permission from Yen SSC. Neuroendocrine regulation of the menstrual cycle. In. Krieger DT, Hughes JC, eds. Neuroendocrinology. Sunderland, Mass: Sinauer Associates, 1980:259–272.) (1010).

the cycle in six normal women. The initial increment of LH and FSH was used to describe pituitary sensitivity while quantitative LH increments to further LHRH injections were used to measure pituitary reserve (508). Treatment with intramuscular injections of estradiol benzoate (EB) 2–8 µg/kg in twice-daily doses for 4 days caused a marked rise of serum E_2 (mean 396 pg/ml) with augmentation of the responses of LH and FSH to LHRH. The addition of progesterone (10 mg i.m.) given with the last dose of EB caused an even more marked amplification of the EB-augmented response to LHRH-induced pulses of LH and FSH (508), and may have been the result of a direct action of P on the gonadotropes. This has been also described by others (685,1017). Progesterone appears to exert a positive feedback on LH and FSH at the preovulatory phase, enhancing the positive feedback effect of estrogens at that particular phase of the menstrual cycle (980). It is unlikely

that P produces an increase in endogenous LHRH.

The most likely mechanism by which disassociation of LH and FSH secretion might occur would involve differential feedback by sex steroids. This feedback represents a complex mechanism, since not only is it exerted both at the pituitary and hypothalamic level, but the pituitary's responsiveness to LHRH also varies with endocrine status and age. Furthermore, exposure of intact animals or cultured pituitaries to steroids prior to LHRH stimulation can either inhibit or stimulate the pituitary responsiveness to LHRH depending on the dose, route of administration and time lapse following steroid administration. However, the nature and ratio of various steroids influence LH and FSH responses to LHRH differently. FSH release due to LHRH appears to be more susceptible to the inhibitory effects of estradiol than LH release, but testosterone and dihydrotestosterone exert a stronger inhibitory action on LH. Contradictory data exist which question the role of progesterone alone in inhibiting the LH and FSH response to LHRH (963). The combination of progestational steroids with estradiol (as in oral contraceptives), however, suppresses LH stimulation more effectively than progesterone or estradiol alone.

Hypothalamic-Pituitary Feedback Sites of Ovarian Hormones

Ovarian E_2 is the crucial feedback signal in the regulation of cyclic gonadotropin release (256,479), exerting negative and positive feedback on both the hypothalamus and pituitary gland. A continuous function occurs for E_2, dependent on its level and duration, to affect positive or negative feedback effect (1018). Approximately 90% of the time, that is, 25 out of the usual 28 days of the cycle, there is negative feedback of circulating sex steroid on gonadotropins. At mid-cycle during the peak of ovarian follicle function and development, positive feedback occurs allowing the gonadotropin surge which results in ovulation. Experimentally induced increased and sustained levels of E_2 in the early follicular phase (1031) also induce a prolonged and augmented release of gonadotropins following a bolus of LHRH (416,832,1022).

Although the exact locus of the positive feedback effect of E_2 is still in doubt, there may well be a dual mechanism whereby estrogens modulate the frequency and magnitude of LHRH pulses and also regulate pituitary sensitivity to LHRH stimulation. During the luteal phase of the menstrual cycle estrogen-induced LH release may fail to occur in normal females due to the inhibitory effects of the elevated circulating progesterone at the hypothalamic as well as the pituitary level (831,980). The positive feedback mechanism involving E_2 may involve increased LHRH receptor concentration on the gonadotrope (478,1031). Yet this is only operable with an increased duration of adequate estrogen exposure (priming) which favors positive feedback. The fact that pituitary responsiveness to LHRH does not always reflect its receptor content on the gonadotrope is well demonstrated by experiments where during estrogen priming,

LHRH-induced release of LH is initially suppressed by estrogen treatment despite the fact that LHRH receptor content of the gonadotropes increase in concentration with increased duration of estrogen exposure (10,257). E_2 probably exerts a negative feedback on the hypothalamus as well as the pituitary gland via different mechanisms (9,142).

The following evidence supports the hypothesis that E_2 modulation can occur at the level of the pituitary gland. Pulsatile infusion of LHRH in castrated monkeys with hypothalamic lesions allows for reestablishment of gonadotropin secretion which responds to the positive and negative feedback effects of E_2 administration (671,725). Similarly, pituitary stalk sections of female rhesus monkeys have yielded similar conclusions (256). Estrogen-induced gonadotropin surges may be seen before and after stalk section and the placement of a Silastic barrier between the cut ends. With pulsatile LHRH replacement in animals with arcuate lesions and intact ovaries, normal menstruation occurs. In summary, these lines of research indicate a permissive, although obligatory role in the hypothalamic control of LH and FSH secretion and that feedback modulation of gonadal steroids acts directly on the pituitary gland (479). The experimental studies which state that the hypothalamus exerts a necessary but passive influence on gonadotropin secretion by the pituitary gland have been based on the assumption that the hypothalamic input was entirely eliminated. This has not always been the case, since Silastic barriers may be permeable to LHRH (691). Studies with Teflon barriers at the transection site of the pituitary stalk failed to demonstrate a gonadotropin surge or ovulation following pulsatile LHRH replacement in monkeys with intact ovaries (691,692). Further studies defining these conflicting experimental studies should be forthcoming.

A pulsatile pattern of LHRH concentration has been demonstrated in the portal blood of rhesus monkeys (117,118). An acute preovulatory rise in LHRH concentrations has been described in portal blood (150,257,675), while, as previously noted, a periovulatory rise in LHRH has also been demonstrated in human peripheral plasma (229). A down-regulation of its own pituitary LHRH receptor occurs in parallel with the preovulatory gonadotropin surge (9,11).

Changes in LHRH receptor concentrations on the gonadotropes may either be mediated by the hypothalamus or result as a direct effect of gonadal steroids. The site of negative feedback to estrogen is exerted by modulating the magnitude (amplitude) and frequency of LHRH secretion at the MBH in the region of the arcuate nucleus (189,788,981), while at the pituitary level the inhibitory effect is probably exerted by decreasing gonadotrope sensitivity to LHRH (189,604). The positive feedback effect of estrogen may elaborate an acute LHRH discharge magnified by a large LHRH receptor concentration at the gonadotrope. Differential effects on LH and FSH secretion may occur as a result of varying the magnitude of each hourly pulse of LHRH (981).

The negative feedback effect of estrogens on gonadotropins are clearly seen in postmenopausal women given estrogens. This may occur as early as two hours following an injection of estradiol-17β (E_2) (685). Injection or infusions of estrogens in the early or mid-follicular phase of cycles results in rapid initial suppression of LH and FSH, with a subsequent rebound surge of LH which may occur anywhere beween 12–72 hours following the termination of estrogen treatment (827,1025). The negative feedback effect of acute E_2 administration is greater for FSH than LH (829,925). The trigger of the LH surge may be related to the decline of the administered E_2, although others (1025) have reported gonadotropin surges while estrogen levels are maintained at constant elevated levels in normal women (116).

Enhanced bioactivity may also play an important role during the mid-cycle gonadotropin surge (589,676). It is tempting to speculate that feedback effects of gonadal steroids may be involved in the bioactivity of the released gonadotropins. The fact that enhanced bioactivity of LH has been demonstrated in patients with PCOD may be of some interest in explaining some of the pathophysiology of this disease (534). A decline in the bioactive but not immunoreactive LH has also been noted in association with estrogen-induced luteolysis (975). This suggests that the luteolytic action of estrogens may be also exerted centrally rather than locally in the ovary.

A progressive increase in hormones other than LH occurs just prior to ovulation. Although their physiologic significance is not clear, the concentrations of prolactin, ACTH, parathyroid and calcitonin and the estrogen-sensitive neurophysin (ESN) rise toward the mid-cycle (741).

Extrapituitary Effects of LHRH

Paradoxical inhibition of human reproductive function has been documented in a number of studies employing LHRH (399). Chronic administration of LHRH agonists has been responsible for new antifertility approaches (162) and LHRH analogues have been used in treating sexual precocity (155) and endometriosis (632). There is a direct inhibitory effect of LHRH and its agonists on ovarian and testicular functions as well as other reproductive organs (401). LHRH and its agonists inhibit steroidogenesis in in vitro cultures of rat ovarian granulosa and luteal cells (152,400,401). Treatment of cultured granulosa-luteal cells with LH causes an increased estrogen and progestin production, while concomitant treatment of these cells with LHRH inhibits LH stimulation of estrogen production (427). In vivo documentation of the extrapituitary action of LHRH and its agonists on ovarian function has also been demonstrated on human chorionic gonadotropin (hCG)-stimulated ovarian growth in hypophysectomized rats (599). These direct gonadal effects of LHRH are blocked by concomitant treatment wth LHRH antagonists (401). Direct effects of LHRH and its agonists have also been shown on ovarian interstitial and/or theca cells (564).

Hsueh and Jones (399) in their review of the extrapituitary effects of LHRH (GnRH) listed inhibition of the following female reproductive functions by chronic treatment with LHRH or its agonists (Table 1-3).

LHRH, similar to other peptide hormones, exerts its effects through binding to specific membrane receptors in specific target cells (150). High affinity and low capacity LHRH binding sites have been found in various ovarian cells (152,599) and testicular cells (826) with a lower binding concentration than that found in the pituitary (152). Local gonadal production of LHRH-like peptides may regulate LHRH by interacting with LHRH receptors in the gonad. It is of interest that a possible decrease in ovarian

TABLE 1-3. The Inhibitory Effects of Chronic Treatment with LHRH or Its Agonists on Female Reproductive Function

1. Implantation delay and pregnancy termination
2. Decreases in ovarian steroidogenesis and gonadotropin receptor content
3. Inhibition of follicular maturation and ovulation
4. Decreases in uterine and oviductal growth
5. Delay of puberty
6. Delay of parturition
7. Inhibition of ovarian-dependent mammary tumorigenesis

From Hsueh AJW, Jones PBC Extrapituitary actions of gonadotropin-releasing hormone Endoc Rev 1981, 2 437–461. (399)

binding sites in the rat may be a contributing factor in the enhancement of puberty (977).

Ying et al. (1030) discovered a small peptide purified from rat follicular fluid which specifically stimulates the secretion of both LH and FSH from the pituitary in vitro as well as in vivo. Preliminary amino acid analysis appears to indicate that its chemical nature is different from that of hypothalamic LHRH, less than 3500 daltons. It thus appears to have LHRH-like activity, and the investigators suggest that the granulosa cells are probably the source of gonadocrinin. The possible importance of this ovarian peptide in the formation of follicular atresia, and in influencing the LH receptors, PRL receptors and steroidogenesis, is an area of research which may lead to a better understanding of ovarian physiology.

Experiments in estrogen-primed hypophysectomized, ovariectomized female rats suggest that LHRH plays a role in the induction of mating behavior, which is not initiated by administration of large doses of either FSH or LH alone. Thus, LHRH may exert additional effects independent of its pituitary effects (721).

LHRH Induced Pituitary Receptor Binding

Realistically, the small concentration of hypothalamic LHRH that is present in the systemic circulation may not be sufficient to cause significant interactions with gonadal LHRH receptor sites (399). It appears that the pituitary gland has the capacity to metabolize the majority of the peptide secreted into the hypothalamo-hypophyseal portal system. A direct action of sex steroids on the pituitary gonadotropes has been demonstrated (671). The mechanisms of these

effects are not fully understood but may involve regulation of the rate of gonadotropin synthesis, packaging and storage, and modulation of the release of stored hormone under both basal and LHRH-stimulated conditions (151).

One of the sites of action of gonadal steroids may be at the gonadotrope plasma membrane receptor level to regulate the extent of binding of LHRH and thus of hormone release. This may occur as a result of an effect on reducing hypothalamic LHRH secretion, thereby reducing pituitary gonadotrope receptors. The removal of the negative feedback action of gonadal steroids in gonadectomized rats and monkeys evokes increased hypothalamic LHRH levels in the pituitary stalk plasma of these animals (675). Another mechanism may be a demonstrable increase in the number of functional LHRH receptors of the pituitary gland which amplifies the LHRH input (151). This is prevented by the administration of an LHRH antagonist that interacts with pituitary receptors.

It is likely that LHRH controls the concentration of its own pituitary binding sites. The LHRH self-priming effect on the pituitary is partly a result of direct receptor induction by the decapeptide, while continuous stimulation of LHRH by infusion methods may cause gonadotrope desensitization by reducing the number of available receptors (150).

It is possible that extrapituitary LHRH binding sites may recognize LHRH-like peptides secreted by gonadal or other tissues (1030). Since maturation of the ovarian follicle is controlled in part by its local microenvironment, future studies in this area will be of vital importance to the understanding of normal and disease states.

Hypothalamic Regulation of Prolactin Release

One of the effects of TRH is its stimulation of prolactin. It is known that prolactin secretion is normally inhibited by a hypothalamic prolactin-inhibitory hormone or factor (PIF). PIF activity has been shown to be present in dilute acetic acid extracts of ovine hypothalamic tissue. Whether this activity is due to the neurotransmitter DA which inhibits prolactin secretion or whether there is a separate PIF is unknown, although most now consider DA as the PIF. Conversely, whether there is a prolactin releasing factor (PRF) separate from TRH is not known.

Anatomical data indicate that tuberoinfundibular dopaminergic neurons terminate in the median eminence adjacent to the portal vessels leading to the anterior pituitary gland. Other dopaminergic neurons originate in the arcuate nucleus and pass through the median eminence. Catecholamines contained in hypothalamic neurons may exert a direct inhibitory effect on pituitary prolactin secretion after being transported to the pituitary gland (967). In vitro data have indicated specific DA binding to receptors on pituitary cell membranes (559). Alternatively, catecholamines have an indirect effect on the pituitary by acting on the hypophysiotropic area of the hypothalamus causing secretion of a second messenger, PIF.

The concentration of catecholamines in the brain is increased by administration of L-Dopa following its metabolic conversion to dopamine and norepinephrine. L-Dopa, within 30 minutes of injection into rats, causes a dramatic decrease in serum prolactin. This effect of L-Dopa is used clinically as a test of pituitary function, in that 500 mg of L-Dopa causes a suppression of serum prolactin with a return to a normal level within 4–6 hours.

The anatomical connection between the median eminence and pituitary gland is critical in maintaining the physiological control of prolactin secretion. Isolation of the pituitary gland from the hypothalamus by stalk section increases serum prolactin concentration. Innervation of the MBH is also important in maintaining normal levels of prolactin because partial or total deafferentation of the MBH results in lowered circulating levels of prolactin in male rats.

A short-loop negative feedback control of PRL secretion has been described whereby PRL controls its own release by enhancing the release of PIF (919). Increased PRL enhances turnover of DA in the medial basal hypothalamus, and the concentration of DA is increased in rat hypophyseal portal blood following PRL administration (368).

There is a nocturnal release of PRL which is sleep-dependent and usually preceded by a sleep-related growth hormone release (1014). Prolactin release shifts completely with shifts of sleep onset (793), and its release cannot accurately be described as a circadian rhythm. No sleep-related rise in PRL occurs in anorexia nervosa, Cushing's disease or in most patients with prolactin-secreting pituitary tumors (920). Maximal levels of PRL in normal subjects usually occur between 5 and 7 A.M. Episodic PRL releases may be of greater amplitude than those occurring during the menstrual cycle. There is an increase of serum PRL during the mid-cycle and to some extent in the luteal phase of the cycle, correlating with the levels of circulating estrogens (946). Such increases are normally difficult to detect in individual cycles since PRL secretion is very labile, and they are probably of minor significance. Such parallelism between endogenous estrogens and PRL is also apparent during pregnancy. PRL is concentrated and may have activity at the ovarian level (626). The significance of these events in the normal menstrual cycle is yet to be clarified.

Neuroendocrinology of Puberty

HYPOTHALAMIC–PITUITARY–GONADAL AXIS. The onset of puberty is not an isolated event, but rather a critical stage in a sequence of complex maturational changes. It appears that the hypothalamic–pituitary gonadotropin–gonadal axis differentiates and functions during fetal life and early infancy, is suppressed to a low level of activity during childhood, and reactivated at puberty. The major restraint on the onset of puberty in the human is the central nervous system (CNS). The LHRH- (or GnRH-)secreting neurosecretory neurons located in the MBH are under tonic suppression in the decade between late infancy and the onset of puberty, resulting in a state of functional LHRH insufficiency at that interval (366).

Hypothalamic-Pituitary-Gonadotropin-Gonadal Axis in the Fetus and Infant. The human fetal hypothalamus synthesizes LHRH by the eighth week, and by mid-gestation fetal serum FSH levels are elevated and comparable to those found in castrated adult women (748). This may be attributed to unrestrained LHRH secretion at mid-gestation, which by stimulating LH and FSH stimulates gonadal growth and sex steroid biosynthesis in the fetal ovary. By the end of the second trimester, however, the serum levels of FSH and LH decline indicative of inhibition of hypothalamic LHRH release. The dominant mechanism at this stage is the development of negative feedback and progressively increasing sensitivity of the hypothalamic–pituitary gonadotropin unit (gonadostat) to the inhibitory effects of placental estrogens (990). Of lesser importance at this time is the maturation of the intrinsic CNS mechanism that suppresses LHRH secretion. At the end of the first week following birth, coincident with the decline of placental sex steroids, serum FSH and LH start to rise in the female infant (991). Responsiveness to LHRH testing elicits a greater FSH than LH response in female, unlike male infants, and the gonadotropin response to LHRH appears to decline gradually after 6 months of age, with a resulting decline in serum gonadotropin and sex steroid levels which persists throughout childhood until the onset of puberty.

Hypothalamic-Pituitary-Gonadotropin-Gonadal Axis During Mid-Childhood (ages 4-11 years).

The marked fall in serum FSH and LH as well as in pituitary gonadotropin reserve to LHRH stimulation between the ages of 4 and 11 years of age reflects an intrinsic CNS inhibitory mechanism independent of gonadal sex steroid feedback that restrains pulsatile LHRH release and inhibits the onset of puberty. This is also demonstrated by a reduction of serum LH and FSH secretion and reserve in agonadal children aged 5–11 years unlike the elevated gonadotropin secretion and response of younger agonadal patients (157). Although the intrinsic CNS mechanism restraining pulsatile LHRH release is dominant, there is also evidence that the hypothalamic–pituitary gonadotropin unit is operative, albeit at a low level with an absence of episodic LH secretion and the presence of marked sensitivity to negative feedback of sex steroids. The fact that the prepubertal child does secrete some FSH and LH and that serum levels of gonadotropins are elevated in prepubertal children with gonadal dysgenesis supports the functional aspect of the hypothalamic–pituitary gonadotropin unit. Furthermore, the low functional aspect of the hypothalamic gonadostat is totally suppressed by administration of small doses of estrogens. This indicates a very high degree of sensitivity

(lower set point) of the hypothalamic-gonadostat to the feedback of sex steroids — more than 5–10 times the sensitivity than that found in the adult (366).

Hypothalamic-Pituitary-Gonadotropin-Gonadal Axis During the Peripubertal Stage.

In the peripubertal period there is increased LH (>FSH) release following LHRH testing (205,780). Increased sensitivity to LHRH indicates a change in the release mechanism of LHRH by the hypothalamus, which results from a change in both the CNS as well as gonadal hormonal restraints of LHRH. This derepression or reactivation of LHRH synthesis as well as increased pulsatile release of LHRH, leads to priming of the pituitary gonadotrope with a resulting increased sensitivity to LHRH resulting in increased elaboration of sex steroids by the gonad. Initially, the onset of puberty is reflected by an increased pulsatile release of LHRH occurring with a sleep-associated increase in serum LH (Fig. 1-11) (93,97,942). The sleep-enhanced LH secretion also occurs in agonadal patients during the pubertal age period (96), suggesting that this is not dependent on gonadal function but is related to changes in tonic CNS control of LHRH release (366). During puberty the CNS maturation coincides with progressive reduction in hypothalamic-gonadostat sensitivity to the negative feedback effect of gonadal steroids (990). This means there is an increased or higher set point of the hypothalamic negative feedback receptors. Thus low concentrations of sex steroids are no longer as effective in suppressing LHRH secretion. The development of positive feedback control of gonadotropins by sex steroids, however, is a late maturational event in the pubertal development of females. Development of the positive feedback action of E_2 requires (1) sufficent E_2 secretion by FSH-primed ovarian follicles, (2) an estrogen-sensitized pituitary gland that can amplify and augment the effect of LHRH sufficient to provide an LH surge, and (3) sufficient LHRH reserve for the LHRH neurons to respond to E_2 with an acute increase in LHRH release (366). A fully functional E_2-induced positive feedback may not occur until 1–2 years after onset of menarche, despite its demonstrable presence as early as the middle of puberty.

Apter et al. (26) reported that up to 80 per-

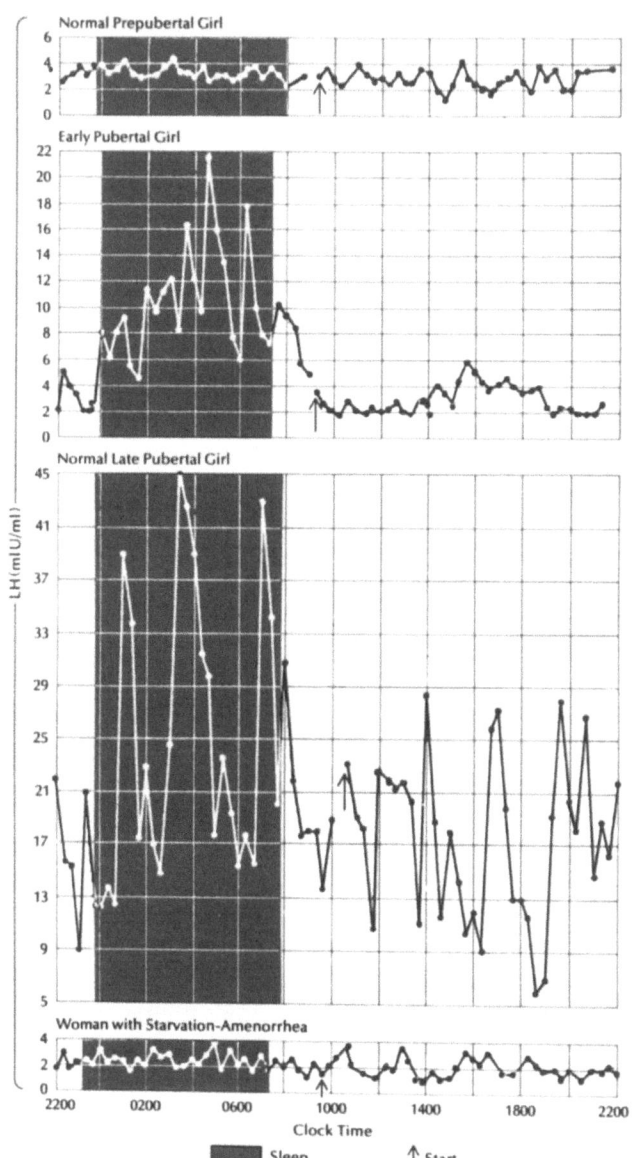

Fig. 1-11. Normal LH secretory patterns at different developmental stages, as determined by Boyar et al. (93) from blood samples obtained every 20 minutes for 24 hours from three normal subjects, are indicated in the top three panels LH secretory pattern at bottom was obtained from a 21-year-old woman with starvation-amenorrhea of 14 months' duration whose weight was 59.5% of her ideal body weight. The patient's LH secretory pattern is strikingly similar to the prepuberal pattern, although she had had normal menarche at 14. (Reproduced by permission from Boyar RM, Katz J, Finkelstein JW, et al. Anorexia nervosa. Immaturity of the 24-hour luteinizing hormone secretory pattern N Eng J Med. 1974; 291:861 – 865.) (93); and reprinted from Vande Wiele RL. Anorexia nervosa and the hypothalamus. In Krieger DT, Hughes JC, eds. Neuroendocrinology. Sunderland, Mass: Sinauer Associates, 1980:205 – 211.) (942).

cent of menstrual cycles are anovulatory during the first year after menarche. Regular cyclical ovulation in adolescents is a slow process. More than one-third of adolescents still have anovulatory cycles in their fifth postmenarchal year, while another third have inadequate corpus luteum function (P < 5 ng/ml). During the sec-

ond year after menarche the response to LHRH appears to be more consistent with an adult pattern of gonadotropin response (516).

In some girls the positive feedback to estrogen culminating with the mid-cycle LH surge may not be established for sometime after menarche, causing persistent anovulation, excessive unopposed estrogen production and adolescent dysfunctional bleeding (339). A clomiphene-induced rise in plasma LH and FSH suggests that the feedback relationship between estrogen and gonadotropins is intact (276). Subsequently, the ovulatory cycles which sometimes appear six months after onset of menarche are frequently associated with a short luteal phase. By the time sexual development is complete, the sleep-related enhancement of LH secretion is no longer apparent, and episodic LH pulses of equal frequency and magnitude occur during waking and sleep periods. A regression to a prepubertal or early pubertal LH pattern has been noted in the majority of patients with anorexia nervosa (93).

The physiological role of prolactin during puberty is unknown. Since estrogen stimulates prolactin secretion, the increased prolactin serum concentration at puberty may induce further pubertal breast development. The first clinical sign of puberty is usually breast enlargement although occasionally this may be heralded by the appearance of pubic hair. Puberty is also associated with growth velocity acceleration. Frisch and McArthur (277) have postulated that attainment of a critical body weight is necessary for the timing of puberty.

ADRENARCHE AND GONADAL MATURATION. At present, the exact role of adrenal androgens in the development of puberty is not clear. Adrenarche is defined as a developmental increase in the adrenal secretion of dehydroepiandrosterone (DHA), dehydroepiandrosterone sulfate (DHAS), androstenedione, testosterone and estrone several years before gonadal maturation (185). It is associated anatomically with differentiation and growth of the zona reticularis of the adrenal cortex. Prolactin levels do not rise at the initiation of the adrenarche (707). The stimulus responsible for the adrenarche is still not known and the possibility of a pituitary adrenal androgen-stimulating hormone has not been proven. Clinically, the changes that occur at this time consist mainly of axillary and pubic hair development. Although some have speculated that in normal puberty the adrenarche and gonadal maturation are closely related (821), the fact that normal puberty can occur in instances of primary adrenal insufficiency suggests that the adrenal gland does not exert a major effect on the timing of puberty. On the other hand, sleep-related LH peaks have been reported by Boyar et al. (95) in two boys aged 6 and 8.5 years with untreated congenital adrenal hyperplasia. Whether this was related to the advanced bone age and associated increased body weight, exposure to increased adrenal androgens resulted in accelerated CNS maturation of the gonadostat and sleep-related LH pulses. In a study of 104 children, ages 7–14 years, by Sizonenko and Paunier (847), elevation of plasma DHA concentration was noted before elevation of those of plasma LH and FSH. The augmented secretion of DHA was present as early as 7 years in girls and 8 years in the boys studied. It was demonstrated that elevation in DHA concentration occurred at an earlier bone age in girls than in boys. The hypothalamic factor(s) inducing the stimulation of adrenal androgens such a DHA and DHAS (392) remains unknown. In 15 girls without pubic hair and with breast development, the mean plasma concentration of DHA and testosterone (T) were 230 and 12 ng/dl, respectively, while with the onset of pubic hair, mean plasma DHAT rose to 395 and 21 ng/dl, respectively. With the appearance of axillary hair, the mean DHA concentration was 490 and that of T 21 ng/dl (847). DHA is a weak androgen, but DHAS, which is secreted in microgram quantities, might be more important. A pattern of DHAS almost similar to that of DHA has been reported by Hopper and Yen (392). The latter investigators found a 7.5-fold increase in DHAS from a mean of 29 to 210 μg/dl from 8-year-old females to their completion of puberty. They speculated that in view of conversion of DHA and DHAS to androstenedione and T, DHAS may perhaps account for androgenic manifestations such as pubic and axillary hair growth during early puberty.

In general, experimental studies indicate an absence of any significant relationship between adrenal function and sexual maturation (185,707). One has to conclude that in view of the clinical dissociation of adrenarche and onset of gonadal development (gonadarche) in such conditions as premature adrenarche, gonadal dysgenesis (Turner's syndrome), hypogonadotropic hypogonadism, and idiopathic precocious puberty, there is strong evidence for an independent role of adrenarche and pubertal development of the gonad (185).

Hormonal Control of Folliculogenesis 2

Primordial Follicle

The primordial follicle is an oocyte whose nucleus is arrested in the diplotene stage of meiotic prophase, following the first maturation division which begins in prenatal life. Conversion of oogonia to oocytes and incorporation of these into primordial follicles are not completed until 6 months postnatally. Those oocytes that fail to be incorporated into primordial follicles degenerate. Studies of fetal rhesus monkeys support a role of the fetal pituitary in supporting follicle growth (371).

Each primordial follicle consists of an oocyte, a single layer of granulosa cells and a basement membrane that separates these two cell types from the adjacent interstitial tissue (Fig. 2-1) (280). These follicles are located in the ovarian cortex beneath the tunica albuginea. Ultrastructural and biochemical studies in animals demonstrate that the earliest change in primordial follicle growth involves a rapid increase in oocyte RNA and protein synthesis.

Preantral Follicle

At the preantral stage the oocyte enlarges and is surrounded by a membrane, the zona pellucida. Proliferation of the granulosa cells is associated with development of the thecal layer from the surrounding stroma. The adjacent stromal cells outside the basement membrane arrange in concentric perifollicular layers, in which the density of the nuclei is less than that of stroma. This layer of differentiated and uniquely or-iented cells constitutes the theca. That portion of the theca adjacent to the basement membrane is called theca interna, while the theca externa is the portion that merges with the surrounding stroma (Fig. 2-1) (280). With increased cytoplasm in the theca interna the cells become more rounded or epithelioid, and capillaries and lymphatic spaces appear among these cells and terminate at the basement membrane (778). The theca with membrane receptors for luteinizing hormone (LH) is normally the major source of follicular androgens. Specific membrane receptors for FSH are located on the granulosa cells allowing for the activation of the aromatase enzyme system which converts androgens to estrogens. The FSH receptor content of granulosa cells limits the quantity of ovarian estrogen production (651,687). The combined effects of FSH and estrogen favor formation of more FSH receptors as well as increased number and proliferation of granulosa cells (Fig. 2-2) (280,749).

The role of androgens in early follicular development is specific and of vast importance. The cytoplasm of granulosa cells has been demonstrated to contain specific androgen receptors (801). The local concentration of androgens is a critical factor in the development of the follicle. Low concentrations of androgens (mostly androstenedione) enhance the effectiveness of FSH-stimulated aromatization (29) and serve as substrate for the FSH-induced aromatization, thus allowing continued follicular growth. In vitro studies of human preantral granulosa cells exposed to an androgen-rich environment favor 5α-reductase activity to

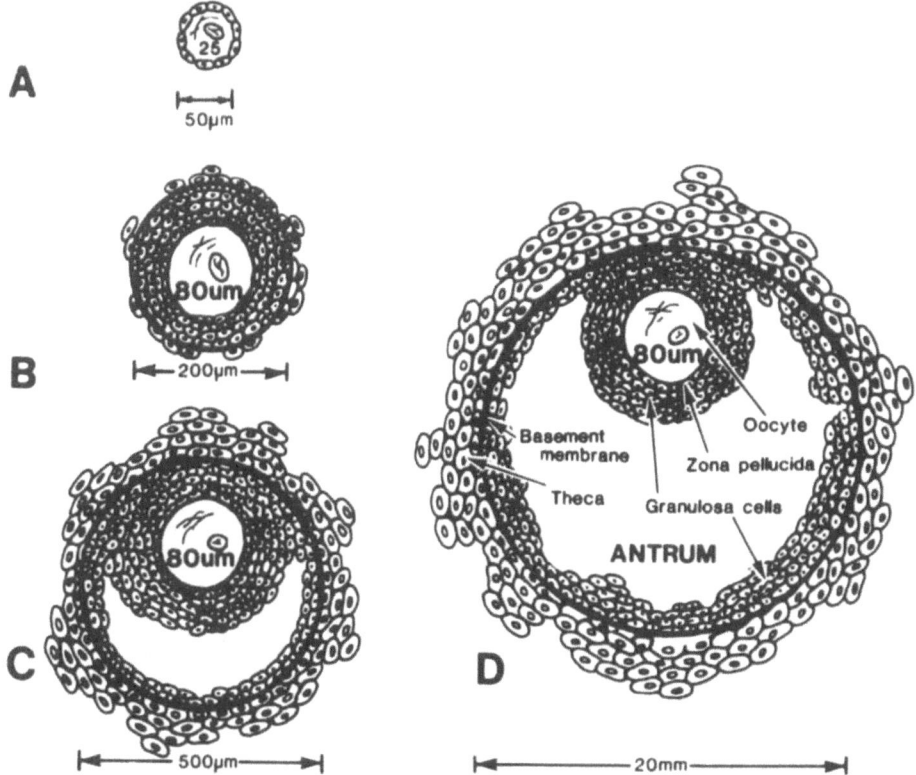

Fig. 2-1. Follicular development (A) Primordial follicle (B) Preantral follicle (C) Antral follicle. (D) Preovulatory follicle (From Fritz MA, Speroff L. The endocrinology of the menstrual cycle the interaction of folliculogenesis and neuroendocrine mechanisms. Fertil Steril. 1982; 38 509–529 Reproduced with permission of the publisher, The American Fertility Society.) (280)

such potent androgens as dihydrotestosterone (DHT) and androstanedione (620). These androgens cannot be converted to estrogens and may indeed inhibit aromatase activity (389). An elevated LH-induced thecal cell proliferation may provide the basis for an androgen-rich environment which may overwhelm aromatization, thereby reducing estrogen production and causing the follicle to become atretic. Follicle development proceeds only in those favored with adequate FSH stimulation which results in sufficient granulosa cell aromatization for the creation of an estrogenic environment.

Although the primordial follicle grows in an avascular ovarian cortex, it migrates to the more heavily vascularized ovarian medulla when the follicle size reaches 150 to 200 μ in diameter (778). At that time, it acquires a theca interna, which consists of a capillary network, small clusters of steroid-secreting cells and connective tissue. Thus the development of a theca interna is an important event in folliculogenesis because the follicle, for the first time, is exposed to the

hormonal milieu of peripheral plasma. At this point the follicle with its complement of FSH, estrogen and testosterone receptors initiates a series of structural and biochemical changes resulting in the formation of the antral follicle. Granulosa cells also have specific estradiol receptors in the cytosol and nuclear fractions. Thus granulosa cells are target cells for estrogen which stimulates mitosis in vivo and increases the sensitivity of their adenyl cyclase system to FSH. Atresia or degeneration of the follicle is rare or nonexistent in primordial follicles. Once a primordial follicle, however, begins to grow and reaches the preantral stage, there is a sharp increase in the percentage of atretic follicles that are found in the ovary. From puberty until menopause, only one of the follicles that develops during each cycle is selected to continue differentiation into a preovulatory follicle; the rest degenerate. During a woman's reproductive life only approximately 400 of the original 2 million primordial follicles develop to the preovulatory stage to undergo ovulation. Thus

99.9% of all the ovarian follicles undergo atresia.

Antral Follicle

The synergistic influence of estrogen and FSH increases the follicular fluid in the intercellular spaces of the granulosa, eventually forming an antrum (Fig. 2-1) (280). The human follicle first forms an antrum when it is between 0.2 – 0.4 mm in diameter. The antral fluid must have estrogen and FSH in adequate concentration to sustain the oocyte, granulosa cell development and continued follicular growth (618). It is the concentration of gonadotropins and steroids within the follicle, rather than in peripheral blood, which correlates with the mitotic and biosynthethic activities of granulosa cells. Antral follicles with the greatest rates of granulosa cell proliferation contain the highest estrogen concentrations and lowest androgen-to-estrogen ratios. This is conducive to further stimulation of granulosa cells, FSH responsiveness and aromatization of androgen precursors to estrogens. An abnormal plasma or intrafol-

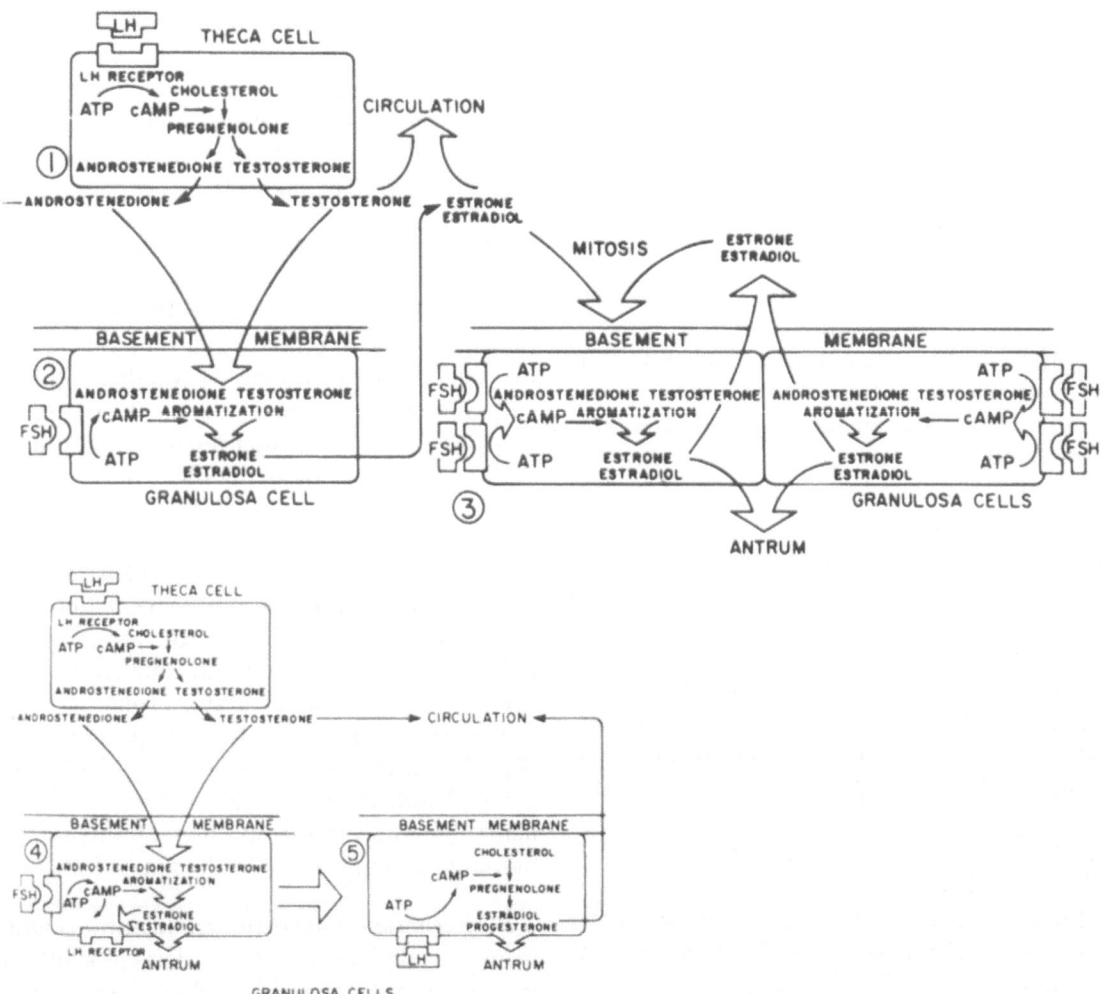

Fig. 2-2. The two-cell theory of follicular steroidogenesis. (1) LH stimulates thecal androgen production. (2) Androstenedione and testosterone are converted to E_1 and E_2 through FSH-induced aromatization in the granulosa cell layer. (3) FSH induces an increase in the development of its own receptor. FSH and estrogen stimulate proliferation of granulosa cells, resulting in an increase in FSH receptors and accelerating estrogen production. (4) FSH induces LH receptors on granulosa cells, which is enhanced by E_2. (5) Acting through its receptor, LH initiates luteinization, resulting in the production of progesterone. (From Fritz MA, Speroff L. The endocrinology of the menstrual cycle. the interaction of folliculogenesis and neuroendocrine mechanisms. Fertil Steril. 1982; 38:509–529. Reproduced with permission of the publisher, The American Fertility Society.) (280).

licular androgenic environment antagonizes estrogen-induced granulosa cell development and may promote degenerative changes in the follicle.

During a 10–15 day follicular phase, the developing follicle accumulates about 50 million granulosa cells and approximately 6.5 ml of antral fluid before it is transformed into a corpus luteum (621). As the antral follicle develops to the preovulatory follicle there is an increase in its size from approximately 200 μ to 20 mm in diameter. This tremendous increase in follicle size is accomplished mostly by the progressive accumulation of follicular fluid in the antral cavity (Fig. 2-1) (280).

Unlike receptors for FSH the number of LH binding sites increases gradually during development of the antral follicle reaching a maximum number in the preovulatory follicle. The increased LH sensitivity of human granulosa cells is correlated closely with an increased concentration of LH in the follicular fluid. In addition to FSH, LH and prolactin receptors, there is some evidence that human granulosa cells also contains specific receptor sites for prostaglandins (PGs — PGF_{2a} and PGE_2).

Although the hormonal concentrations perfusing the two ovaries are similar, ovulation only occurs in one of them during each menstrual cycle (209). Therefore some process is acting at the level of each follicle to determine its fate (ovulation or atresia). Studies of antral fluid levels demonstrate two populations. In one, estrogens and progestins predominate, while in the other androgens predominate. Estrogen predominance is commonly found in follicles measuring 8 mm or more in diameter, while androgens, such as androstenedione and testosterone, are present in higher concentrations in smaller follicles (622,624). Similarly, antral FSH is present in larger follicles and absent in smaller androgen-predominant follicles (621). Differences in the intraovarian hormonal milieu in human ovaries is regulated follicle by follicle, and it is this that determines the occurrence of maturation or atresia of the follicle.

PITUITARY HORMONES IN ANTRAL FLUID. There appears to be a careful regulation of gonadotropins in the developing antral follicle (621). Small follicles are described as those 4–8 mm in diameter, while large follicles are those greater than 8 mm in diameter.

FSH. FSH is more frequently detectable in large follicles than in small follicles. At no time during the cycle is antral fluid FSH more than 60% higher than peripheral FSH levels, and these levels remain constant despite fluctuating plasma FSH levels. The highest FSH concentrations are found in the largest follicles during the late follicular stage. Some FSH may be found, however, even in small follicles (621).

LH. LH is more readily detectable in larger than smaller follicles. Moreover, LH is found most frequently in antral fluid at a time when LH levels are elevated in the plasma. Only antral follicles with FSH in antral fluid contain LH. The concentrations of LH are highest in large follicles during the late follicular phase and are virtually absent in small follicles. Antral fluid LH concentrations are less or equal to 30% of LH peripheral plasma levels. Thus as the follicle develops, the antral LH level remains low until the mid-cycle LH peak (621).

PRL. PRL is detected in all follicles at concentrations greater than 1.5 ng/ml. Antral fluid concentrations vary with the different stages of follicular growth; unlike FSH, they are highest in small follicles during the early follicular phase and lowest in large follicles during the late follicular phase. With follicular enlargement during the late follicular phase, the PRL concentration in the antral fluid declines (621).

OVARIAN HORMONES IN ANTRAL FLUID. The steroids in antral fluid have been identified as pregnenolone, P, 17α-hydroxyprogesterone (170HP), dehydroepiandrosterone (DHA), androstenedione, dihydrotestosterone (DHT), testosterone (T), estradiol-17β, (E_2) and estrone (E_1). All antral follicles contain relatively high levels of androgens. Retention of steroids in follicular fluid may be due to a high-affinity steroid binding protein present in the antral follicle.

Pregnenolone. The major contribution comes from granulosa cells. LH stimulates its synthesis from cholesterol. Large follicles have increased concentrations of this steroid, and the largest concentration occurs at the late follicular phase (mean level of 8000 ng/ml).

Progesterone (P). During the follicular phase large follicles contain higher concentrations of P than small follicles. Unlike a peripheral plasma concentration of 0.5–25 ng/ml, the level of P in the antral follicle may be 2–2000 times higher than plasma (mean level of 1350 ng/ml) during the late follicular phase. In contrast to the follicular phase, small follicles contain a larger concentration of P than larger follicles during the luteal phase. In the preovulatory follicles, P concentration increases coincidentally with increasing hypertrophy and delta^5-3β-hydroxysteroid dehydrogenase activity of the granulosa cells. The major source of P in antral follicles are the granulosa cells (621).

Androstenedione. Androstenedione is the major androgen present in antral fluid and its concentration is 100–500 times higher than its peripheral plasma concentration. The levels of androstenedione do not vary between small and large follicles (approximately 500 ng/ml), except during the late follicular phase when small follicles have an even greater antral concentration (mean, 700 ng/ml) than larger follicles (mean, 300 ng/ml). The major source of androstenedione in antral fluid appears to be the theca cells, and to a lesser extent, the granulosa cells.

Testosterone (T). The concentration of testosterone in antral fluid is much less than that of androstenedione (mean T level varies from 25–100 ng/ml) in both small and large follicles with peak concentrations in small follicles during the late follicular phase.

Dihydrotestosterone (DHT). An interesting observation is that the DHT concentration in follicular antral cells of this potent androgen is 2–10 times higher than that of T (mean DHT level, 150–700 ng/ml) (618).

Estradiol-17β (E$_2$). E$_2$ is the major estrogen in antral fluid and its concentration is 40–40,000 times higher than that in plasma. During the follicular phase large follicles have a 7 to 10-fold increased E$_2$ concentration than smaller follicles, with no differences between small and large follicles in the luteal phase (75–200 ng/ml). The preovulatory follicle may have E$_2$ concentrations of 1–2 μg/ml. In antral fluid most of the E$_2$ comes from the granulosa cells. However, in ovarian venous plasma, E$_2$ probably reflects secretion both of granulosa and thecal cells. P and E$_2$ in fluid from recently rup-

tured follicles demonstrate a 100–1000 times higher concentration than peripheral plasma. Postovulatory corpus luteal fluid P concentration increases from approximately 1500 to 10,000 ng/ml, while the E$_2$ concentration drops from approximately 2000 to 200 ng/ml (621).

Estrone (E$_1$). The pattern of E$_1$ follows that of E$_2$ although there is about 18 times less E$_1$ present in most follicles. Similar findings have been reported by Baird and Fraser (42). While peripheral values of E$_1$ vary from 40–300 pg/ml, the concentrations of E$_1$ in antral fluid are between 5–15 ng/ml. A late follicular 10-fold increase in E$_1$ concentration occurs in large follicles. It is presumed that E$_1$, like E$_2$, is mostly of granulosa cell origin.

Prostaglandins and cAMP. Very little of PG and cAMP are detected in antral fluid of the follicular phase. Their major cellular source is as yet not clear.

Quantitative Relationships Between Hormones in Antral Fluid. A common feature of human antral follicles greater than 4 mm is that most contain more androstenedione than E$_2$ except for the few which are greater than 8 mm in diameter (621). This also occurs in small follicles throughout the menstrual cycle, and in larger follicles (greater than 8 mm diameter) throughout the luteal phase. When FSH is detectable in antral fluid, there is an increased ratio of E$_2$ to androstenedione, irrespective of the stage of the menstrual cycle. Similarly, with increasing levels of FSH in antral fluid there is more granulosa cell proliferation and aromatization of androstenedione to E$_2$. It is also of interest that prolactin levels are lowest in those follicles with the highest E$_2$ concentration (621).

Significantly higher P concentrations are found in large follicles containing LH. LH appears to enter the follicle for the first time during the late follicular phase. The appearance of LH into the follicle leads to inhibition of granulosa cell mitosis (196,625), the resumption of oocyte maturation (526), initiation of granulosa cell luteinization (41) and probably PG synthesis (726).

Despite the high incidence of follicular atresia in the human ovary, little is know about the functional state of the follicles undergoing atresia or how they differ from the population that has the potential for further development (625). The vascularized thecal tissues of every antral follicle are probably exposed to similar concentrations of hormones; however, the cells within the avascular regions of each follicle (i.e., the granulosa cells and the oocyte) are exposed to a hormonal milieu differing from that in serum or in adjacent follicles (625). As already stated, it is the hormonal microenvironment of the follicle (concentrations of gonadotropin and steroids) which is a key factor in determining its subsequent growth and maturation.

The diameter of each follicle and its number of granulosa cells and the concentrations of P, androstenedione, T, E_1, E_2, and DHT in antral fluid of individual follicles have been reported by McNatty et al. (618). The meiotic nature of the oocyte was noted at time of recovery and after 48 hours in culture from hysterectomies of 59 women aged 25 – 48 years (618). The nongrowing primordial follicle is about 0.05 mm in diameter. At the onset of menstruation the largest follicle with a full complement of granulosa cells has been found to be 4 mm in diameter, an already relatively late stage of maturation.

Regardless of the stage of follicular maturation, the steroids present in highest concentration are E_2, androstenedione, and to a lesser extent DHT. Progesterone is not a major steroid in follicular fluid except in the late follicular phase. In noncystic follicles (i.e., in follicles containing adequate granulosa cells), P, T, E_2 and E_1 are mainly derived from granulosa cells, while androstenedione is probably derived from both granulosa and theca cells.

Those follicles with a greater than 75% of their full complement of granulosa cells have the highest antral fluid content of E_2 and FSH. The presence of both FSH and E_2 is necessary for permitting the granulosa cells to aromatize theca-cell and/or granulosa-cell androgens to estrogens (619,650), with a resulting estrogenic microenvironment. Those follicles with severely deficient granulosa cells (less than 25% of their optimum number) have a greater than 100-fold change in the androgen to estrogen ratio, mostly due to a reduction in estrogen. As the amount of estrogen in the antral fluid is reduced, so does the granulosa cell population become reduced. The androgenic environment, without FSH, is incapable of supporting granu-

losa cell proliferation, leading to follicular atresia and eventually to oocyte degeneration.

The data of McNatty et al. indicate that 9 out of 10 antral follicles greater than 1 mm in diameter in any ovary are undergoing some atretic changes (618). Since the average number of antral follicles greater than 4 mm in diameter in women of reproductive years averages 14 or less (621), and only 12% of follicles contain a full complement of granulosa cells, it is probable that only 1 or 2 antral follicles continue to generate a full complement of granulosa cells after reaching a diameter of 4 mm or greater during each cycle; a rather limited number.

TWO-CELL THEORY FOR STEROID SYNTHESIS. There appears to be some functionally compartmentalized synthesis of steroid hormones within the follicular granulosa and theca cells. Although each cell type has the ability to produce estrogens, androgens and progestins, the aromatase activity of the granulosa cell far exceeds that of the theca where no FSH receptors are detectable (388,619). Estrogen production is preferentially produced by the granulosa cells (214,650) while androgen biosynthesis predominates in the theca (615,650). LH stimulates thecal cells to produce androgens which are converted by FSH-induced aromatization to estrogens by granulosa cells of larger antral follicles (Fig. 2-2) (269,280,620,650). FSH induces a further increase in the development of its own receptors on proliferating granulosa cells. The effects of FSH as well as LH are associated with dose-dependent increases of cyclic AMP (927). The combined interaction of the granulosa cell and thecal compartments becomes fully functional during the later phase of antral development with resulting acceleration of estrogen production. By day 7 of the cycle, E_2 concentration is greater in the ovarian vein from that ovary containing the preovulatory follicle (42). The increased estrogen production occurs as a result of the synergism of both granulosa and theca cells (650). LH receptors in the theca interna respond to circulating LH by producing primarily androgens with perhaps a limited amount of estrogens. In contrast, granulosa cells have a limited capacity to synthesize androgens on their own, but contain an active FSH-stimulated aromatization capacity to utilize the thecal androgens substrates (mainly androstenedione) and convert them to estrogens (29). Cultured granulosa cells are limited in their production of androgens from C_{21}-precursors without the addition of C_{19} substrates, because of a probable deficiency of 17α-hydroxylase and/or $C_{17,20}$-lyase enzymes (29). Thecal androgens diffuse across the basement membrane and enter the granulosa cells. Under normal conditions however, the follicular fluid bathing the granulosa cells contains androstenedione and testosterone (622), both of which are readily convertible to estrogens by FSH-induced aromatization activity. Thus both FSH and LH are necessary for adequate estrogen synthesis utilizing both granulosa and theca cells in the process (30). This has been termed the "two-cell" theory of estrogen production (Fig. 2-2) (280). Unlike the facilitation of estrogen synthesis by the larger antral follicles, the granulosa of small antral follicles, similar to the preantral granulosa cells, exhibit an in vitro tendency to convert androgens to the more potent 5α-reduced forms. The androgenic microenvironment interrupts further significant estrogen production by the granulosa cells, leading to an irreversible atretic change in the follicle (620).

Although the "two-cell" theory is a fairly simplistic approach to an understanding of the steroidogenesis of the developing follicle it is more realistic to appreciate that the ovary contains granulosa cells, thecal and stromal tissue which are all capable of the biosynthetic capacity to produce estrogens, androgens and progestins (619). None have the exclusive capacity to produce any steroids at any stage of the menstrual cycle or at any stage of antral follicle growth or atresia. During the follicular phase, granulosa cells produce large amounts of E_2 and smaller amounts of androstenedione. During atresia of the follicle, it has already been stated that the ratio of E_2 to androstenedione declines. With luteinization of the granulosa cells there are high tissue levels of P and androstenedione with reduced levels of E_2, due to progressive loss of aromatase activity and mitotic activity (619). Unlike granulosa cells, thecal cells produce mainly androstenedione and relatively small amounts of E_2 (269,649,650,927). It is of significance that although thecal tissue from atretic follicles loses its ability to produce estrogens, the capacity to produce androgens remains. In the presence of a vascular environment, the thecal

secretions may enter the ovarian blood stream without ever entering the follicular compartment, thus exerting their effects at distant sites. Steroid production by the stroma is gonadotropin-dependent, but in view of its large mass, stromal tissue may secrete a significant amount of steroids. During low plasma gonadotropin levels, in vitro steroid production by the stroma is reduced. At higher levels of FSH in plasma (during early follicular phase) the stromal tissue produces E_2. At mid-cycle with peak levels of LH and FSH, stromal tissue produces more P, androstenedione and T. Compared to thecal tissue the amounts of stromal steroids produced in vitro are low. However, it is difficult to assess what the relative contribution of the stroma is in vivo.

FEEDBACK MODULATION OF FSH. While estrogen exerts a positive role on FSH action inside the maturing follicle, the negative feedback relationship with FSH at the hypothalamic–pituitary level withdraws FSH support from other less developed follicles (208,1036). A consequence of a decline in aromatase activity limits estradiol production and results in conversion to an androgenic microenvironment in all but the more mature follicles. At this time a selected or *dominant* FSH-dependent follicle must complete its preovulatory development despite a declining level of plasma FSH at the midfollicular phase (Fig. 2-3) (280). The dominant follicle must have a rate of granulosa cell proliferation with greater FSH receptor content and capacity for aromatization than that of its cohorts of less developed follicles. By day 7 of the cycle, peripheral levels of E_2 rise significantly and the dominant follicle also develops marked increased thecal vasculature, affording preferential delivery of FSH to allow its continued preovulatory development despite a reduction of circulating FSH (209).

FSH induces membrane receptors for LH in granulosa cells of large antral follicles which is facilitated by high local estrogen concentrations particularly in the dominant follicle (Fig. 2-2) (280,750,1037). In contrast to the suppression of FSH by estrogen, when a plasma E_2 elevation exceeds 200 pg/ml, a transition from negative to positive feedback of LH occurs. Once this critical E_2 threshold level in the human is achieved it must be maintained for up to 50

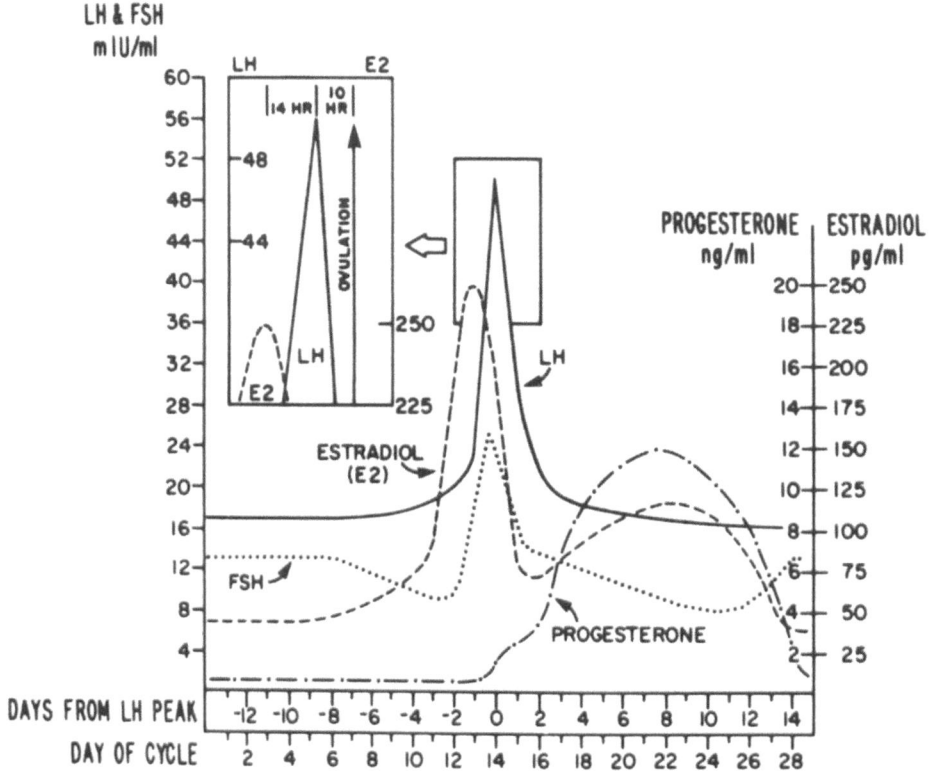

Fig. 2-3. The temporal relationship of FSH, LH, estradiol and progesterone in the normal menstrual cycle. (From Fritz MA, Speroff L. The endocrinology of the menstrual cycle: the interaction of folliculogenesis and neuroendocrine mechanisms. Fertil Steril 1982; 38:509–529. Reproduced with permission of the publisher, The American Fertility Society.) (280).

hours or more to be effective for the preovulatory LH surge (1031). With increasing peripheral levels of LH, thecal androgen production increases and is utilized as a substrate for further accelerated estrogen production by the dominant follicle.

Feedback modulation of FSH may also occur as a result of a nonsteroidal peptide inhibitor, inhibin, present in the follicular fluid (141). It is synthesized by the granulosa cells and secreted into the follicular fluid and ovarian venous effluent. Steroid-extracted follicular fluid from medium and large follicles in porcine ovaries significantly suppresses serum FSH of rats in a dose-dependent manner (577). Since porcine follicular fluid suppresses FSH levels in ovariectomized animals, it must act at the level of the hypothalamic–pituitary axis. It appears that FSH is under dual control of estradiol and a nonsteroidal inhibitory substance. The concept of an inhibitory substance in follicular fluid is well documented (192,577). The presence of inhibin within human follicular fluid has also

been noted to have the ability to suppress pituitary FSH but not LH. This has been performed by infusion of human follicular fluid (143) directly into the anterior pituitary gland of ovariectomized rhesus monkeys. A second method demonstrating the effect of inhibin on FSH has been noted by a pituitary cell culture system previously treated with LHRH. Inhibin has been demonstrated in human follicular fluid of women only in the follicular phase and not during the luteal phase of the menstrual cycle. Inhibin concentrations may soon be able to be measured in ovarian venous blood, and those findings should be of great interest in the understanding of FSH regulation in health and disease.

ROLE OF DOMINANT FOLLICLE. In monkeys, in the presence of the dominant follicle, which usually occurs on the fifth day of the cycle, follicles on the same and contralateral ovaries have reduced responsivity to exogenous human menopausal gonadotropin (hMG)

(210). Using a hypophysectomized, immature, estrogen-treated rat, diZerega el al. (207) identified a heat and trypsin-labile substance from human ovarian venous blood containing the dominant follicle. This substance inhibited the response of the rat ovaries to injected hMG as determined by ovarian weight and peripheral serum E_2 concentration. This inhibitory substance was absent in ovarian venous effluents of anovulatory women. This potential intra- and/ or interovarian regulator of folliculogenesis may mediate dominance of the preovulatory follicle. This would be accomplished once the preovulatory follicle has been selected, causing suppression of gonadotropin responsiveness of other follicles on the same and contralateral ovaries (207).

Preovulatory Follicle

Meiosis resumes in the dominant preovulatory follicle nearing completion of its reduction division. The size of the preovulatory follicle is approximately 20 mm (Fig. 2-1D) (280). The granulosa cells enlarge with lipid inclusions and the theca becomes vacuolated and vascular. The levels of E_2 rise rapidly and peak 24–36 hours prior to ovulation (Fig. 2-3) (280,554,712). Sustained elevated levels of E_2 stimulate the LH surge, which causes atresia rather than luteinization of the remaining FSH-suppressed follicles. In view of the FSH-primed LH receptors in the dominant follicle, LH promotes granulosa cell luteinization with production of P (Fig. 2-2) (280). The resulting small but significant preovulatory rise in circulating P, which can be demonstrated on the day of the LH peak, facilitates the positive-feedback estrogen-induced LH surge. There is also good evidence in the human that the preovulatory rise in P is necessary for induction of the mid-cycle FSH peak (576).

Ovulation and Oogenesis

Accurate prediction of time of ovulation is now of even greater importance with the advent of in vitro fertilization. Considerable variation exists from cycle to cycle even in the same patient. Most studies estimate ovulation 10–12 hours after the LH peak and 24–36 hours after the estradiol peak is achieved (Fig. 2-3)

(280,305,712). A recent study by Taymor et al. (904) reveals that ovulation does not generally occur until 36–38 hours after the onset of the LH surge. These investigators found the onset of the LH surge to be a better marker than the LH peak in timing ovulation.

The LH surge results in a rise of tissue concentrations of cAMP (686) which (1) initiates completion of meiosis and maturation of the oocyte; (2) favors luteinization of the granulosa cells, possibly by overcoming local nonsteroidal inhibitors of meiosis and luteinization in the follicular fluid (141); and (3) together with progesterone, enhances activity of proteolytic enzymes which digest follicular wall collagen and increases its distensibility (233,718). The LH surge also promotes granulosa cell synthesis of P and PGs, prostaglandins E (PGE) and prostaglandins F (PGF), which may act in the digestion of the follicular wall, or possibly stimulate "contractions" of smooth muscles fibers located in the theca externa, causing oocyte expulsion (958). The functional significance of the ovarian contractions for ovulation is controversial.

As circulating LH reaches its peak, levels of E_2 plunge due to "down-regulation" of the LH receptors. (In a number of endocrine target organs prolonged exposure of high concentrations of hormone results in a decreased response of such tissue.) The preovulatory rise of P also may aid in terminating the LH surge via its negative-feedback effect. The P-dependent mid-cycle rise of FSH also insures sufficient LH receptors for adequate P production in the subsequent luteal phase.

Corpus Luteum

It is important to stress again the importance of optimal FSH-primed preovulatory follicular development for adequacy of the luteal phase. Following ovulation the follicular wall becomes convoluted and its antrum filled with blood and lymph. Luteal cells are derived mainly from the granulosa cells which enlarge and become lipid laden with lutein pigment.

Following the LH and FSH peak the granulosa cells hypertrophy and ultrastructurally are typical steroid-secreting cells. These luteinized granulosa cells produce large amounts of P, E_2, as well as androgens (mostly androstenedione) between the 13th and 17th day of the cycle, but their production is markedly reduced after the 22nd day. The factors that regulate the production of androgens and estrogens by the corpus luteum (CL) are unknown, but it is possible that a theca-granulosa luteal cell synergism exists similar to that in the preovulatory follicle. Theca-lutein cells may differentiate from the surrounding theca and stroma to become part of the corpus luteum (719). Marked vascularization from branching thecal vessels penetrates the granulosa layer. The luteal cells of the CL produce P in view of the extensive number of LH receptors on the granulosa cells predetermined during the follicular phase of the cycle. Steroidogenesis of the CL is dependent on tonic LH secretion. The postovulatory increased vascularization of the CL allows low-density lipoprotein (LDL) to reach the luteinized granulosa for use as a substrate in P biosynthesis (119).

Progesterone levels rise sharply after ovulation and peak approximately 8 days after the LH surge (Fig. 2-3) (280). P acts at an ovarian and antral level to suppress new follicle growth. At the ovarian level P may act to suppress aromatization, while via the negative-feedback mechanism it inhibits gonadotropin release, causing a low peripheral gonadotropin level at the height of the progesterone peak. As the CL ages it becomes less sensitive to LH and the steroidogenic capacity of luteal cells gradually declines (888). Although estradiol from the CL rises to another peak at the midluteal phase, P production begins to decline (447), and when a low basal level of P is reached, menstruation occurs. It does appear that estrogens cause a decline in the CL. The mechanism of estrogen-induced luteolysis may involve inhibition of LH binding of

luteal tissue (672). Thus a decrease of LH receptors would explain the loss of LH sensitivity and reduced steroidogenesis which is seen in the latter half of the luteal phase. Although the CL is capable of synthesizing local PGs, an increase of the PGF/PGE ratio in the latter half of the luteal phase may be luteolytic (45,892). Estrogen itself may alter the balance by favoring the local luteolytic action of $PGF_{2\alpha}$ (44). Additional studies indicate that luteal tissue contains a nonsteroidal LH receptor binding inhibitor (LHRBI) which increases in concentration during the luteal phase (108). In vitro inhibition of P by LHRBI has been implicated in the process of luteolysis (108). In the presence of human chorionic gonadotropin (hCG), the CL regression is transiently halted (31). PG synthesis is inhibited by placental hCG, while augmenting the production of progesterone. The point at which the fetus becomes independent of luteal function is variable. Down-regulation of LH/hCG receptors does appear to play a role in the refractoriness of the CL to high concentrations of hCG. The role of PRL in the luteal phase is discussed in Chapter 8.

The largest antral follicle sizes occur during the middle to late luteal phase. These undergo atresia perhaps secondary to declining gonadotropin levels. The follicle destined to ovulate in the next cycle is drawn from a "pool" of smaller preantral follicles present during the luteal phase whose size may be 100μ or greater. Hormonally dependent maturation of these follicles may be initiated by estrogens, followed by FSH and then LH, beginning late in the luteal phase and continuing into the follicular phase of the next cycle.

Androgen Transport and Plasma Levels in the Normal Female

3

Testosterone and Androgen Transport in Plasma

In normal women, 99% of circulating T is bound and biologically inactive. Testosterone is bound in the plasma to testosterone-binding globulin (TeBG), also called steroid-hormone-binding globulin (SHBG), a specific beta-globulin produced by the liver with a high affinity for T, and it is also bound to albumin. In normal women, the TeBG level is approximately double that of men. TeBG binds 78% of T, while albumin binds approximately 20% of T. Albumin has a lower affinity for T but has a larger binding capacity. In a study by Nisula and Dunn (689) total testosterone bound to albumin was 57.4% while the TeBG bound total T was 41.2%. These differences reflect different methods for characterization of testosterone binding to both albumin and TeBG. DHT and 5α-androstane-3α, 17β-diol (3α-diol), 5α-androstane-3β,17β-diol (3β-diol) and E_2 are also bound to TeBG. It appears that steroids with a 17β-hydroxyl group are tightly bound to TeBG (Table 3-1) (773).

The binding affinity of E_2 to TeBG is about 30% that of T, while the binding affinity of DHT is 2.5 times greater than that of T. In women the concentration of TeBG is increased by estrogens and thyroid hormone and decreased two-fold by androgens. An androgenic progestogen, such as norgestrel, also depresses TeBG. Markedly elevated serum prolactin levels such as those observed in patients with prolactinomas may suppress TeBG (949).

Growth hormone has also been described as possibly suppressing TeBG (198). Estradiol is bound much more strongly than E_1 to TeBG (546). There is minimal if any binding of androstenedione, DHA and P to TeBG.

The postulate that free testosterone is the biologically important fraction of blood androgens is supported by correlating clinical androgenicity with free testosterone in the blood (775,954). However, studies by Vermeulen et al. (955) first suggested that the rate of testosterone metabolism in humans correlated directly with the quantity of free plus albumin-bound testosterone and inversely with TeBG concentration in the plasma. It appears that TeBG-bound androgens are not readily active or available for in vivo metabolism. Thus for testosterone metabolism to express its biologic activity in reproductive tissues and skin argues that both free and albumin-bound testosterone enter tissues where they are available for full biologic activity (51). Although some data indicate that TeBG may enter androgen-responsive cells such as prostate, the fact that TeBG is not present in the plasma of all species suggests that this binding protein does not play an essential role in the mechanism of androgen action (173).

New insights into the complexities of the secretion and metabolism of steroid hormones has been brought forward by the application of isotopic dilution methods of the secretion rates of gonadal hormones. The formulation of the concepts of secretory rates as opposed to production rates and metabolic clearance rates requires defining.

TABLE 3-1. Competition of Selected Steroids with Testosterone for Binding Sites on TeBG (Testosterone = 100%).

C_{19},17β-HYDROXYSTEROIDS	PERCENT
Dihydrotestosterone	250
Androstane-3β,17β-diol	121
Androstane-3α,17β-diol	108
Testosterone	100
Delta^5-Androstenediol	90
5β-Dihydrotestosterone	8

Reprinted with permission from Rosenfield RL. Studies of the relation of plasma androgen levels to androgen action in women J Ster Biochem 1975, 6 695–702, Pergamon Press, Ltd (773)

Secretion Rate (SR) = the total of the secretion rate from an endocrine gland per unit of time.

Production Rate (PR) = the sum of rates of de novo entry of the hormone from peripheral (extraglandular) sites and from endocrine gland secretion. (When a hormone is derived exclusively from glandular secretion the secretion rate and production rate are obviously the same. When a hormone originates from extraglandular conversion as well as from glandular secretion, the PR will exceed the SR.)

Metabolic Clearance Rate (MCR) = the apparent volume of whole blood or plasma from which a substance is irreversibly cleared (by metabolism, or by excretion via any route) per unit of time. It equals the hepatic and extra-hepatic clearance, and is expressed in liters of plasma per 24 hour.

Under steady-state conditions where the quantity of steroid metabolized per unit time is compensated by the secretion of an equivalent amount of hormone, the product of the MCR and the mean plasma concentration over the period considered gives the blood production rate per unit time.

Blood Production Rate (PR)
= MCR × plasma concentration
of the hormone (C).

It must be remembered that reported values for MCR and PR are only approximations obtained under strictly controlled conditions, and that physiologic variables such as period of day, dietary patterns and activity markedly alter these values (948).

The splanchnic (hepatic) system is the major contributor to steroid metabolism and thus of the MCR of steroids. The extrasplanchnic (extrahepatic) clearance is frequently a parameter of target tissue metabolism. The two clearances are difficult to determine separately. In normal women it has been estimated that 10% of T metabolism occurs extrahepatically, while extrahepatic clearance of androstenedione approximates 50% of its total clearance (43). Metabolism of androgen prehormones results in the formation of more potent hormones at target tissues (e.g., androstenedione → T and T → DHT). On the other hand, in hepatic tissues active androgens are usually converted to less active substances.

The formation of less active and inactive hormones from androgens involves 5α- and 5β- reduction of the A ring, reduction of the 3-oxo group (3α- or 3β) and generally 17β-hydroxyl group oxidation (948). Following reduction of ring A, the androgen metabolites are conjugated predominantly by the liver (glucuronic ≫ sulfuric acid) making them water soluble for urine excretion. Etiocholanolone and androsterone glucuronide represent 65% of the urinary metabolites of T or androstenedione. The lesser metabolites may be noted in Fig. 3-1 (948). DHAS may be excreted as such, metabolized to delta^5-androstenediol, or hydrolyzed to DHA which become conjugated with either sulfuric or glucuronic acid.

TeBG binding capacity is an important determinant of the metabolic clearance rate (MCR) of T, DHT and 3α-diol, and it is apparent that TeBG binding is an important mechanism in the distribution of androgens. An inverse correlation occurs between an androgen's MCR and the strength of its binding to TeBG. Those steroids with a high affinity for TeBG have a relatively low MCR (773) while a decrease in TeBG binding of T is paralleled by an increased MCR. The MCR of T has been shown to be related to the amount of free T as well as the albumin-bound T (323). The albumin-bound steroids appear to be more available than TeBG-bound steroids for hepatic degradation (773).

Elevated plasma levels of testosterone in pregnancy or hypothyroidism do not cause virilization and are generally accompanied by a low MCR. This again suggests that TeBG-bound testosterone is not biologically active, and not as readily metabolized as the free and the albumin-

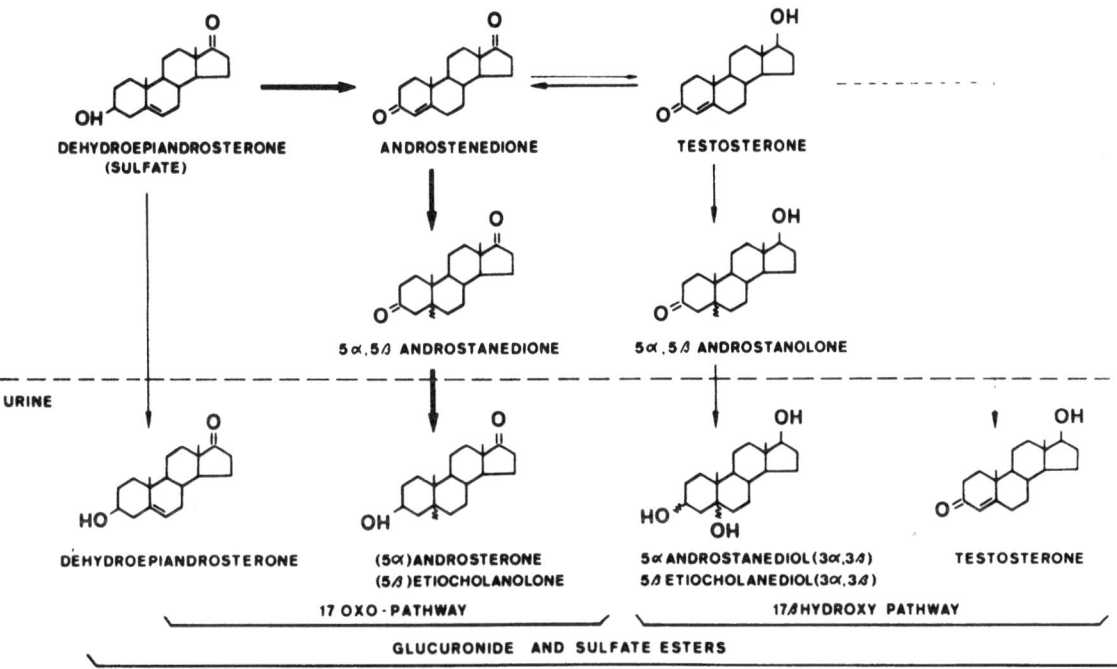

Fig. 3-1. Degradative metabolism of androgens. (Reproduced with permission from Vermeulin A. Androgen secretion by adrenals and gonads In Mahesh VB, Greenblatt RB, eds. Hirsutism and Virilism. Boston. John Wright, PSG Inc , 1983 17–34). (948)

bound fraction. The increased MCR observed in hirsute women by Bardin and Lipsett (54) might be the consequence of decreased TeBG (capacity) by the persistent, although slight, increase of plasma T levels.

The effect of changes in TeBG concentration on unbound E_2 is relatively small, while the effect on unbound T is quite significant. An increase in E_2 secretion leads to an increase in the unbound E_2. This leads to an increase of TeBG and a subsequent reduction of unbound T as

well as a proportionate reduction in the MCR of testosterone (21). On the other hand, increased androgens increase the unbound T, which leads to a reduction of TeBG and an alteration of the unbound T/E_2 ratio.

A method based on equilibrium dialysis of diluted plasma, by which the apparent free T concentration (AFTC) is obtained, has been reported by Vermeulen et al. (Table 3-2) (954).

Additional studies of mean plasma-free testosterone concentrations (474) and the %-free

TABLE 3-2. Mean Plasma Values of the %-Free Testosterone, Free Testosterone, and Total Testosterone.

GROUP	%-FREE TESTOSTERONE	(AFTC) FREE TESTOSTERONE (NG/DL)	TOTAL TESTOSTERONE (NG/DL)
PCOD	1.91	3 19	159
(n = 4)	(range 1.50–2 22)	(range 1 58–5 61)	(range 105–255)
70 Normal Females	0.96 ± 0.07 (SE)	0.35	36 0 ± 15 0 (SE)
(15–44 yrs) (n = 70)		(range 0.20–0.75)	
Men (20–50 yrs)	2.08 ± 0.08 (SE)	II 6 ± 0.7 (SE)	—
(n = 44)		(range 5.5–20)	
Pregnancy	0.23 ± 0.02 (SE)	0 22 (± 0.02) (SE)	99 0 ± 9.0 (SE)
(n = 18)			

Reproduced with permission from Vermeulen A, Stoica T, Verdonck L The apparent free testosterone concentration, an index of androgenicity J Clin Endocrinol Metab 1971, 33 759–767) (954)

TABLE 3-3. Mean Plasma Free Testosterone and %-Free Testosterone in Normal Adult Men and Women and in Various Clinical States.

GROUP	AGE (YEARS)	% FREE TESTOSTERONE MEAN ± S.D. (646)	% FREE TESTOSTERONE MEAN ± S.D. (263)	MEAN PLASMA FREE TESTOSTERONE CONCENTRATION (NG/DL) (646)
Normal men		2 50 ± .035	1.71 ± 0.29	12.80
Hirsute women		2 21 ± 0 62	1.68 ± 0 52	1.61
Normal women		1 38 ± 0 28	1 02 ± 0 17	0 54
Pregnant women	20 – 40	0.58 ± 0 06		0.46
Women on BCP		0.86 ± 0.05	0.67 ± 0 06	0 66
DXM females	19 – 28	1 36 ± 0 32		0 42

BCP = birth control pills
DXM = dexamethasone treated, 2 mg daily × 2 – 30 days
Modified from Moll GW Jr, Rosenfield RL Testosterone binding and free plasma androgen concentrations under physiological conditions characterization by flow dialysis technique J Clin Endocrinol Metab 1979, 49 730 – 736 (646) And from Fisher RA, Anderson DC Simultaneous measurement of unbound testosterone and estradiol fractions in undiluted plasma at 37 degrees C by steady-state gel filtration Steroids 1974, 24 809 – 824 (263)

testosterone levels in normal men and women, hirsute and pregnant women and women on oral contraceptives are listed in Table 3-3 (263,646).

Androgen and Estrogen Levels in Normal Menstrual Cycle

Several days before the LH surge, serum levels of androstenedione, T, and 17α-hydroxyprogesterone (170HP) begin to rise (Fig. 3-2) (741). Coincident with the LH surge, serum P and 170HP rise and E_2 decreases. This is associated with a decrease of the transient preovulatory rise of androstenedione and T.

Serum estrone parallels the E_2, although to a lesser extent. While almost all of the E_2 is of ovarian origin, less E_1 is of ovarian origin, while the remaining estrone is derived from peripheral conversion of androstenedione and to a much lesser extent E_2. In normal men and women 1% of secreted androstenedione is converted peripherally to E_1. Since the PR of androstenedione is approximately 3000 μg/day, about 20 – 40 μg of estrone is produced daily from extraglandular conversion of androstenedione. P output reaches a maximum 8 days after the LH peak, with smaller parallel increases of E_2, E_1 and 170HP.

P. During the follicular phase (prior to the LH surge), most of the P in the circulation is derived from extraglandular conversion of adrenal pregnenolone and pregnenolone sulfate to P and also from the secretion of small amounts of P from the adrenals. The ovary containing the dominant follicle then secretes increased amounts of P. In vitro studies of antral fluid reveals that P is secreted by granulosa cells of preovulatory follicles which respond to LH. During the luteal phase the progesterone production may exceed 25 mg/day.

170HP. The rising peripheral level of 170HP during ovulation and in the luteal phase of the cycle reflects almost entirely the secretory activity of the ovary containing the corpus luteum. During the follicular phase most of the 170HP is derived from extraglandular conversion of 17α-hydroxypregnenolone, which is almost exclusively adrenal in origin.

ANDROGENS. There are four main steps to androgen action (419): (1) the entrance of unbound T and DHT into the cells; (2) the binding of these androgens to specific cytoplasmic androgen-receptor proteins which are transferred to the nuclei; (3) an interaction of the steroid-receptor complexes with acceptor sites on the chromatin that is associated with synthesis of precursors of different RNAs (948); and (4) the translation of steroid-specific RNAs on the polyribosomes which results in the formation of hormone-specific proteins along with other cellular components required for altered target cell function (419). The two main factors that regulate androgen responses in individual tissues are (1) the steroid-recognition machinery which includes the concentration and steroid-binding specificity of androgen receptors and (b) the structure of chromatin determined during differentiation so as to allow the androgen-receptor complex to activate tissue responses selectively (419). One of the mechanisms by which antiandrogens such as spironolactone and cyproterone acetate act is by direct competition and interference for the cytosol-receptor binding sites.

One of the effects of testosterone is induction of 5α-reductase activity. The 5α-reductase enzyme is present in most androgen-sensitive tissues, where T is rapidly converted to DHT upon entering the cells of these target organs. The high affinity binding cytosol receptor protein preferentially binds DHT rather than T (Fig. 3-3) (886). Furthermore, the steroid–cytosol receptor interaction produces a conformational change in the androgen receptor protein which is a prerequisite for the rapid translocation of the steroid-receptor complex to the cell nucleus. It must be emphasized that not all tissues require 5α-reduction of T for androgenic activity. These include the anabolic action of skeletal muscle, bone marrow stimulation, sexual and behavioral changes in the brain, differentiation of the wolffian ducts and others, where androgen expression is either through T, or metabolic products of T other than DHT.

The ovary produces primarily three androgens: androstenedione, T, and DHA. DHAS is produced almost entirely by the adrenal cortex. Androstenedione appears to be the major prehormone for blood DHT in the adult female, while T is the major source of plasma DHT in the male.

The adrenal cortex can sulfurylate 3β-ol steroids by means of the enzyme 3β-hydroxysteroid sulfokinase (948). In view of the large quantities of secreted DHA and DHAS by the adrenal cortex, it appears that the delta[5] pathway is the major pathway for androgen biosynthesis in the adrenal. The sequence of the delta[5] pathway

goes from pregnenolone $\rightarrow$ 17αOH-pregnenolone $\rightarrow$ DHA (Fig. 3-4) (354). The minor delta[4] pathway occurs from pregnenolone $\rightarrow$ progesterone via 3β-ol isomerization $\rightarrow$ 17OHP $\rightarrow$ androstenedione (Fig. 3-4) (354).

Androstenedione. Androstenedione is the major androgen secreted by the ovary. It has very little affinity for TeBG (6.6%) and 85% binds loosely to albumin. A relative mid-cycle increase in androstenedione and T (10–20%), which remains even after adrenocortical suppression with dexamethasone, is consistent with the ovarian origin of the mid-cycle increase (5,436,459,953). Adrenal androstenedione has a diurnal rhythm similar to that of cortisol. The adrenal contribution does not vary with the menstrual cycle. An approximate doubling of androstenedione level may occur near mid-cycle with a subsequent drop, and the luteal phase level is somewhat higher than that of the follicular phase (5). The finding of increased plasma T

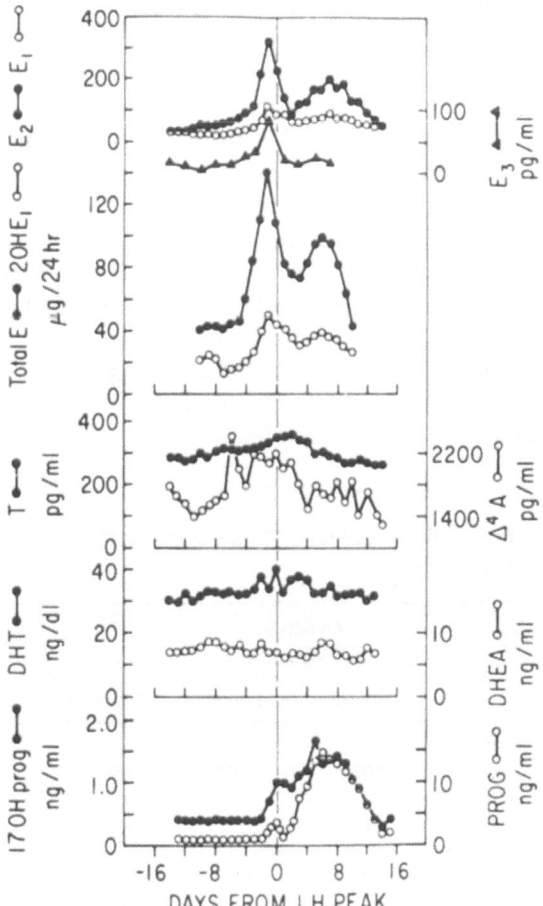

Fig. 3-2. Steroid patterns during the menstrual cycles. Total E = total urinary estrogens, 20HE₁ = 2-hydroxyestrone, E₃ = estriol; PROG = progesterone (Reproduced with permission from Rebar RW, Yen SSC Endocrine rhythms in gonadotropins and ovarian steroids with reference to reproductive processes In: Krieger DT, ed. Endocrine Rhythms. New York: Raven Press, 1979 259–298) (741).

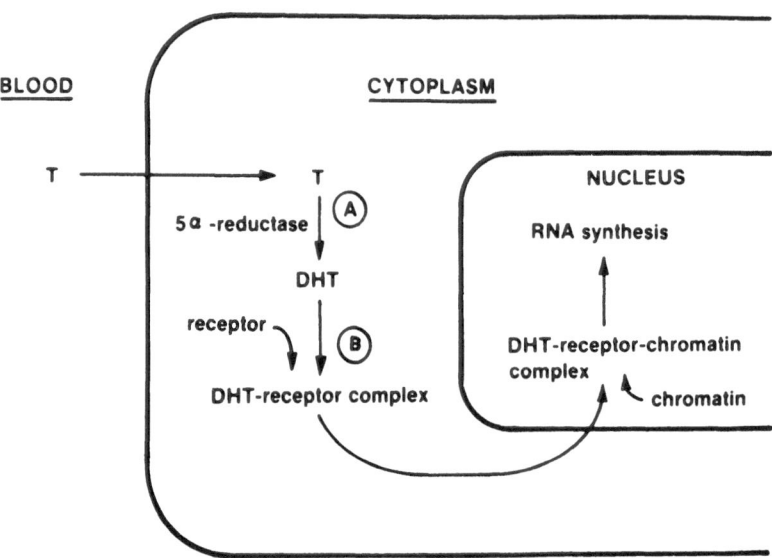

Fig. 3-3. Testosterone is converted to DHT in the target organ cell. DHT is then bound by a specific cytosolic DHT-receptor complex. This enters the cell nucleus where it stimulates RNA synthesis. Abbreviations: A = point of inhibition by antiandrogens which inhibit 5α-reductase, B = point of inhibition by antiandrogens which block receptors. (Reproduced with permission Stewart ME, Pochi PE. Antiandrogens in the skin. Int J Derm. 1978; 17:167–179). (886).

and androstenedione at mid-cycle has also been confirmed by Judd and Yen (436).

T. Most of the T in normal adult women comes from peripheral conversion with little coming from the adrenals or ovaries. In normal females, 50–70% of T is mainly derived from the peripheral conversion of androstenedione (54,397), and to a lesser extent (<15%) from DHA and DHAS (395,397). Horton and Tait (397) demonstrated a peripheral conversion rate of 14% for androstenedione to T. In the normal nonhirsute female, only 15–35% of T is produced from ovarian and adrenal glandular secretions (250,397). Fluctuations during the menstrual cycle are minimal. Reports of higher

mid-cycle T levels (5,436,953) may be due to peripheral conversion of androstenedione which is cyclically secreted by the ovaries.

Horton et al. (396) determined the concentration of T and androstenedione in peripheral and ovarian venous blood in five patients with metastatic breast cancer and found an ovarian-peripheral venous ratio of 1.58 for T and 6.5 for androstenedione. They concluded that T is a minor secretory product of the ovary as compared to androstenedione (396).

DHT. DHT is the intracellular effector of T action. Small or negligible amounts come from the normal ovary (820). Approximately 80% is

TABLE 3-4. Mean Androgen Levels of Normal Women (ng/dl) during the Follicular and Luteal Phase of the Menstrual Cycle.

	ANDRO-STENEDIONE		T		DHA		DHT	
	Follicular	Luteal	Follicular	Luteal	Follicular	Luteal	Follicular	Luteal
Ovarian vein	1972	1238	81	76	1670	1471	17	17
Peripheral vein	161	256	20	36	618	617	12	14

Reproduced with permission from Serio M, Dell'Acqua S, Calabresi E, et al. Androgen secretion by the human ovary: measurement of androgens in the ovarian venous blood. In: James VHT, Serio M, Giusti G, eds. The Endocrine Function of the Human Ovary. New York: Academic Press, 1976 471–479. (820)

derived from peripheral conversion of androstenedione, much more so than T (410). Its concentration in the peripheral venous plasma of normal women is about 15–17 ng/dl (410,924). The production rate in normal women is about 40–60 μg/24 hrs, while the MCR is about 170–238 l/day (410,786,924). Only a small fraction of DHT enters the blood (580), since most of the DHT synthesized in tissues is reduced in situ to 3α- and 3β-androstane-

diols (499). DHT may also be further metabolized to androsterone in splanchnic (hepatic) tissues (948).

The mean concentration of steroids in ovarian venous blood obtained from the ovary containing the ripe follicle and corpus luteum were reported by Serio et al. (Table 3-4) (820).

Insignificant gradients of DHT between ovarian and peripheral plasma (Table 3-4) (820), are in agreement with the data of ovarian

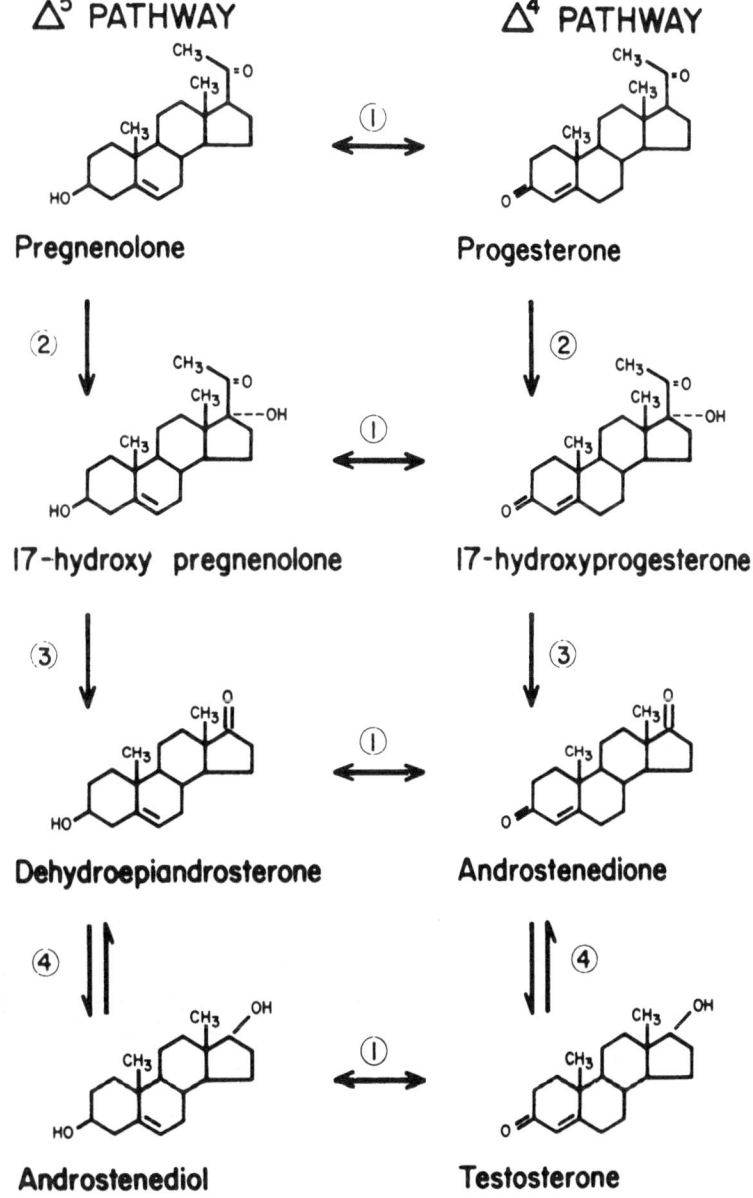

Fig. 3-4. Alternate pathways in the synthesis of androgens. (1) = delta^5-3β-ol-dehydrogenase delta^5-isomerase; (2) = 17-hydroxylase; (3) = 17,20-desmolase (lyase); (4) = 17β-hydroxysteroid dehydrogenase (oxireductase) (Reproduced with permission from Granoff AB, Abraham GE. Peripheral and adrenal venous levels of steroids in a patient with virilizing adrenal adenoma. Obstet Gynecol. 1979; 53:111–115, Elsevier Science Publishing Co., New York.) (354).

TABLE 3-5. Metabolic Clearance Rates, Production Rates and Sources of Steroidal Sex Hormones in Normal Women

	MCR plasma (liter/day)	Mean plasma concentration (range—ng/dl)	Mean PR (mg/day)	SOURCES OF CIRCULATING STEROID			Ovarian secreting rate (both ovaries—mg/day)
				Ovarian secretion %	Adrenal secretion %	Extraglandular formation % (from)	
Androstenedione (A)	2010 Premenop	160 (90–290)	3.2	30–70	30–70	15 (DHA)	1 0–2 2
	Postmenop	70	1 4	<30	70–100	15 (DHA)	<0 4
Testosterone (T)	690 Premenop	40 (30–50)	0.18	<30	20–40	50–60 (A)	<0.05
	Postmenop	20	0.09	15–35	25–45	40 (A)	0.01–0 03
DHA	1640 Premenop	500 (300–700)	8.0	<20	>30	<60 (DHAS)	<3 0
	Postmenop	200	3.3	<20	>30	<60 (DHAS)	<1 0
17OHP	2000 Early foll	50	1 0	20–80	—	20–80 (17OH5P)	0 2–0 8
	Late foll	150	3 0	>90	—	—	2 7–3 0
	Mid-luteal	200	4 0	>90	—	—	3.6–4 0
	Postmenop	30	0 6	0	—	100	0
Progesterone (P)	2400 Follic	40	1 0	10–70	5–65	25 (5-P)	0 1–0 7
	Luteal	1500	36 0	>90	—	1 (5-P)	32–36
	Postmenop	20	0.5	0	>90	5 (5-P)	0
20a-OHP	2300 Follic	5	1 1	80	—	20 (P)	0 8
	Luteal	25	5 8	50	—	50 (P)	3 3
DHT	170 Premenop	12	0 02	<5	<5	95–100 (A > T)	0
DHAS	8	170 µg/dl	13 6	—	100	—	0
Androstenediol	1000	80 (73–90)ng/dl	0.75	<5	<5	>90–95 (DHA, DHAS)	—
Estradiol (E₂)	1350 Early follic	40 (20–100)pg/ml	0.05	85	0	5(A),10 (E₁)	0.04
	Late follic	300 (250–700)pg/ml	0.40	>90	0	<10(A),(A,E₁)	0.36–0 40
	Mid-luteal	150 (50–300)pg/ml	0.20	>90	0	<10(A),(A,E₁)	0.18–0 20
	Postmenop	15 pg/ml	0.01	0	0	>90(A)	0
Estrone (E₁)	2210 Early follic	50 pg/ml	0.11	70	0	20(A),10 (E₂)	0.08
	Late follic	150 pg/ml	0.33	70	0	7(A);25 (E₂)	0.23
	Mid-luteal	80 pg/ml	0.18	60	0	13(A);23 (E₂)	0 11
	1610 Postmenop.	25 pg/ml	0 04	0	0	>90(A),	0

MCR = metabolic clearance rate
PR = production rate
5-P = pregnenolone
17-OH5P = 17α-hydroxypregnenolone

venous samples obtained by Ito and Horton (410).

Although DHT is probably the active peripheral androgen, its utilization as a useful marker for peripheral androgen action has been disappointing (529).

Delta⁵-Androstenediol. Small amounts of delta⁵-androstenediol are secreted by the adrenals and to a lesser extent, the ovaries. Most comes from secreted DHA. A minimal ovarian gradient for delta⁵-androstenediol was noted in five hirsute subjects by Kirschner (460). The PR has been reported as 530 μg/day (464) and as 969 μg/day (82), with a metabolic clearance rate of 584 l/day (464) and 858 l/day (82). The plasma concentration is approximately 90 ng/dl (464). As with DHA and DHAS, delta⁵-androstenediol is not a significant prehormone of plasma T in women (464). Some increase in plasma delta⁵-androstenediol and in its production rate has been reported in hirsute females (464).

DHA and DHAS. Quantitatively DHA and DHAS are the principal androgens secreted in the normal female. Both are mainly of adrenal origin (>80–95%, respectively) (385), and therefore little, if any, menstrual cycle fluctuations occur (6,193). DHAS is probably not directly secreted by normal ovaries but in view of its partial origin from the peripheral conversion of DHA, a small fraction may therefore indirectly originate from the ovaries. Abraham (5) has estimated that 4% of peripheral DHAS is ovarian in origin. Kirschner (460), however, found no ovarian gradient for DHAS in ovarian vein effluents of women with idiopathic hirsutism. In women most DHA and DHAS is converted to delta⁵-androstenediol, rather than to

androstenedione. The concentration of DHA appears to be in synchrony with cortisol. DHA and DHAS are interconverted peripherally, with the half-life of DHAS 20–40 times longer than DHA. This accounts for the general absence of circadian fluctuation of DHAS (768). DHAS is the major constituent of the plasma 17-ketosteroids (1006), and its plasma measurement is an ideal index of adrenal androgen secretion (582). Suppression with dexamethasone reduces DHAS levels below 40 ng/dl (2,1006).

Using four days of dexamethasone (DXM) suppressive doses of 0.5 mg 4 times daily, Abraham (5) found that this regimen had no effect on the levels of P, 17OHP, and E₂ throughout the menstrual cycle of normal women. Dexamethasone treatment did not effect the pattern of testosterone or of serum androstenedione but lowered the mean levels approximately by 15–25 ng/dl and 60 ng/dl, respectively. DXM suppression caused a decline of the mean DHT level of 15–20 ng/dl to 5–10 ng/dl. The latter data suggest that adrenal and ovarian contributions to peripheral DHT levels are 10 ng/dl for each gland (5). The ovarian contribution to peripheral DHT and DHA is not influenced by the menstrual cycle.

Summary of Sources, Metabolic Clearance Rates and Production Rates of Sex Hormones in Normal Women

Table 3-5 is a compilation of data indicating the sources of steroidal sex hormones in normal women, including the MCR, plasma concentrations and mean PR. (The data include personal communications from Dr. E. Gurpide and Dr. C. Longcope and from references 372, 373,545,579,778,896).

The Pathologic Anatomy of Polycystic Ovarian Disease

4

Gross Pathology

The ovaries may be normal sized (238,852,905) but they are usually enlarged occasionally up to five times normal size. The enlargement is usually bilateral and symmetrical, but rarely may be unilateral (194,206,222,945). Unlike the slightly flattened ovaries of normal adult women, the ovaries of those with polycystic ovarian disease are usually ovoid or globular. They tend to have an oyster-gray color and a smooth glistening tense surface overlaying a thickened pearly gray capsule. The capsule often has characteristic telangiectasia. Numerous small subcapsular (subcortical) cysts are present, measuring 2–15 mm (averaging 2–6 mm) in diameter (909), and numbering 10 to more than 100 in each ovary (Fig. 4-1). Larger macrofollicular subcortical cysts with clear or yellow fluid may also be present. The cysts may cause bulging of the surface but are often not fully appreciated prior to sectioning because of the thickened ovarian capsule. Many atretic follicles and occasional corpora albicantia may be present but recent corpora lutea or corpus luteum cysts are infrequent.

Histopathology

The tunica albuginea is characteristically widened by a fibrous thickening of dense eosinophilic hyalinized collagen tissue. Forming wide bridges or columns the cortex may penetrate deeply into the ovary. Unlike the normal ovary whose tunica is thin and often indistinct (100 μ

or less), the capsule in patients with PCOD is increased in thickness up to 10- to 15-fold (150–600 μ) (86,359,905). Numerous microfollicular cysts of varying size are evenly distributed beneath the tunica albuginea (Fig. 4-2). There are many different sized follicles in all stages of maturation and atresia with numerous corpora fibrosa. The walls of the follicular cysts consist of usually one or occasionally several layers of granulosa cells, beneath which is a wider layer of theca interna cells (Fig. 4-3) (909).

Luteinization of hypertrophic perifollicular theca interna cells may occasionally be extensive (Fig. 4-4) (909) and may be present with hyperplasia and vascularization of the adjacent theca externa. The most common type of luteinized theca interna cells are those with clear cytoplasm. Less common types of luteinized theca interna cells include those with a hazy lightly pink eosinophilic cytoplasm, and another type consisting of smaller deep-staining red-pigmented cells (902). The presence of all three cell types in normal ovaries negate their usefulness as a characteristic finding of PCOD (902). It is clear that attempts to quantitate the degree of thecal cell luteinization about an atretic follicle is most difficult.

Theca cell hyperplasia may be noted occasionally in the ovarian stroma. Clusters of large luteinized theca cells with finely vacuolated cytoplasm and a round vesicular nucleus may be dispersed irregularly within the cortex and medulla. Initial reviews on Stein-Leventhal syndrome (SLS) considered the pronounced theca cell luteinization and hyperplasia as characteristic histopathological features. This, however,

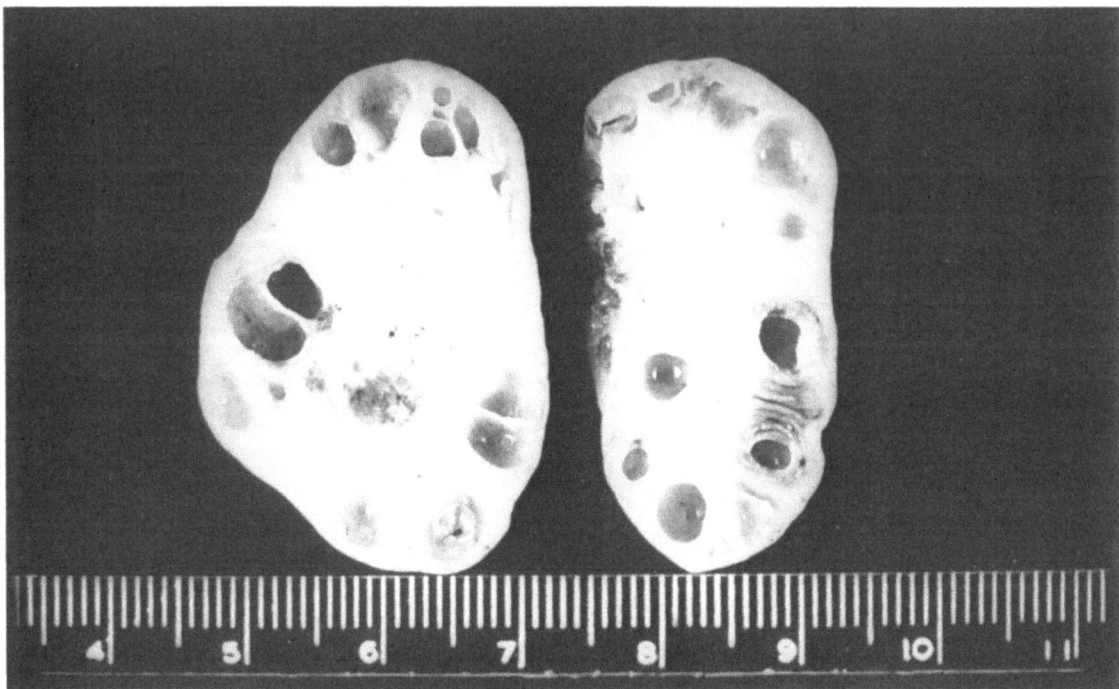

Fig. 4-1. Multiple cystic follicles are present in the subcapsular zone. No corpora albicantia are noted The stroma appears compact.

has not proven to be frequent, specific or characteristic. Although stromal hyperplasia with luteinization is infrequently observed in PCOD (359,491,905), the presence of individual islets of luteinized stromal theca cells may be associated with more severe masculinizing features (309).

The hypothesis that the thick sclerotic tunica albuginea acts as a barrier to ovulation is apocryphal. In this connection it is noteworthy that

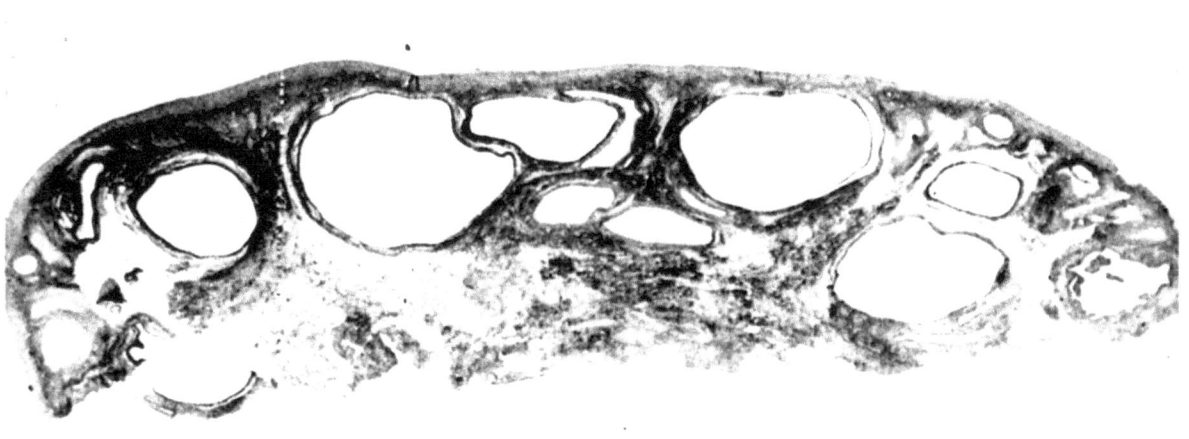

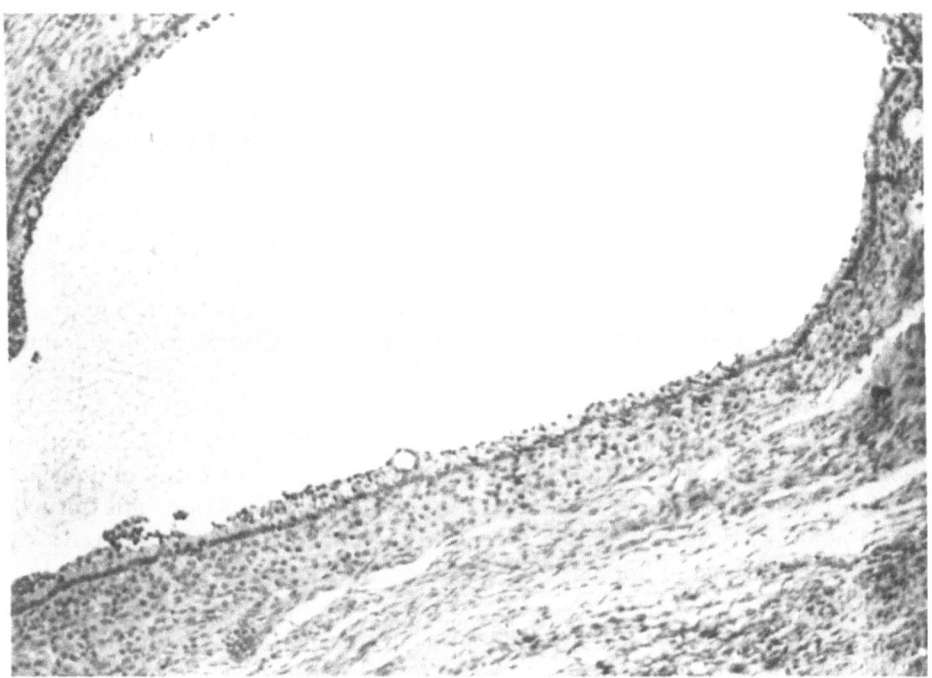

Fig. 4-3. The wall of the follicle cyst is lined by granulosa cells, beneath which is a thickened layer of theca interna cells (×40).

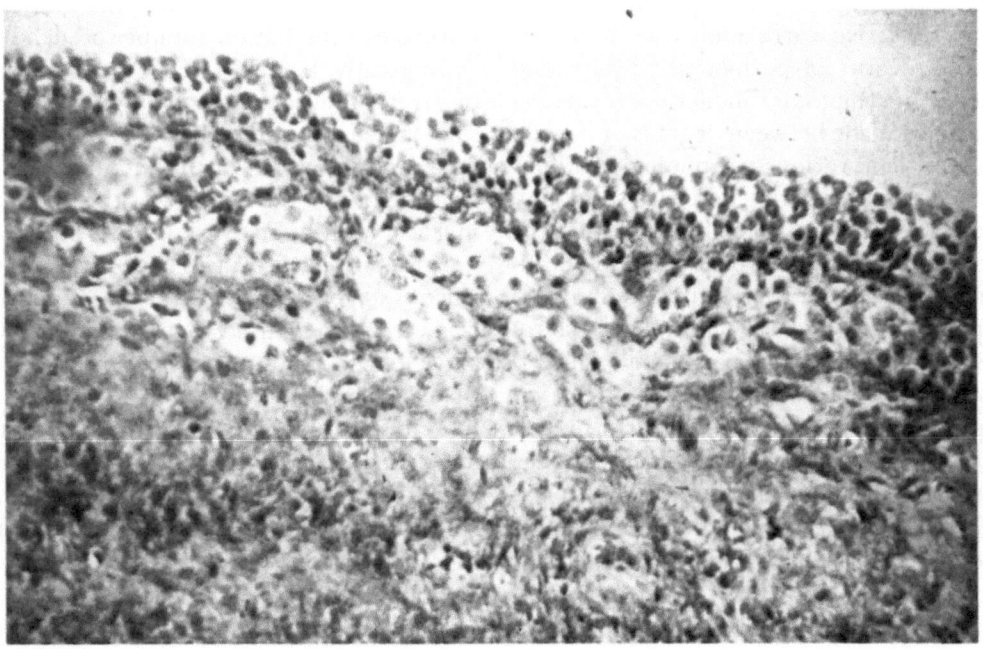

Fig. 4-4. Luteinized theca interna cells appear to have a clear vacuolated cytoplasm These are surrounded by theca externa cells (×250)

Greenblatt observed that performing unilateral oophorectomy in five patients with the classic Stein-Leventhal syndrome resulted in cyclic ovulation from the contralateral ovary despite its thickened capsule (361). Since clomiphene, gonadotropin therapy, steroids and other forms of treatment may induce ovulation, the sclerotic capsule is obviously no deterrent to ovulation. Similarly a number of investigators have studied the significance and frequency of stromal thecal cell hyperplasia in patients with polycystic ovaries. Its incidence is less than 10% of patients with PCOD (359). Furthermore, a number of stromal thecal cells may be found in some presumably normal post-menopausal ovaries without PCOD (808). It is clear that stromal theca cells may be found in ovaries without PCOD, and are nonspecific histological findings.

Significance of Peripheral Sclerosis

The frequent finding of a thickened capsule in patients with PCOD has interested a number of investigators. A retrospective study was made in patients aged 15 – 48 years, of the role of peripheral sclerosis in ovarian dysfunction (380). Cases were selected from pathology records of patients diagnosed as having peripheral sclerosis of the ovaries. In 61 patients PCOD was suspected with bilateral wedge resections performed from 1963 to 1967. No correlation was found between the severity of peripheral sclerosis and prevalence of symptoms. Similarly, no correlation could be made between degrees of peripheral sclerosis and various morphologic and histologic signs of ovarian function or dysfunction. A close correlation was noted between multiple follicle cysts and symptoms of anovulation. Multiple small subcapsular cysts were noted in 80% of the patients with significant peripheral sclerosis (380). It appears that peripheral sclerosis does not interfere mechanically with ovulation but represents a sign of hyperandrogenism. Administration of testosterone to animals can cause thickening of the ovarian capsule (349). It has been shown in animals that a thick ovarian capsule does not result in polycystic changes nor does it prevent ovulation in response to gonadotropins or clomiphene (349).

There appear to be no differences in the degree of thecosis and other morphological characteristics between ovarian sections from women with evidence of overproduction of ovarian androgens and those without (756, 909). In PCOD the microscopic appearances vary from one ovary to another in the same patient, and from one to another part of the same ovary (349). Goldzieher and Axelrod noted that polycystic changes in the ovaries may be reversible (348). This has also been noted by Gambrell by administration of estradiol (301), and by Wortsman et al. (997) with medroxyprogesterone acetate treatment for 6 – 9 months.

Taymor et al. (905) studied the capsules of 40 patients with PCOD undergoing ovarian wedge resection. Variability of capsule thickness was evident in the same ovary and even within the same histological section. The normal ovary has little tissue that can be considered a capsule, and if so it rarely exceeds 0.1 mm in thickness. These investigators only studied patients whose mean capsule thickness exceeded 0.1 mm and who demonstrated thecal cell hyperplasia. A mean capsular thickness of 0.2–0.4 mm was found in 26 of their 40 patients (65%), while 6 of 40 (15%) had a mean capsular thickness exceeding 0.4 mm. Further conclusions may be noted from their study of the degree of theca luteinization which was prominent even in atretic follicles. Thirty-four of 40 patients had some degree of theca interna luteinization (85%) (905). The degree of theca luteinization appeared to be no greater, however, than that normally seen in normal ovaries, but the number of such follicles were greatly increased. Each individual follicle or atretic follicle was indistinguishable from a similar structure found in a normal ovary (359). The range in width of the thecal cells and the morphology of these cells was the same in normal as in polycystic ovaries (359, 756).

Since polycystic ovaries have more follicles at various stages of growth and atresia, more follicles with a condensed theca are found. Green and Goldzieher in a study of 45 patients with PCOD, found no evidence of marked theca cell luteinization and hyperplasia (359). An interesting feature of polycystic ovaries is the fact that the degree of luteinization of the theca interna cells is approximately the same in all follicles. Electron microscopic studies have shown no ultrastructural difference between normal ovarian follicles and corresponding follicles in polycystic ovaries (359). Only occasional small clusters of round clear luteinized cells may be found in the abundant stroma. Hilus cells are found along the line of insertion of the mesovarium into the ovary; however, it is unusual to find them in markedly increased numbers or hyperplastic.

It appears that the major differences which may be found in ovaries of subjects with PCOD as opposed to normal ovaries are (1) the more frequent presence of a thickened capsule, (2) the presence of more numerous follicles in various stages of growth and atresia and (3) the more frequent presence of theca cell hyperplasia and luteinization.

Hyperthecosis

The term *hyperthecosis* was introduced by Fraenkel in 1943 (271) to describe theca interna hyperplasia of the ovary. Since the hyperplastic theca interna frequently was luteinized, the luteinization was accepted in the concept of hyperthecosis. In 1942, Geist and Gaines (309) reported two patients with diffuse luteinization of ovaries who on exploratory laparotomy had numerous small follicle cysts at the periphery of enlarged ovaries, while the solid portions of the ovaries appeared yellowish. Although extensive proliferation of theca cells was noted around atretic follicles with well-defined luteinization, many clusters of similar large luteinized hyperplastic theca cells were irregularly scattered throughout the parenchyma, giving the yellow spotted appearance on gross section. Clinically these patients appeared to be more obese and masculinized than those described earlier by Stein and Leventhal. The authors suggested that the ovarian effects were probably secondary to increased gonadotropin stimulation. Subsequently, Sohval (858) suggested that "diffuse luteinization of the ovary" and "ovarian hyperthecosis" were findings which represent varying degrees of a fundamentally similar endocrine disturbance (858) (see Chapter 9). Shippel further described clinical and pathological aspects of the "hyperthecosis syndrome" (838).

Many of the clinical and histologic features of ovarian hyperthecosis overlap those of PCOD (13), and may represent a different spectrum of the same pathophysiological process (335,858) (see Chapter 9). *Hyperthecosis* is the term presently applied to a masculinizing syndrome associated with nests of luteinized hyperplastic theca cells or stromal cells in the ovarian stroma. In PCOD, the luteinized theca cells are usually confined to areas around the cystic follicles, whereas in the hyperthecosis syndrome islands of luteinized theca or stromal cells are gathered in clusters or scattered diffusely in the ovarian stroma, away from follicles and extending to include the hilar region (Fig. 4-5). In hyperthecosis the ovaries are usually enlarged 2–3 times normal size, but may occasionally be normal sized. Although infrequent, the presence of follicle cysts in some areas and characteristic collagenization of the outer cortex supports the possible pathological overlap between hyperthecosis and polycystic ovarian disease (124).

Scully associated hyperthecosis with an excess of ovarian stroma and focal yellowish areas (809). Within the hyperplastic ovarian stroma are nests of stromal lutein cells with abundant, clear lipid-rich cytoplasm and round prominent nuclei (the hallmark of ovarian hyperthecosis). As Scully noted in his discussion of a patient with hyperthecosis (123), "if one reviews the literature on the subject of polycystic ovarian disease on the one hand and hyperthecosis on the other, it is very hard to sort out which of these two disorders many authors are reporting. There are several reasons for this confusion. Although the term *hyperthecosis* was coined in 1943 by Fraenkel to designate the presence of theca or lutein cells within the ovarian stroma — in other words, stromal hyperthecosis — many authors have since used the term *hyperthecosis* for follicular hyperthecosis — i.e., prominence of theca cells around the follicles, and this change is found commonly in polycystic ovarian disease without stromal hyperthecosis. So unless there is careful pathological documentation one never knows whether the author is referring to the stromal hyperthecosis of Fraenkel (271) or the follicular hyperthecosis that may be seen in polycystic ovarian disease. Another problem has been that many authors have not searched for these cells in the stroma." In cases of PCOD where only wedge resections are submitted for examination, there may be only limited amounts of stroma to analyze. Although there are clinical differences between "classic" cases of PCOD and hyperthecosis the two disorders do appear to merge both clinically and pathologically (14,858).

Combined ovarian and adrenocortical biopsies were obtained in six hirsute and/or obese

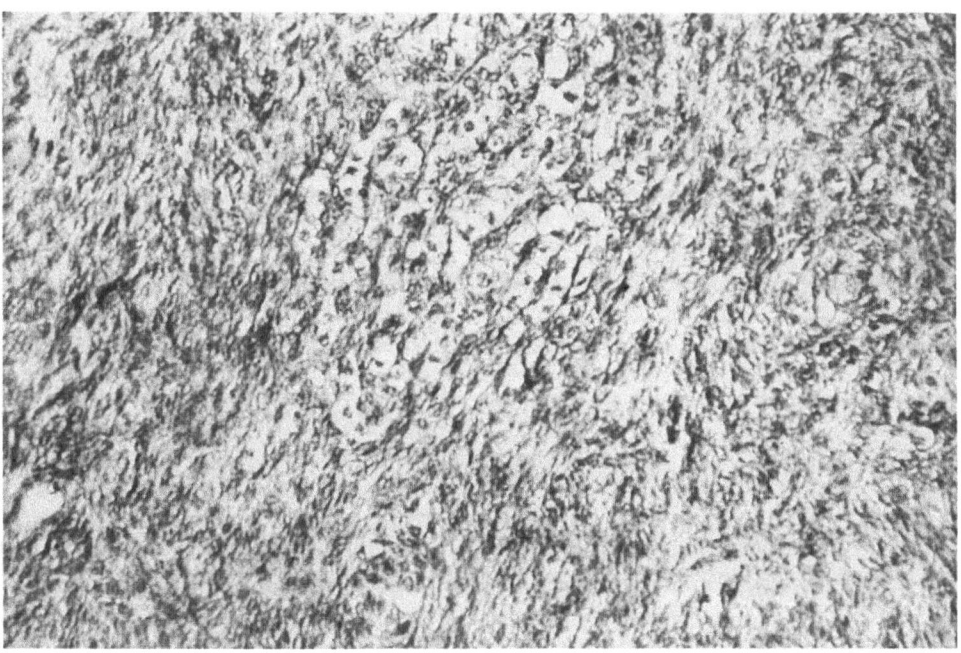

Fig. 4-5. Nests of luteininized theca cells with a clear cytoplasm may be seen in a compact stroma (×150)

and amenorrheic patients by Benedict et al. (71). Significant adrenocortical hyperplasia was noted in only two patients. One patient had hyperthecosis while another was an 8-year-old girl with sexual precocity and a luteinized theca interna. A lack of uniformity was noted in the biopsies of the adrenals, but those with hyperthecosis tended to be associated with some degree of adrenocortical hyperplasia, unlike patients with enlarged ovaries where this was not evident (71).

It is of some interest that some female-to-male transsexuals have documented evidence of polycystic ovaries as well as clinical manifestations suggestive of PCOD prior to treatment with testosterone (289). Histopathological studies of the ovaries following treatment with testosterone may be of some interest.

Genetics of Polycystic Ovarian Disease

5

PCOD, and particularly hyperthecosis, can occur as an inherited disorder (17,127,160, 238,335,435,568,609,918,922,985). At the present time the frequency of PCOD occurring as a genetic disorder is not known. Givens studied the incidence of oligomenorrhea and/or hirsutism in 48 sibships of 18 families having one or more member with diagnosed PCOD (324,325). Twenty-eight of 48 sibships had maternal transmission only and the incidence of oligomenorrhea and/or hirsutism was 47%. The 28 sibships had 93 females, 39 of whom had oligomenorrhea and/or hirsutism (an incidence of 42%). Paternal transmission was noted in 15 sibships and the incidence of oligomenorrhea and/or hirsutism was 41 of 47 females, an incidence of 87%. Five sibships had both paternal and maternal transmission and the incidence was 90% (9 of 10 sibships). These data suggest X-linked dominant inheritance but do not exclude autosomal dominant inheritance. X-linked transmission of PCOD is also suggested by dermatoglyphic data (864). Analysis of the latter data demonstrate that women with PCOD have hand dermatoglyphic characteristics similar to those of normal men. Mothers of women with PCOD demonstrate no abnormal pattern while the fathers have a combination of "male" and "female" dermatoglyphic characteristics of the hand. There appears to occur a premature balding incidence of 8–25% among male relatives of hirsute PCOD patients (260). The relative prevalence of premature balding among fathers and brothers also suggests a genetically determined disorder with a modified dominant form of inheritance (260).

In support of X chromosome involvement are sporadic reports of abnormalities of the X chromosome in PCOD. Reports have demonstrated deletion of the long arm of the X chromosome and mosaicism involving abnormalities of the number or the structure of the X chromosome. Women with the somatic abnormalities of Turner's syndrome have been observed infrequently in association with polycystic ovaries (331,983). However, most women with PCOD have a normal 46,XX karyotype. Random inactivation of an abnormal X chromosome bearing a mutant gene (Lyon hypothesis) responsible for PCOD could account for the broad spectrum of findings observed in the sibships of PCOD subjects (555).

PCOD is the most common endocrinopathy causing familial hirsutism, and one must agree with Givens that it may well be the most frequent cause of hirsutism (324). All women with a family history of hirsutism and/or oligomenorrhea should be investigated for PCOD.

Involvement of male kin has been suggested (154,335). In two families with PCOD an increase of LH/FSH ratio and a reduction of T was noted in three brothers (335). In a study by Cohen et al. (154) brothers of PCOD patients had low or lower than normal FSH, one had maturation arrest, while a third brother had Klinefelter's syndrome. Studies of semen and hormonal analyses for FSH may be of interest in selected male family members of patients with PCOD. Other abnormal features in the family included precocious adrenarche, beardless males, eunuchoidism and prepubertal grand mal seizures (154). Thirteen of 27 women in five generations were hirsute, an incidence of 48%. Hirsutism occurred on the maternal side of the hirsute women except for one instance where it was paternal. Menstrual irregularity was noted in three patients. Only three women over 21 years of age were childless. Three instances of PCOD were noted, and were associated with prepubertal grand mal seizures. Eight males of three generations were beardless. Only two beardless men fathered children. The mode of inheritance in this family could be X-linked dominant, since in 48% of females maternal transmission was involved, while male to male transmission was not noted.

Four families in whom at least two siblings had evidence of PCOD had HLA genotyping performed on peripheral blood lymphocytes (573). Similar studies were also performed on patients with nonfamilial PCOD. Neither group of patients with PCOD were linked to HLA. Congenital adrenal hyperplasia (CAH) due to 21-hydroxylase deficiency was exluded by intravenous administration of 0.25 mg of ACTH with no patient having a plasma 17OHP response greater than 300 ng/dl at 60 minutes. There were no biochemical differences between familial and nonfamilial PCOD (573).

Cooper et al. (160) studied 18 families in which the Stein-Leventhal syndrome occurred and concluded that the transmission of the hereditary potential for the disease is consistent with a dominant mode of inheritance, probably autosomal. A typical and consistent chromosomal abnormality was not associated with PCOD (160) and confirmed similar observations of other investigators (112,939). The study of Cooper et al. (160) stressed the frequency of affected menstrual abnormalites in 10 out of 22 sisters of patients with PCOD. Pronounced hirsutism was present in 5 of 24 sisters while mild hirsutism was present in another 9 sisters. Infertility was present in 5 sisters of the propositi. Culdoscopy was performed in 12 sisters of the patients with known PCOD, and 8 of the 12 subjects "exhibited Stein-Leventhal type ovaries" (160). In conclusion, the data of

Cooper et al. (160) suggest that approximately one-half of sisters of patients with PCOD may be similarly affected.

Occasional abnormal chromosomal studies were noted in several studies of patients with PCOD (83,191,307,331,383,519,677). Chromosomal studies performed on 41 patients with the Stein-Leventhal syndrome and 21 normal controls were performed by Stenchever et al. (885). All but one patient with the Stein-Leventhal syndrome exhibited normal karyotypes. An apparent abnormality in a G-group chromosome in one patient was felt not to be significant.

While some patients show various sex-chromosome abnormalities the majority have a normal karyotype (Table 5-1) (112,160,307,708, 885,939).

TABLE 5-1. A Summary of Cytogenetic Analyses of PCOD.

KARYOTYPE	NO. OF CASES	REFERENCE
46,XX	164	112,160,307, 708,885,939
46,XXq-	1	307
46,XX/46,XXq-	2	191,677
45,X/46,XX	6	83,307,331,383
46,XX/47,XXX	3	307,677
45,X/46,XX/47,XXX	1	677
45,X/48,XXXY	1	307
46,XX/47,XXY	3	191,307,519
45,X/46,XY/46,XXq-	1	307

Reproduced with permission from Parker R, Ming PML, Rajan R, et al Clinical and cytogenetic studies of patients with polycystic ovary disease Am J Obstet Gynecol 1980, 137 656–659) (708)

Parker et al. (708) found 5 of 15 patients with PCOD and normal phenotype to have trisomy 14 in 2–4% of the cells analyzed. The phenotype was normal in these patients, and the implication of this cytogenetic finding remains unclear.

Despite some evidence of a genetic factor of inheritance, further large scale studies are necessary to define the frequency of a genetic basis for PCOD.

Pathophysiology of Polycystic Ovarian Disease 6

Inappropriate Gonadotropin Secretion

Most patients with polycystic ovarian disease (PCOD) have inappropriately elevated LH release and low or a low normal FSH secretion, namely, an elevated LH/FSH ratio (24,39,74, 138, 202, 203, 242, 302, 327, 332, 434, 443, 529, 530, 647, 711, 733, 742, 830, 934, 973, 998,1015,1028,1029). The mean normal mid-follicular LH/FSH ratio is 1.3 (1.0–1.6) (24, 39,332). The high circulating LH level is maintained by exaggerated pulsatile LH discharge, either in the form of enhanced amplitude or increased frequency (oscillations) (Fig. 6-1) (39, 742,973). The serum LH has no consistent pattern in magnitude or interval in PCOD (473). Daily LH excursions are frequently so great that they may resemble those of normal cycling women, or to the magnitude seen in a spontaneous mid-cycle LH surge (1015). It has been demonstrated that surges of LH in patients with polycystic ovaries may be preceded by a rapid increase of endogenous circulating E_2 (1015).

FEEDBACK CONTROL OF LH SECRETION IN PCOD. Rebar et al. confirmed the fact that the elevated LH levels are not related to a defect in the negative-feedback effect of estrogen on gonadotropin release (742). This was suggested by an appropriate fall of LH in four patients with PCOD who were given an acute infusion of E_2. An E_2 infusion of 50 μg/hr for 4 hours resulted in a rapid decline of serum LH with an attenuation of LH pulses (Fig. 6-2) (742). The E_2 infusion had no effect on FSH levels. Similar results of estrogen infusion on serum LH in PCOD patients with associated reduced frequency of LH pulsatile release have been demonstrated in normal women and in hypogonadal subjects (926,1015,1023). Resumption of increased LH levels with increased pulse amplitude occurred 3–4 hours after cessation of the E_2 infusion (742). This quantity of estrogen infusion resulted in levels of 300–800 pg/ml, a concentration seen in normal cycling women during the late follicular phase of the menstrual cycle. In addition, 100 mg clomiphene citrate a day for 5 days elicited increases of both LH and FSH in PCOD patients qualitatively and quantitatively comparable to those observed in normal cycling women given the same treatment (742). The latter study suggested that the positive-feedback mechanism of estrogen on LH release was also intact since the preovulatory elevation of E_2 induced an LH surge as well as a lesser but significant FSH elevation in patients with PCOD. The increased E_2 in normal cycling women, however, was 2–3 times greater than that of patients with PCOD. The positive-feedback effect of the rise of endogenous E_2 induced an appropriate gonadotropin surge with a mean of 7 days (range 5–12 days) following completion of clomiphene treatments for both PCOD and normal subjects. A luteal phase rise of progesterone usually occurred in both groups suggesting, but not necessarily proving, ovulation. Corroborative data of intravenous (24,1029), intramuscular (830) or oral (39) estrogen provocation tests to patients with PCOD by other investigators confirm the conclusions drawn from the ovulatory response to clomiphene that both negative- and positive-feedback responses to es-

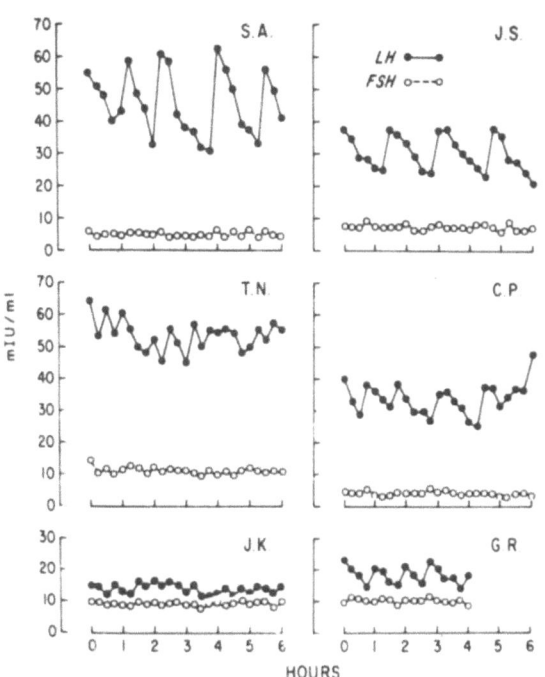

Fig. 6-1. Representative patterns of pulsatile LH release (but not FSH) in six patients with PCOD (Reproduced from Rebar R, Judd HL, Yen SSC, et al. Characterization of the inappropriate gonadotropin secretion in polycystic ovary syndrome J Clin Invest 1976, 57 1320–1329, by copyright permission of the American Society for Clinical Investigation.) (742).

trogens are usually intact (742,830,1029). Shaw et al. (830) noted that 4 of the 19 patients with PCOD who failed to demonstrate a rebound elevation of LH following intramuscular injection of 1.0 mg of estradiol benzoate also failed to respond to clomiphene, indicating failure of positive feedback in the 4 patients. A 24-hour earlier onset of positive feedback to oral estrogen administration (200 μg ethinyl estradiol for three days) to patients with anovulatory PCOD as compared to control subjects has been noted by Baird et al. (39), which may reflect anterior pituitary sensitization to chronic estrogen exposure (508).

Earlier studies in the late 1950s by McArthur et al. (600) as well as by Keettel et al. (452) demonstrated an inappropriately elevated LH secretion with a relatively low FSH release. The urinary findings of the above investigators were corroborated by later studies of serum LH and FSH which demonstrated the inappropriate elevation of LH in PCOD. The pathogenesis of the inappropriate gonadotropin secretion (IGS) in PCOD (24) is not yet fully defined but may arise as inappropriate feedback due to abnormal steroidogenesis (571,965), or a primary hypothalamic-pituitary defect (36).

LHRH RESPONSIVENESS IN PCOD. The response to LHRH testing in patients with PCOD is greater than that seen in normal cycling women, with both groups, however, achieving maximum LH and FSH response at 30 minutes (39). The degree of pituitary response to LHRH appears to depend on the basal level of serum LH. The higher the basal LH the greater is the LH release following LHRH (647,742). Even a small bolus of 10 μg LHRH induces an LH release in PCOD which is four times greater than that seen in normal women during the early follicular phase of the menstrual cycle (1017). Yen et al. (1017) and Rebar et al. (742) demonstrated a progressive decrease of pituitary LH response to five sequential 10 μg pulses of LHRH administered at 2-hour intervals to two patients with PCOD (Fig. 6-3) (742). This may reflect a partial depletion of pituitary gonadotropin store occasioned by the enhanced release which occurs as a result of increased pituitary sensitivity. Thus the pituitary reserve when viewed as the availability of releasable LH pool may be actually increased in these patients. These interpretations are derived from observations noted in similar experiments during the early and mid-follicular phase of the normal menstrual cycle where pituitary sensitivity is much lower and LH increments in response to successive pulses of LHRH are found to be stable (508,1017). The demonstration of a heightened pituitary sensitivity to LHRH may offer an explanation for the occurrence of the exaggerated pulsatile LH release in polycystic

Fig. 6-2. The negative-feedback effect of E_2 infusion (50 μg/hr for 4 hrs) on the pulsatile release and the decline of basal concentrations of LH in four patients with PCOD No FSH changes were noted (Reproduced from Rebar R, Judd HL, Yen SSC, et al. Characterization of the inappropriate gonadotropin secretion in polycystic ovary syndrome J Clin Invest 1976, 57 1320–1329, by copyright permission of the American Society for Clinical Investigation.) (742).

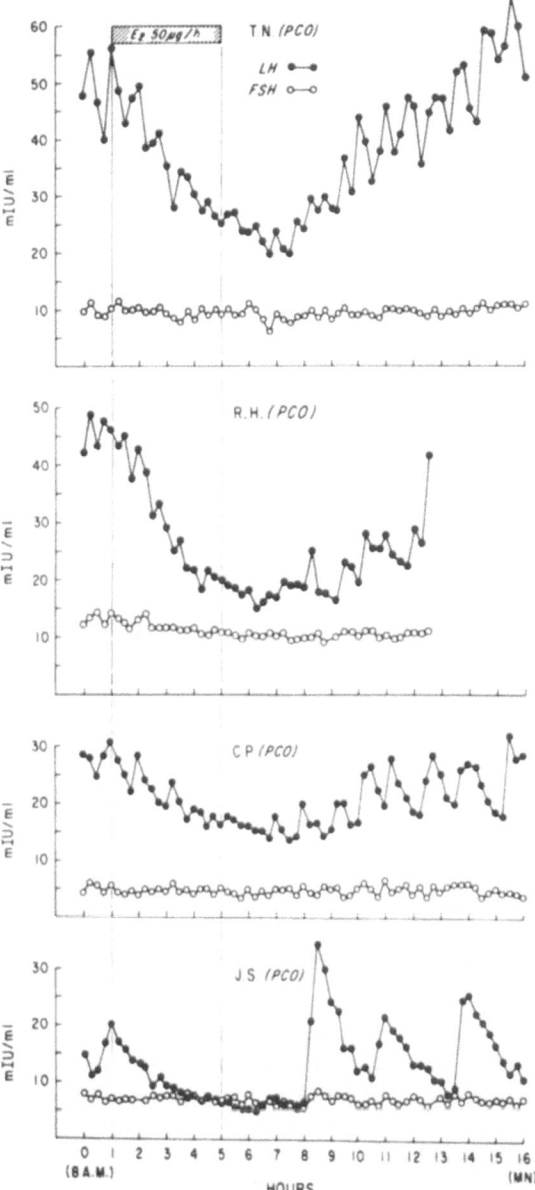

ovarian disease without implicating an associated increase in endogenous LHRH secretion. Unlike the response of the two PCOD patients to 10 μg of sequential LHRH described previously (742,1017) Moltz et al. (647) administered two doses of 25 μg LHRH intravenously 2 hours apart to 26 patients with PCOD. All 26 patients demonstrated a further augmented LH response following the second dose of LHRH as compared to their initial response. Those with elevated basal levels of serum LH (12 of the 26 patients with PCOD) demonstrated the most augmented response of LH. Basal serum FSH levels were normal (202,219,451) and the response to the LHRH was similar to that of normal control subjects (647). The authors suggest that increased synthesis as well as sensitivity to LHRH occurs in PCOD and is related to peripheral estrogen levels. There is firm evidence that increased pituitary sensitivity to LHRH may be related to chronically inappropriate estrogen levels of patients with PCOD (203,742). A positive correlation between levels of E_1 and/or E_2 and the basal LH concentrations has been reported (203,443,451) and a significant correlation between E_1 and LH increments to LHRH has also been demonstrated (203,742). Lobo et al. (539) have also observed a correlation between an elevation of unbound serum E_2 and LH in 23 subjects with PCOD, possibly induced by a reduced TeBG. The duration of estrogen exposure appears more important than the dose in determining pituitary gonadotropic activity (416).

The elevated LH levels in PCOD may be related to a heightened pituitary sensitivity to LHRH. With a maximum dose of 100–150 μg LHRH, PCOD patients have a net increase of serum LH and FSH greater than that observed in normal women during the early and late follicular phase (Fig. 6-4) (24,596,711,742,828, 938,1020). The peak increment of LH to 150 μg LHRH correlates with the mean preinjection LH level. Thus the level of serum LH mirrors the sensitivity of the pituitary to LHRH-mediated release of LH. Basal E_1 and E_2 levels correlate with serum LH levels and are also positively correlated with peak increments of LH induced by 150 μg LHRH in patients with PCOD (203,742). Some studies indicate that when LH levels are normal (at time of sampling) a relatively normal or less hyperresponsive LH rise occurs, rather than the exaggerated LH response following LHRH injection (451, 711,1033). In a study by Duignan (218) only 2 of 34 patients with PCOD had elevated serum LH levels. The response to LHRH was similar to that of normal women in the luteal phase of the menstrual cycle (218). The response of serum

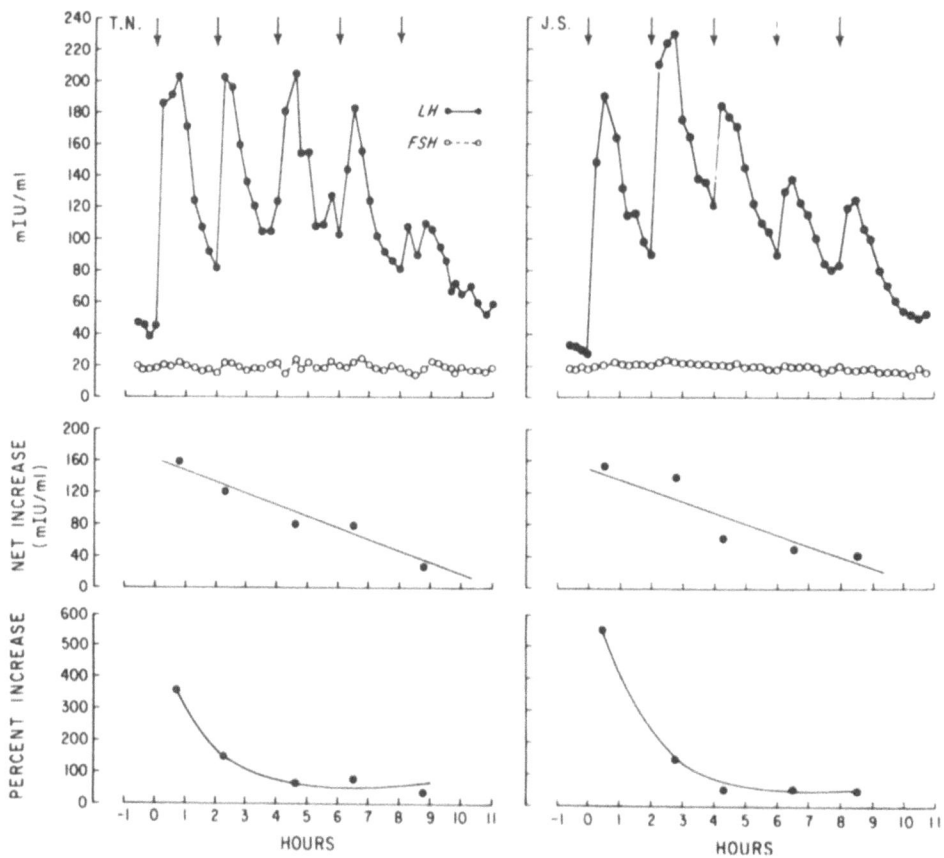

Fig. 6-3. Changes in the serum concentrations, the net increase and the percent increments of LH and FSH in response to pulses of 10 μg LHRH at 2-hr intervals (Reproduced from Rebar R, Judd HL, Yen SSC, et al. Characterization of the inappropriate gonadotropin secretion in polycystic ovary syndrome. J Clin Invest. 1976, 57.1320–1329, by copyright permission of the American Society for Clinical Investigation.) (742).

FSH to LHRH has been variable, with reports of a normal or slightly enhanced response (24, 647,828,938,1020,1033). Other investigators, however, have reported a relative insensitivity of FSH to LHRH (711,742,973,1017). With a small dose of 10 μg LHRH (742), no effect on the basal, virtually maximally suppressed, serum FSH was noted in 2 PCOD subjects while LH release was four times greater than that seen in normal women during the early follicular phase. This disparity between LH and FSH secretion may be explained by a preferential inhibitory action of estrogen on FSH release (1019) associated with a relative insensitivity of FSH release to low-dosage LHRH stimulation (742,1017). The LH response of patients with PCOD to a small dose (10 μg) of LHRH is practically similar to their response to 150 μg LHRH, and indicates near maximal release even with the smaller dose. In normal women a near maximal response requires 150 μg LHRH (1020).

Baird et al. (39) noted that the basal values of LH and FSH and their response to LHRH were almost identical in patients with ovulatory PCOD and normal women. Basal serum concentrations of FSH were similar in the anovulatory PCOD group and control group (mean, 5.8 mU/ml, and 5.7 mU/ml, respectively), as was the peak value following LHRH (12.5 and 11.6 mU/ml, respectively). The peak concentration of LH, however, was significantly higher in the anovulatory PCOD group than in the control group (mean, 60.4 vs. 24.8 mU/ml, respectively).

The data from Rebar et al. appear to favor an absence of an inherent defect in hypothalamic–pituitary regulation of gonadotropin secretion in PCOD (742). A number of investigators also conclude that it is unlikely that anovulation in PCOD is due to an intrinsic hypothalamic abnormality in that both negative and positive feedback responses to estrogen are present (24,

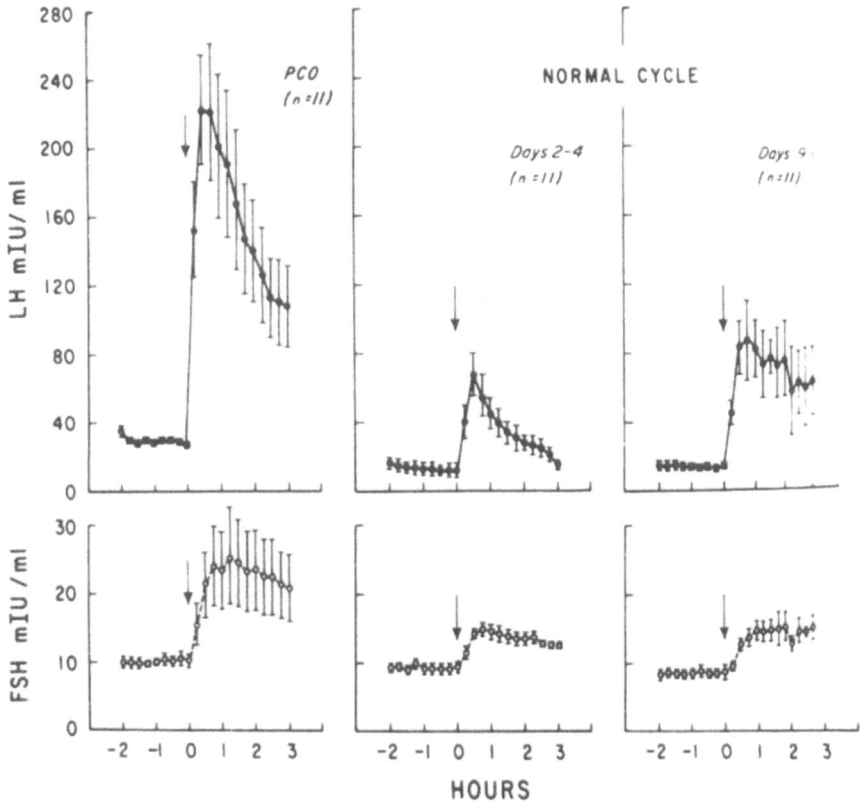

Fig. 6-4. Comparison of quantitative LH and FSH release in response to a single bolus of 150 μg of LHRH in PCOD patients and in normal women during the early and late follicular portions of their cycle (Reproduced from Rebar R, Judd HL, Yen SSC, et al. Characterization of the inappropriate gonadotropin secretion in polycystic ovary syndrome. J Clin Invest. 1976, 57.1320–1329, by copyright permission of the American Society for Clinical Investigation.) (742).

39,742). FSH is more sensitive to the negative-feedback effect of estrogen in PCOD and is inhibited by levels of estrogens which may stimulate LH (1019). Defective secretion of FSH appears to be crucial in the pathogenesis of PCOD since administration of FSH (441,738, 800) or clomiphene (39,742) frequently results in ovulation. Perhaps a functional derangement consequent to inappropriate estrogen feedback leads to a cycle of chronic anovulation and inappropriate gonadotropin secretion. It is clear that heightened pituitary sensitivity to LHRH resulting in increased serum LH/FSH is augmented by estrogen administration in normal and hypogonadal women (36,416,508,737, 940,964,1017,1018,1019). The estrogen-induced pituitary sensitivity to LHRH may result in an altered feedback set-point. It is of interest that LH augmentation to LHRH in PCOD appears to be enhanced further by the administration of progesterone than estradiol benzoate (828).

ROLE OF EXTRAGLANDULAR SOURCE OF ESTROGEN. The demonstration of increased pituitary sensitivity to LHRH during the late follicular phase as well as an augmented response to LHRH following estrogen administration in normal and hypogonadal women (416,508,940,964,1017,1018,1019) offers further evidence for an estrogen induced, increased pituitary sensitivity in PCOD patients resulting in an altered feedback set-point. More than half of estrone production is derived from peripheral conversion of androstenedione in PCOD (844). The extraglandular source of estrogen is related to body weight and may be of etiologic importance in the maintenance of chronic anovulation (203). In a study of six anovulatory women with PCOD by MacDonald and Siiteri (557), the secretion of androstenedione was 10.6 mg/day or 3–5 times that of normal ovulatory women. The extent of conversion to estrone was normal, 1.3%, but the production of estrone was elevated 3–4-fold to

$140-160$ μg/day. Extraglandular aromatization of androstenedione to E_1 in normal cycling women is only 40 μg/day, and less than the quantity of E_2 and E_1 secreted by the ovary. The extraglandular production of androstenedione accounts for almost all the E_1 production in PCOD. The high E_1/E_2 ratio in PCOD (203) is compatible with extensive production of estrogen by extraglandular aromatization of androstenedione (844). It is important to stress that one of the major influences on the hormonal milieu of PCOD is the elevated androstenedione which is peripherally converted to estrone (227). As stated previously, one must conclude that estrogens alter the sensitivity of the anterior pituitary to LHRH (456). The raised level of LH in PCOD further stimulates the secretion of androstenedione from the ovaries. The constant extraglandular production of estrogen from androstenedione selectively inhibits the secretion of FSH so that normal follicular development is impaired (40). Some women who have anovulatory cycles due to failure of positive feedback may subsequently present with PCOD. Probably a variety of factors which interfere with the finely regulated control of gonadotropin secretion by ovarian steroids predispose to PCOD (40). The increased extraglandular production of estrone in PCOD may also account for the fact that the majority of women under the age of 40 who develop endometrial cancer have PCOD (227). The incidence of PCOD associated with endometrial cancer in patients under 40 years old has been variably reported from $19-25\%$ (357,860). In another report by Chamlian and Taylor (135), 25% of young women with endometrial hyperplasia had associated sclerocystic ovaries.

It is probable that alterations in gonadotropin secretion in PCOD may be a reflection of feedback response to chronic acyclic extraglandular estrogen production which is derived from increased ovarian androgen production. Circulating E_1 in PCOD is usually elevated (39,138, 203,429,733), while E_2 may be normal or at the lower limit of normality when compared to normal cycling women (350,434,539,733). Chang et al. (138) assessed the role of E_1 on gonadotropin release. Seven patients with proven PCOD were compared to five normal women. Estrone benzoate in a dosage of 5 μg/kg intramuscularly every 12 hours for 4 days was given from days $3-6$ of the cycle in normal women and also to patients with PCOD. LHRH was adminis-

tered 10 μg intravenously at zero and 2 hours before and after estrone benzoate treatment. The PCOD patients had estrone treatment extended to 14 days at which time the LHRH test was repeated. In normal subjects, serum LH and FSH were unaltered by treatment with estrone benzoate, and LHRH testing revealed no difference beween the basal and post-treatment response of serum LH and FSH. In PCOD patients, however, administration of estrone benzoate caused a decrease of serum FSH in all subjects without an effect on serum LH (138). Progressive enhancement of the LH/FSH ratio occurred so that the baseline ratio of 2.3 increased to 2.7 after one week and to 3.2 after 14 days of estrone benzoate treatment to PCOD subjects. Responses to LHRH were unaffected before and after treatment with estrone benzoate in patients with PCOD, with similar hyperresponsiveness noted before treatment as well as on days 4 and 14 (138). Certain assumptions may be drawn from this study: (1) a $2-3$-fold increase of circulating estrone exerts no suppressive effect on serum LH in normal women or patients with PCOD; (2) the length of treatment of E_1, perhaps, may have been insufficient to cause an effect on LH; and (3) the lack of a positive-feedback effect of E_1 on patients with PCOD may have been due to the fact that LH was already maximally stimulated by endogenous LHRH. Thus exogenously administered estrogens were unable to augment basal LH release or enhance LH responsiveness to LHRH. Yet the disparity between LH and FSH was enhanced by estrone administration in patients with PCOD, unlike normal subjects. Whether this was due to the continued estrone administration for 14 days or the mildly increased levels of E_2 secondary to conversion from E_1 cannot be ascertained. An approximate 5% extraglandular conversion of E_1 to E_2 has been reported by Longcope et al. (545). It is quite clear that inhibition of FSH assumes a primary role in the pathogenesis of PCOD (230). The study by Chang et al. (138) supports the hypothesis of Rebar et al. (742), who suggest that the IGS in PCOD reflects preferential inhibitory feedback action of estrogen on FSH as compared to LH release.

POSSIBLE ROLE OF INHIBIN IN REDUCTION OF FSH. Feedback modulation of FSH may also occur as a result of a nonsteroidal peptide inhibitor, inhibin, which is synthesized by the granulosa cells and secreted into the follicular fluid and ovarian venous effluent (141). Steroid extracted follicular fluid from medium and large follicles in porcine ovaries significantly suppresses serum FSH of rats in a dose-dependent manner. Since porcine follicular fluid suppresses FSH levels in ovariectomized animals, it must act at the level of the hypothalamic–pituitary axis (577). The presence of inhibin within human follicular fluid has also been noted to have the ability to suppress pituitary FSH but not LH. This has been performed by infusion of human follicular fluid (143) directly into the anterior pituitary gland of ovariectomized rhesus monkeys. A second method demonstrating the effect of inhibin of FSH has been noted by a pituitary cell culture system previously treated with LHRH. Inhibin has been demonstrated in human follicular fluid of women primarily in the follicular phase and to a much lesser extent during the luteal phase of the menstrual cycle.

A possible role of inhibin in PCOD is appealing in that the inappropriate gonadotropin secretion is not fully explained by a greater negative feedback of estrogens on FSH, or relative insensitivity of FSH to LHRH, since ovarian wedge resection transiently alleviates PCOD. Inhibin-F (FSH-suppressing substance) has been demonstrated in human follicular fluid and has been correlated with the follicular androgen/estrogen ratio, which is a reflection of follicular viability (140). Inhibin-F activity was examined in human follicular fluid of 13 follicles collected from wedge sections of five patients with PCOD and 31 control follicles from normal women in the follicular phase of the menstrual cycle (900). A rat anterior pituitary cell monolayer cell culture technique was utilized to measure inhibin-F activity (140). The inhibin-F activity of the PCOD follicles were similar to those of viable follicles of normal control follicles (intrafollicular androstenedione/estrogen ratio <10), but were significantly greater than atretic follicles of normal women in the early follicular phase (intrafollicular androstenedione/estrogen ratio $>10/1$, containing $<50\%$ of the maximum number of granulosa cells for that follicle diameter). The majority of PCOD follicles varied from 3–4 mm, and was similar to the size of the majority of control early-follicular-phase follicles. The numbers of granulosa cells in PCOD follicles were significantly lower than the granulosa cell numbers found in normal follicles.

These data suggest that PCOD follicles contain normal inhibin-F activity in their follicular fluid despite a reduced granulosa cell concentration for the follicle diameter. The presence of increased numbers of antral follicles in PCOD over normal ovaries probably is responsible for the increased inhibin-F activity in PCOD. Nine of 10 antral follicles in a normal ovary are atretic and may thus contribute less inhibin since inhibin-F activity in normal ovaries depends on follicular viability rather than follicle size (618). Since PCOD follicles contain fewer granulosa cells per follicle compared to normal follicles with comparable levels of inhibin-F, it is probable that the inhibin-F secretion per granulosa cell is greater in PCOD than in normal ovaries (900). This occurred in spite of a reduced number of granulosa cells per follicle diameter in PCOD. Katz et al. (450) noted increased FSH following wedge resection in two cases of PCOD, suggesting that reduction of inhibin-F may have been causal. Studies of inhibin-F activity in ovarian venous blood of PCOD patients are in progress (900).

Elevated levels of LH may down-regulate LH receptors on granulosa cells (739) and cause thecal hypertrophy. This leads to increased thecal androgen and increased inhibin-F secretion from the granulosa cells thereby inhibiting pituitary FSH. Increased intraovarian androgens contribute to follicular atresia (551). The reduction of FSH and down-regulation of granulosa cell receptors also favor poor follicular growth. The increased androgen elaboration is peripherally converted to estrogen which augments pituitary sensitivity to LHRH thereby perpetuating the cycle by causing more LH secretion.

Franchimont et al. (273) have demonstrated that the addition of both aromatizable (androstenedione and T) and non-aromatizable (DHT) androgens to the culture medium of granulosa cells stimulates inhibin production without any change in progesterone (P) secretion. Aromatization of androgens to estrogens is not necessary for inhibin stimulation since DHT (which is not aromatized) is the most potent stimulus of inhibin secretion. The addition of E_2 and E_1 to the culture medium exerts no influence on inhibin production, whereas P decreases inhibin secretion.

Six women with longstanding unexplained infertility and regular menses were studied by Dmowski et al. (211). Serial studies of FSH, LH,

E_2 and P were performed and compared to normal controls. All had pelvic laparotomies during the luteal phase of the cycle which demonstrated no abnormal findings grossly. None had known endocrinopathies, hirsutism or local factors which could explain the infertility. The E_2 and P values were similar to those of control subjects throughout the menstrual cycle. Grossly abnormal FSH and LH patterns were detected in five of the six women. Four patients demonstrated persistently elevated plasma LH concentrations, and in three subjects the LH was elevated throughout the menstrual cycle, but with clearly identifiable mid-cycle surges. The LH/FSH ratio was abnormally elevated in the four patients with an abnormally low level of FSH. Dmowski et al. (211) claimed that these patients probably did not have PCOD, but it must be remembered that some patients with PCOD have normal ovulatory cycles with occasional absence of gross changes on laparoscopy, or evidence of clinical hyperandrogenism. Although these investigators state that plasma androgen studies were normal, their discussion noted that two of the patients had abnormal androgen levels (one with an elevated plasma DHA and another with an elevated plasma DHAS). The mechanism for the inappropriate gonadotropin secretion in these patients is speculative, but an increased LH/FSH ratio may not be incompatible with ovulation and perhaps several patients in this study did indeed have occult PCOD. (Again, could some of these patients have had increased inhibin from multifollicular ovaries?).

VARIABILITY OF ELEVATED LH LEVELS IN PCOD. The preferentially augmented LH release exhibits marked daily variation in a random fashion. Alternating periods of secretion are seen which at times result in LH levels that are comparable to those seen in normally cycling women (1011) and which on other occasions are similar to those observed in postmenopausal women (1023). In PCOD patients who have been sampled either randomly or daily for up to 14 days, serum LH levels are elevated above the normal range for ovulatory women (except at the mid-cycle surge) in 42–77% (74, 202,203,302,711,742,1028,1029). In a study of 36 proven cases of PCOD with bilaterally enlarged ovaries, Gambrell et al. (302) performed daily serum LH and FSH levels for 3–14 days. Wide fluctuations of serum LH were noted with 46 of 75 determinations of serum LH above the

normal mean (61%) and 29 of 75 determinations (39%) below the mean. The significance of their study confirms the fact that not only may random sampling demonstrate serum LH to be in the normal range, but even in the low–normal range (219,302). Mean serum FSH values were generally lower than those found in the early follicular phase of the menstrual cycle (302).

Baird et al. (39) studied 12 patients with PCOD and 6 controls. Serial measurements of steroids and gonadotropins were performed over a 12-week period prior to testing. Nine of 12 PCOD patients had values of 24-hour urinary pregnanediol less than 1.2 mg/24 hr, indicative of anovulation. Three of 12 patients had increased pregnanediol values, but 2 of these 3 had prior wedge resection of the ovaries. Total urinary estrogens in anovulatory women with PCOD were similar to those of normal cycling women during the early follicular phase of the cycle (39). A comparison of mean basal values (24–36 observations) in six control subjects and nine anovulatory patients with PCOD is shown in Table 6-1 (39).

As may be seen in Table 6-1, patients with anovulatory PCOD tended to have elevated serum levels of LH, androstenedione and E_1 as compared to normal control subjects.

LH LEVELS AND CIRCULATORY ANDROGENS IN PCOD. Judd et al. (434) suggested that the high intraovarian levels of androgens may decrease the follicle sensitivity to FSH. Most investigators have demonstrated no correlation between serum androgen and LH levels (24,

TABLE 6-1. Serum Hormone Levels in Patients with Anovulatory PCOD and Control Subjects.

SERUM HORMONE	CONTROL (N = 6)		ANOVULATORY PCOD (N = 9)	
	Mean ±	SE	Mean ±	SE
LH (mU/ml)	10.3	0 8	15 8	1.2
FSH (mU/ml)	8.4	1 0	6 5	0.3
Androstenedione (ng/dl)	113.0	13.0	357.0	23.0
Estrone (pg/ml)	80 0	4 0	139.0	16.0
Estradiol (pg/ml)	57.0	4 0	75 0	7.0

Modified from Baird DT, Corker CS, Davidson DW, et al. Pituitary–ovarian relationships in polycystic ovary syndrome. J Clin Endocrinol Metab 1977, 45 798–809 (39)

203,443). On the other hand, Duignan et al. (219) found an inverse relationship between basal testosterone and LH levels, suggesting possible suppression of LH at the hypothalamic–pituitary level. In Japanese women with PCOD, however, with mean testosterone levels less than those described in the USA and Europe, mean LH values are also significantly elevated, with a mean LH/FSH ratio of 3.2 (± 0.9 S.D.) (24).

The fact that the LH/FSH ratio remains abnormally high with a value of 3.6 when gonadotropin secretion and androgen levels (testosterone and androstenedione) are suppressed by norethindrone 2 mg-mestranol 0.1 mg, 65 and 58%, respectively, also suggests that the gonadotropin abnormality is not entirely due to increased amounts of circulating androgens (332).

The pattern of a picture of episodes of ovulation with anovulation emerged in a study of four subjects with PCOD (39). In general they show a lessened serum LH level (mean, 10.6 mU/ml ± 2.2) at those times when they are spontaneously ovulatory. The other parameters, including FSH, E_1, E_2 and androstenedione, do not differ significantly among these patients when they are ovulatory or anovulatory. It must be stressed that although the mean basal LH value in PCOD is increased above that found in normal control subjects during the early follicular phase, the LH concentration is variable from patient to patient and in the same patient from day to day (39). This variability is due to increased amplitude rather than frequency of pulsatile release (742) and is probably related to the increased sensitivity of the pituitary to LHRH. The FSH concentration may be reduced in PCOD patients when compared to normal cycling women during the early follicular phase of the cycle (302,1029). Analysis of samples collected at 15-minute intervals indicate that the reduced FSH levels in patients with PCOD are associated with reduced frequency of pulsatile FSH release. The magnitude of the LHRH-induced FSH pulses, however, is frequently similar to that found in controls.

LH LEVELS AND OVARIAN SIZE; PROBLEMS OF CLASSIFICATION OF PATIENTS WITH PCOD ON THE BASIS OF SERUM LH LEVELS AND OVARIAN SIZE. In patients sampled frequently for two days, Berger et al. (74) classified a group of patients with PCOD on the basis of ovarian enlargement and called those with ovarian enlargement Type I PCOD and those without ovarian enlargement Type II PCOD. No significant clinical differences were noted between the two groups in the degree of hirsutism, age, length of amenorrhea, urinary 17-ketosteroid excretion and serum testosterone. Although mean serum FSH levels were similar in both groups (8.8 mIU/ml in Type I as opposed to 7.6 mIU/ml in Type II patients), the mean serum LH levels were markedly elevated in Type I as opposed to Type II patients, 49.2 and 10.1 mIU/ml, respectively. Ovarian tissue obtained for histologic examination in both groups of patients revealed mainly capsular thickening in Type II with few if any subcortical cysts or cystic follicles. Luteinization and stromal hyperplasia was infrequent. All Type I patients had subcortical cysts with varying degrees of luteinization and stromal hyperplasia. A thickened capsule was present in most subjects of both groups except for one subject in Type II. Based on these findings, the authors suggest that PCOD patients with normal LH levels may represent a separate group of patients. Additional studies by the same group (711) demonstrated a lessened hyperresponsiveness of LH to 150 μg LHRH intravenously in the Type II patient with PCOD. Another report by this group (736) again revealed no laboratory differences between Type I and Type II PCOD in total and free T and TeBG (711). In some PCOD patients sampled daily for 2–4 weeks the marked daily variation of LH levels oscillating from normal to elevated levels (39,742) suggest that patients with normal LH levels are women who are probably studied during a period of reduced pituitary secretion of LH who are therefore not necessarily a distinct group of patients with polycystic ovaries (327,341,1011).

Givens et al. (327) reported 10 patients with PCOD with menstrual disturbances and hirsutism. The patients were divided into five subjects with high 24-hour urinary LH levels and five subjects with low urinary LH levels. The mean plasma LH of the high-LH group was 43 mIU/ml while that of the normal-LH group was 12 mIU/ml. Mean plasma FSH levels of each group ranged from 6–10 mIU/ml and did not differ in the two groups. The mean plasma LH/FSH ratio was 5.8 in the high-LH group and 2.1 in the normal-LH group. The latter ratio was higher than that found in the follicular phase of the menstrual cycle of normal women. Their findings agreed with the data of Berger et al.

(74) in that there was no difference in age, degree of hirsutism, severity of menstrual dysfunction, urinary 17-ketosteroids, plasma FSH or testosterone levels of women with PCOD who have normal-sized ovaries as opposed to those with enlarged ovaries. Similarly, no difference was found in the clinical features of those with normal versus elevated LH levels. Givens et al. (327) differed from Berger et al. (74) by finding no correlation between the presence or absence of enlargement of the ovaries and LH levels. The application of three days of 24-hour studies of urinary LH by Givens et al. (327) was done to minimize random fluctuations of plasma LH which are usually found in PCOD. One must conclude from an analysis of their data, that a three-day interval study may not always be sufficient to characterize subjects with PCOD into a high- or normal-LH group. The study of Baird et al. (39) suggests that spontaneous fluctuations of the clinical state of patients with PCOD is common. Intervals of anovulation may alternate with ovulatory cycles, and frequent observations are necessary for an accurate assessment of each individual patient. Similar observations have been made by Goldzieher (341).

An analysis of available data does not allow a differentiation of subgroups of PCOD based on ovarian enlargement and/or elevated serum LH levels. The marked variability of LH levels during the day, or over a period of weeks, makes this criterion questionable in clinical assessment, and an absence of an elevated LH or of an elevated LH/FSH ratio does not exclude PCOD. The observations of Berger et al. (74), who classified patients with PCOD on the basis of ovarian enlargement and noted a correlation of enlarged ovaries with elevated LH levels, has been disputed by other investigators (24,39,327, 341,647,742).

Rebar et al. (742) found no relationship between the size of the ovaries in PCOD and serum concentration of LH. In all 14 PCOD patients studied, the mean serum FSH level was in the low normal range for cycling women (9.4 mIU/ml) while the mean LH level was 36.8 mIU/ml (742). Ten of the 14 patients had elevated serum LH levels greater than 25 mIU/ml. The frequency of LH pulses ranged between 1–5 with a mean of 3.1 pulses over the six-hour study interval. The four patients with normal LH levels demonstrated a pulsatile LH pattern similar to that found in normal women during the early follicular phase of the cycle (1024). Three of the latter four patients with normal LH levels had enlarged ovaries. FSH levels remained relatively constant with an absence of a pulsatile FSH pattern in all 14 patients (742). Similar findings were reported by Wentz et al. (973).

Baird et al. (39) demonstrated that basal plasma LH and its response to LHRH was related to the hormonal environment of each patient six weeks prior to testing. Gross enlargement of the ovaries in "typical" PCOD may reflect prolonged anovulation and probably is not diagnostic of a specific subgroup of PCOD. In the two patients in whom serial daily measurements were made following clomiphene-induced ovulation, the LH concentration fell progressively during the luteal phase of the cycle. It appears that the raised basal level of LH is related to continued unopposed estrogen stimulation of the pituitary, with reduced progesterone levels — the latter usually enhances negative feedback (384).

ROLE OF THE HYPOTHALAMUS IN THE IGS OF PCOD. As previously noted, chronic estrogen levels in PCOD can augment the LH sensitivity to LHRH by a direct action on the pituitary gland (74,742,828,1017). An additional mechanism to account for the exaggerated pulsatile pituitary release of LH in PCOD may occur as a result of a reduction of an inhibitory influence of dopamine (DA) in PCOD (733, 1011). Quigley et al. (733), noted prompt suppression of elevated serum LH in eight normoprolactinemic patients with PCOD with infusion of DA (4 μg/kg/minute for 4 hrs). When this was compared to the response of women studied during the early follicular phase of the menstrual cycle, the maximal suppression of LH due to DA infusion was significantly greater in the PCOD group. This enhanced sensitivity of LH to DA inhibition in PCOD suggests that the inappropriate LH release and exaggerated LH pulses may be related, in part, to a reduction of endogenous DA inhibition of LH secretory activity (733). The maximum suppression of LH occurred in those patients with PCOD who had the highest mean basal LH levels. The mean net decrement in serum LH was 10 times greater, and the mean maximum percent decrease in LH was also significantly greater in patients with PCOD than normal women (59% vs. 38%, respectively; P < 0.05) (733), or ovariectomized subjects on estrogen therapy (429). The decline in serum PRL was equal in both groups. Although the mechanism for the DA inhibition is not entirely clear, experimental data support the concept that the tuberoinfundibular dopaminergic system inhibits LHRH neuronal activity in the lateral palisade zone of the median eminence by a different mechanism from that regulating PRL secretion (295). These DA neurons are subject to estrogen modulation, and the chronically elevated estrogen levels in PCOD may possibly cause a reduced endogenous DA inhibition of LHRH (733).

A possible hypothalamic mechanism resulting in the persistent anovulation in PCOD has been proposed (332,441,997). The resulting increased serum LH and hyperandrogenemia leads to increased conversion of androstenedione to estrogens with resulting suppression of FSH. The fact that the sequence of events in PCOD leading to anovulation may be reversed by pure FSH as well as by clomiphene citrate strengthens this contention (441).

Administration of a combination estrogen-progestin for 17–21 days to seven patients with PCOD who had a mean elevated LH/FSH ratio of 3.7 revealed that the ratio was unchanged during the treatment period (332). The persistence of inappropriate gonadotropin secretion (IGS) even during suppression of LH and FSH suggests a possible primary hypothalamic–pituitary abnormality in PCOD (332).

The association of pituitary tumors in some patients with PCOD (284,290) may be more than coincidental and its pathophysiology may perhaps indicate an inherent abnormality of the hypothalamic–pituitary axis. Sommers and Wadman (859) studied the pituitaries of seven patients with PCOD and noted unusual numbers of heavily granulated basophils collected into hyperplastic nodules. Pituitary basophile hyperplasia was noted in all patients with PCOD. The association of hyperprolactinemia and galactorrhea in some patients with PCOD may be causally related to chronic hyperestrogenemia, which in turn may be associated with lactotrope hyperplasia and adenoma formation (412,413,610,837,906,956). The frequency of hyperprolactinemia in PCOD may also result from reduced dopaminergic tone (733). Indeed, abnormalities of hypothalamic–pituitary testing have been noted in normo- and hyper-prolactinemic patients with PCOD (246,417). Jaffee et al. (417) have described abnormalities in L-dopa responsiveness and a paradoxical rise in growth hormone following chlorpromazine in PCOD. Prolactin hyperresponsiveness to thyroid-releasing hormone (TRH) (164,246) and an exaggerated response to dopamine blockade with haloperidol has also been described and may be due to enhanced sensitivity and priming of pituitary lactotropes to chronic hyperestrogenemia (246). TRH hyperresponsiveness may also reflect increased pituitary PRL reserve. Hyperresponsiveness of PRL to metoclopramide stimulation in PCOD has been described by Baranowska et al. (49). The thyroid-stimulating hormone (TSH) response to TRH, however, is normal in PCOD (218).

Administration of medroxyprogesterone acetate (MPA) 400 mg intramuscularly every 12 weeks for 9 months to 21 patients with proven PCOD revealed a mean decrease of serum LH and testosterone of 70% and 40%, respectively, after 3 months of therapy (997). Following completion of treatment the ovaries were not palpable and the hirsutism improved in 13 of 19 patients. Laparoscopic observation in 5 patients revealed normal sized ovaries without external evidence of cysts. Laparoscopy had previously been performed on all patients, with criteria of PCOD consisting of the demonstration of a smooth glistening capsule with loss of surface crenations, abnormal vascularity and one or more subcapsular cysts (998). The regression of polycystic ovaries grossly and the reduction of LH and T with MPA suggested to the authors that a primary hypothalamic abnormality involving the cyclic release of gonadotropins is the primary cause for the sequential changes leading to the polycystic ovary syndrome (997). The oral administration of MPA 10 mg 4 times a day for 4–6 weeks to 6 patients with PCOD also caused a reduction of serum LH, a mean reduction of the plasma T by 43%, and a mean drop in the production rate of T of 33% (350). Gordon et al. (350) noted that the MCR of T increased on treatment by a mean value of 23%. MPA appears to inhibit LH secretion by the pituitary, reducing the LH-dependent hyperandrogenism. As already stated, it may again be argued, however, that the inappropriate gonadotropin secretion in PCOD is a result rather than a cause of excessive and prolonged extraglandular production of estrogen from androstenedione (39).

As noted previously, FSH appears to be more sensitive to the negative-feedback effect of estrogens and is inhibited by levels of estrogen which actually stimulate LH (39,1019). Experimentally increased magnitude of LHRH pulses results in a decline of FSH secretion due to "down-regulation" of FSH while LH concentrations are unaltered (478). Intrinsic hypothalamic abnormalities in PCOD, however, have been questioned by Baird et al. (39) in view of the demonstration of the presence of negative and positive feedback in PCOD.

It must be stressed again that an intrinsic hypothalamic abnormality which may result in an increased pulsatile release of LHRH cannot as yet be entirely excluded. Direct sensitive measurements of LHRH in subjects with PCOD may ultimately yield an answer. Until the latter studies are performed one must conclude that the elevated levels of serum LH and/or elevation of the LH/FSH ratio as well as the enhanced responsiveness to LHRH in patients with PCOD may be related to changes in circulating estrogens which result from extraglandular conversion of androgens to estrogens. The augmentation of the pituitary response to LHRH by estrogens as well as the changes in LHRH responsiveness during the normal menstrual cycle favors such a mechanism. The response of LH is preferentially enhanced in PCOD more so than that of FSH. The resultant elevated circulating LH level further stimulates ovarian androgen production, and the abnormal cycle continues.

The levels of bioactive LH were assessed by Lobo et al. (531) and correlated with various laboratory parameters in 20 patients with PCOD. All women were obese or overweight as defined by a Ponderal Index (PI) of less than 12 (812). Ten women in the early follicular phase of their menstrual cycle were used as controls. The mean levels of immunoreactive LH and bioactive LH and LH/FSH ratio were elevated in patients with PCOD. Thirteen of the 20 patients with PCOD had an LH/FSH greater than 3.2, while 19 of the 20 patients had elevated bioactive LH. The bioactive LH correlated with the immunoreactive LH, T and DHAS in PCOD, and did not correlate with weight nor the PI, unbound E_2, androstenedione, delta[5]-androstenediol, or DHA.

An elevated LH/FSH ratio probably is found in no more than 70% of patients with PCOD

(531). Although immunoreactive LH showed no correlation with DHAS, the bioactive LH did show a positive correlation. The normal ovary does not secrete DHAS and the correlation between bioactive LH and serum DHAS cannot be explained. The ratio of bioactive LH/immunoreactive LH is also increased in postmenopausal or oophorectomized women. The increase in bioactive LH may occur in states of increased biosynthesis and release of LH such as occurs in PCOD (531).

Lobo et al. (530) demonstrated that psychological stress is more prevalent in women with PCOD than in control subjects or women of similar weight with hypothalamic–pituitary dysfunction. The instrument that was used for the evaluation of psychological stress was the Modified Life Events Inventory, which has been shown to have a useful prognostic value in indicating the relationship between stress and the onset of illness. Many more items were scored above 60 (Major Life Events) among the 23 patients with PCOD, which suggests that these women either have experienced the items as being more stressful or they perceive them as being so. Since this was a retrospective study of a relatively small group of patients and only the mean score was presented, the data on the significance of psychological stress in patients with PCOD must be confirmed. The investigators found no differences in plasma ACTH and urinary-free cortisol in patients with PCOD, normal controls subjects and women with hypothalamic–pituitary dysfunction. The same group of investigators also studied urinary 3-methoxy-4-hydroxyphenylglycol (MHPG) which primarily reflects CNS norepinephrine (NE), 3-methoxy-4-hydroxymandelic acid (VMA), which is a peripheral NE metabolite, and platelet serotonin levels. (The latter is of questionable validity in assessing brain serotonin levels.) Platelet serotonin levels were elevated in PCOD patients, but the authors did not address that issue further. Although the mean 24-hour urinary MHPG was significantly elevated in patients with PCOD as compared to the other two groups, only 3 of 15 patients with PCOD had levels that exceeded 2 S.D. above the mean of control subjects. The urinary VMA levels were similar in all three groups. The data of Lobo et al. (530) suggest but do not prove that women with PCOD have increased catecholamine turnover derived from the brain, which may perhaps be a factor in enhancing LH secretion. The authors hypothesize that perhaps the increased CNS NE may modulate adrenal androgen-secretion since both MHPG and VMA were positively correlated with serum DHAS while MHPG was positively correlated with serum LH. One must conclude that although these findings were novel and should invite further studies of the possible role of psychological stress and elevated neurotransmitters (NE and serotonin) in PCOD, these must be confirmed in a larger group of patients of varying weights and different degrees of hirsutism. The latter two factors alone may cause significant psychological stress which may in turn be associated with abnormal stress indices.

Soffer and Fogel (855) described a gonadotropin inhibitory factor which was reduced in patients with Stein-Leventhal syndrome. This inhibitor is found in the urine of normal adult subjects and exerts a specific LH-inhibitory effect in mice and rats (294) and may perhaps warrant reevaluation.

Experimental hypothalamic lesions in the anterior hypothalamus have led to persistent estrus with failure of ovulation and the production of polycystic ovaries (201). Raised intracranial pressure has also been occasionally associated with polycystic ovaries as have clinical instances of brain damage, encephalitis and trauma (59). There are reported cases in which patients with polycystic ovaries also have tumors of the hypothalamus (102). These associations are tenuous, at best, and a possible hypothalamic derangement leading to PCOD in these instances is speculative.

Androgenization of hypothalamic centers may produce polycystic ovaries. Similarly, a single injection of testosterone to neonatal female rats may lead to permanent anovulation with persistent estrus syndrome (57,58). The pioneering work of Barraclough and his group has demonstrated the importance of the androgen and estrogen environment of the CNS at a critical period in development. Alterations of this environment may delay or permanently alter cyclic secretion of LH and FSH resulting in polyfollicular ovaries (57). Administration of androgen to female neonatal rats produces subsequent anovulation with inability of estrogen (and progesterone) to exert a positive feedback on the neurons involved in the cyclic release of LH and FSH. (This subject is reviewed in detail in Ref. 57.) The importance of the nature of

aromatization of androgens into estrogens by the hypothalamus (669) and its effects on LHRH secretion (as well as sexual behavior) appears to be a promising area of research.

A review of the pathophysiology of IGS in the polycystic ovary syndrome has been attempted. Not all patients with PCOD manifest IGS, but frequent plasma sampling may alert the clinician to its existence. There is no clear evidence which enables one to completely exclude the possiblity of a hypothalamic derangement as the initial event which triggers IGS. The role of the hormonal milieu, extraglandular source of estrogens, selective inhibition of FSH by estrone, as well as the role of endogenous dopamine and other factors on LH, must be further reevaluated. Direct measurement of LHRH would, of course, yield much needed information, and until such time that this technique is applicable to a wide spectrum of patients with PCOD the exact pathogenesis will remain elusive.

Steroidogenesis of Polycystic Ovarian Disease

In Vitro Studies of Ovaries in PCOD. With the advent of tissue culture techniques to study the steroidogenesis of isolated granulosa and theca cells, further insights into the steroidal capacity of polycystic ovaries was made possible. These techniques were later combined with the development of specific radioimmunoassays which allowed microquantitation of various steroids and peptides in biological tissue.

It was previously stated that low concentrations of FSH and estrogens are present in the antral fluid of most small antral follicles in the early follicular phase of the menstrual cycle. Subsequently, the FSH-induced granulosa cell proliferation of the preantral follicle secretes estrogens. With further induction of FSH receptors, aromatase activity is enhanced, allowing for the formation of estrogens from thecal androgen substrates (187,616,620,650). The intrafollicular concentrations of steroids and gonadotropins correlate with the mitotic and biosynthetic activity of the granulosa cells much more so than plasma hormone levels (619). The concomitant increased intrafollicular estrogen and FSH levels causes induction of LH receptors in the granulosa cells. LH inhibits further mitosis of granulosa cells, and a reduced intrafollicular prolactin concentration is noted. LH stimulates the enzymes converting cholesterol to pregnenolone (Pe), P to 17OHP, and the latter to androgens. Although the theca produces androgens under the influence of LH and converts androstenedione to 5α-reduced androgens, it is also capable of estrogen production, particularly in larger-sized follicles. Prostaglandins may inhibit steroid biosynthesis by blocking the ability of LH to activate cAMP (623). McNatty et al. (620) demonstrated that the three ovarian tissue compartments (granulosa cells, thecal cells and stromal tissues) preferentially metabolize androstenedione to DHT, with the exception of the estrogen-secreting cells from large antral follicles (> 10 mm in diameter) and possibly also luteal tissue from mid-luteal phase ovaries. The three types of ovarian tissues also have the capacity to synthesize P, T, as well as androstenedione, DHT, and the estrogens E_1 and E_2. It has also been previously stated that androgens enhance follicular atresia by antagonizing estrogen-induced follicular development (551). Some of the antagonistic effects of androgens on folliculogenesis may be expressed by the actions of the nonaromatizable 5α-reduced androgens such as DHT and 5α-androstanedione. The enlarging thecal cell envelope, as well as the large stromal (medullary) mass, contribute to an androgen-enriched follicular microenvironment which suppresses granulosa cell numbers and activity resulting in follicular atresia (613).

Studies of steroidal content of ovarian cyst fluid and in vitro incubations of polycystic ovarian tissue in the 1960s indicated (1) an aromatization deficiency and (2) excessive production of androstenedione as well as other androgens by PCOD ovaries (35,36). Short and London (842), in 1961, found elevated levels of androstenedione present in the follicular fluid of polycystic ovaries, but no estrone (E_1) or E_2. Some investigators concluded that polycystic ovaries have a defect in aromatase activity which prevents conversion of C_{19} steroids to C_{18} steroids (841,842). Furthermore, the follicular cysts in the PCOD ovaries may not mature fully, resulting in relatively low estradiol production and increased conversion of precursors to androstenedione (32,34,36,571,841,842). Confirmatory results using in vitro tissue incubations were reported by Axelrod and Goldzieher (36), who also found an enhanced capacity for delta[4]

production with little if any aromatization ability. Ovarian incubation studies of nine patients with PCOD revealed defects in 17-hydroxylation and aromatization and in 3β-ol dehydrogenase activity, while in a normal ovary testosterone was a better precursor for aromatization than androstenedione (35). The presence of a 3β-ol dehydrogenase deficiency in some patients with polycystic ovaries may account for an increased ovarian DHA concentration. On the other hand, no evidence of a 3β-ol-dehydrogenase deficiency was noted by Jeffcoate et al. (422) in their in vitro studies of polycystic ovarian tissue. PCOD patients demonstrate an accumulation of T, DHA and other C_{19} metabolites (35), while additional reports also have found increased DHA, androstenedione and 17α-hydroxyprogesterone (170HP) from ovarian wedges of patients with PCOD (360,569,571). A partial deficiency in aromatase activity was generally proposed (571,863), whereby androgens such as androstenedione and testosterone were inadequately converted to estrogens (32,36).

Studies in rats (231) and humans (650) have shown that FSH plays a crucial role in stimulating ovarian estrogen secretion by acting on specific FSH receptors on the granulosa cells to increase aromatase activity. Erickson et al. (230) reported in vitro studies of granulosa cells obtained from four anovulatory patients with polycystic ovaries. The isolated granulosa cells from medium-sized follicles measuring 4–7 mm in diameter were pooled, and controls obtained from follicles measuring 4–15 mm in diameter from four normal women at different stages of the menstrual cycle. The medium sized follicles from polycystic ovaries contained multiple layers of granulosa cells, an oocyte and a prominent theca interna with 5–7 layers of theca cells with a high cytoplasmic to nuclear ratio. Granulosa cells were sparse in the 10 mm or greater cysts and were therefore not used, since only a single layer of flattened squamous epithelial cells was noted. The addition of aromatase substrate (androstenedione) caused only a minimal increase in estrogen production when added in vitro to granulosa cells of PCOD patients (230), confirming the previously noted aromatase deficiency in PCOD. However, when appropriately stimulated in vitro with FSH, the granulosa cells of PCOD patients were capable of aromatizing androstenedione. Treatment of these women with purified FSH (300–600 IU × 2–3 days) also caused a marked increase of E_2 to over 300 pg/ml in vivo, and ovulation following FSH treatment has been noted by others (441,800). This agrees with previous findings of marked sensitivity of PCOD subjects to FSH (647,738,800). It is of interest that granulosa cells isolated from normal medium-sized follicles (4–6 mm) of normal subjects do not have an active aromatase activity, but this may be induced by administration of FSH. Moon et al. (650) confirmed this in normal human granulosa cells studied in vitro with an increase in aromatase activity following FSH. The aromatase deficiency in PCOD resides in the granulosa cell, and the absence of aromatase activity is related to a defect in quality and/or quantity of available FSH in PCOD (230). Thus granulosa cells of follicles under 8 mm lack aromatase activity, but this may result from an inadequate concentration of FSH in the follicular fluid. Although granulosa cells from patients with PCOD have an inherent ability to respond to FSH induction of aromatase activity, the Graafian follicles never develop to the size at which the aromatase enzyme becomes active. Folliculogenesis generally ceases at the mid-antral stage, and insufficient estradiol is secreted to reach the preovulatory peak necessary for the LH surge, resulting in anovulation. FSH administration reverses the defect with formation of estrogen and preovulatory follicle formation (647,738,800). McNatty el al. (624) noted that the FSH concentration in follicular fluid of normal follicles under 8 mm is very low. On the other hand, follicles over 8 mm in diameter have a higher FSH concentration, enhanced granulosa cell aromatase activity and a higher concentration of estrogens resulting in increased ovarian vein estrogen levels (622,624). An active aromatase activity usually present in follicles greater than 8 mm (230,785) may be considered to be a reflection of the previous in vivo induction of aromatase enzymes by endogenous FSH.

Wilson et al. (986) compared two normal ovaries to two with PCOD. One patient with polycystic ovaries had clusters of large epithelioid cells with eosinophilic cytoplasm scattered throughout the medullary stroma, suggestive of hyperthecosis. No obvious differences between the de novo steroidogenic potentials of isolated cultured theca and granulosa cells of mid-antral follicles (4–7 mm in diameter) of normal and polycystic ovaries were demonstrated. Wilson et al. (986) suggest that since follicle development up to the mid-antral stage is normal in PCOD, cessation of follicle maturation at that stage may not be related to an inherent developmental abnormality in the theca or granulosa cells of the polycystic follicles. Defective secretion of FSH in PCOD may, however, be the likely cause for the cessation of follicle development in PCOD. The granulosa cells from mid-antral follicles of both normal and PCOD ovaries undergo morphologic luteinization and secrete increased P in response to LH, FSH and cAMP in vitro. The thecal tissue of normal and polycystic ovaries are quite similar and secrete primarily androstenedione, and little estrone or estradiol. The in vitro capacity to secrete androstenedione in both normal and PCOD ovaries appears to be equal.

In vitro studies of polycystic ovaries have produced conflicting results. Some patients with PCOD have demonstrated two defects: (1) an aromatase deficiency and (2) a 3β-hydroxysteroid dehydrogenase deficiency which leads to increased production of delta-[5] steroids such as DHA or DHAS. In contrast, others have been unable to define defects of steroid enzymes in PCOD and suggest that the increased androgens result from an increased amount of ovarian tissue or from the hyperactivity of certain ovarian cell types (448). Reports of 11β-hydroxylase activity (592) and glucocorticoid production in polycystic ovaries (1) have been sparse, and no consistent trophic effects of ACTH have been noted on granulosa or thecal cells of polycystic ovaries (986).

The effect of severe hyperandrogenemia on ovarian steroidogenesis was reported by McNatty et al. (616), who studied the ovaries of a 15-year-old girl with ovarian hyperandrogenism, acanthosis nigricans and insulin resistance. The patient had primary amenorrhea, severe hirsutism, and apparent hyperthecosis with an increased T > androstenedione ovarian output. In vitro steroidogenic studies were carried out and compared to those of comparable tissues in normal ovaries. Ovarian stromal tissues, thecal tissues and granulosa cells were studied by tissue culture techniques as well as status of oocytes, and steroid concentrations in follicular fluid. Most of the 1–6 mm follicles of the hyperandrogenic ovaries had a deficiency of granulosa cells, with only 5% containing healthy oocytes. No follicles greater than 6 mm were noted. The 1–4 mm follicles of the hyperandrogenic ovaries had antral fluid concentrations of E_2 similar to that of normal ovaries, while there was a 30 to 200-fold increase of T and a 4 to 10-fold increase of androstenedione. In vitro, the granulosa cells, thecal cells and stromal tissues from the hyperandrogenic ovaries were all capable of producing estrogens as well as androgens. This suggests that there was no obvious enzymatic block in the biosynthetic pathways to androgens and estrogens . The thecal tissues of the patient with hyperthecosis were more active than normal ovarian thecal tissues producing 2–5 times more androstenedione and 4 times more testosterone than normal ovarian tissue. In addition, the stroma from the hyperandrogenic ovaries produced between 49 and 250 times more T in vitro on a per unit basis than the stroma from normal ovaries. When it is considered that the entire mass of stromal tissue may exceed the total mass of thecal tissue by 5000-fold, it is likely that the stromal compartment is a major source of androgen within the follicles as well as in ovarian and peripheral blood. Indeed, high levels of androstenedione and T were found in the antral follicles from this patient. The levels of DHT in the antral fluid from the hyperandrogenic ovaries were, however, significantly lower than that found in normal ovarian follicles, indicating a lower follicular level of 5α-reductase activity in some hyperandrogenic ovaries. The major source of DHT in normal antral fluid is not known, but may arise from the oocyte-cumulus cell complex and/or the granulosa cells. The levels of DHT in stromal and thecal tissues and ovarian venous blood is at least 1000 times lower than those in antral fluid (579,618,820). In contrast to the androgens, the antral fluid levels of E_2 and E_1 in the hyperandrogenic ovaries were comparable to those of normal ovaries. In healthy follicles less than 12 mm in diameter, E_2 was synthesized by the granulosa cells de novo, and also in vivo and in vitro by the hyperandrogenic ovaries. Since the granulosa cells of the hyperandrogenic ovaries secrete estrogens, it is probable that preantral follicular development proceeds normally. After antrum formation, the fluid-filled cavity develops increased androgens from stromal- and thecal-derived sources. This decreases the

number of granulosa cells with progressive degenerative changes in the oocyte. Although large amounts of androgens were secreted in vitro by the theca and stroma of this patient, the intrafollicular LH and FSH concentrations were low (2 mIU/ml for both LH and FSH) (616).

In a study by Mori et al. (655), slices of follicular and stromal tissues obtained by wedge resection of five patients with PCOD were analyzed for their ability to incorporate radioactive acetate into androgens. Stromal tissue was found to incorporate radioactive acetate into androgens less efficiently than follicular tissues. Androstenedione formation by the atretic follicles exceeded that of T and DHA (655).

Evidence for a role of androgens in follicular maturation has been presented by Louvet et al. (551), and may perhaps apply to polycystic ovaries. The inhibition of ovarian weight response with small doses of hCG in hypophysectomized immature female rats may result from local intraovarian effects of androgens secreted by the ovary in response to gonadotropins (551). Thus ovarian androgens produced locally by the LH-like effect of hCG appear to inhibit the effect of estrogens on follicular growth, and therefore have some control in the process of follicular maturation. The observations of Louvet et al. (551) also suggest that granulosa cells may have specific androgen as well as estrogen receptors which help regulate oogenesis in the rat. The inhibition of the effect of small doses of hCG in estrogen-primed hypophysectomized immature female rats by antiandrogens indicates an inhibition of the receptor binding and nuclear retention of DHT. FSH injection, however, has no effect on inhibiting the estrogen effect on ovarian weight (551).

The demonstration of normal LH binding to membrane receptors on the follicles of patients with PCOD, and the finding of a reduced concentration of LH receptors in these patients, suggests a possible down-regulation effect of LH in developing follicles (739).

To summarize, the inappropriate secretion of gonadotropin in PCOD results in cessation of follicle growth. With the elevated LH/FSH ratio, there is excessive androstenedione production by the theca interna cells. Thus despite the presence of aromatase substrate, the FSH-dependent aromatase deficiency does not allow the granulosa cell to form adequate estrogens, and folliculogenesis ceases at the mid-antral stage, resulting in anovulation. Goldzieher (341) has noted in perspective that the studies performed in the early 1960s were basically correct in focusing on the role of defective estrogen biosynthesis in PCOD. The proper role of FSH deficiency in the development of impaired aromatization (231) also appears quite clear.

OVARIAN AND/OR ADRENAL SOURCE OF HYPERANDROGENEMIA IN PCOD.

Ovarian and/or Adrenal Source of Hyperandrogenemia. Controversy exists as to the source of increased androgen secretion in hirsute women. Using differential catheterization of the adrenal and ovarian veins, Kirschner et al. (463), concluded that 95% of hirsute women have excessive T secretion from the ovary. On the other hand, Abraham et al. (2) concluded that the adrenal cortex is a major source of androgens alone or in combination with an ovarian source of hyperandrogenism in 85% of hirsute women.

Theoretically a simplistic approach to an adrenal source of increased androgens would be the determination of an enhanced responsiveness of adrenal androgen precursors to ACTH stimulation and suppression of the adrenal source of androgen with a glucocorticoid such as dexamethasone (DXM) (1,5). Unfortunately such short-term studies generally do not clarify the source of androgen (see later in this section). Although a number of such studies have purported to yield information on the possible role of the adrenal cortex in PCOD and/or undefined hirsutism, it appears that ACTH stimulation studies may be primarily of benefit in possibly defining occult partial enzymatic defects in adrenal steroidogenesis. (See Chapter 9.) Some investigators, however, even question the specificity of ACTH hyperresponsiveness in PCOD since this effect may be secondary to increased ovarian steroid production. This entire question is more than of academic interest since specific glucocorticoid therapy may be successfully employed in patients with a significant adrenal factor in the treatment of the menstrual dysfunction, infertility and hirsutism. Furthermore, attenuated forms of adrenocortical hyperfunction leading to hyperandrogenism may be associated with polycystic ovaries. The latter

may subsequently result as a consequence of inappropriate gonadotropin secretion which has been generated by increased steroids of adrenal origin.

The measurement of urinary 17-ketosteroids (17-KS) is a poor index of hyperandrogenism (527) since in ovarian disorders significant hirsutism may be present despite normal levels of urinary 17-KS (909). The levels of urinary 17-KS in patients with PCOD are usually similar to those of normal menstruating control subjects (502,527). Weak androgens such as DHA and DHAS contribute more than 90% to the total urinary 17-KS of adult women (580). Urinary 17-KS correlate poorly with plasma androgen concentrations (580,582). Significant elevation of urinary 17-KS, however, suggests an adrenal etiology, such as congenital adrenal hyperplasia or adrenal neoplasms. Urinary testosterone determinations have been of greater value than the urinary 17-KS in correlating with the degree of hirsutism (272,292,525,701,909). Urinary levels of testosterone and epitestosterone have been found to be elevated in instances of hirsutism and PCOD (114,292,293,525, 701). However only 1% of the T production rate is excreted in the urine as testosterone glucuronide (114,395). Normal women excrete $2-8$ μg per 24 hours of T-glucuronide (114, 292). The discrepancy between plasma and urinary T may be explained by the observation that plasma steroids, other than T, serve as precursors of T-glucuronide. Androstenedione and DHA are converted to T in the liver and skin, which is then conjugated to glucuronic acid before entering the plasma T pool. Thus urinary T does not accurately reflect the plasma T production rate (465). There is usually good correlation, however, between the total and particularly the free testosterone levels in hirsute women, with a discrepancy noted in only a minority of hirsute women (883).

In the hirsute female the primary abnormality is an increase in the androgen production rate (52,54,465). Increased circulating androgens increase 5α-reductase activity of the skin (370). Genetic factors may modify the effects of increased androgens in that some women with increased androgen levels may not be hirsute (54, 206). A possible potentiation of the effects of T on hair growth may be a reduced E_2/T ratio (931).

Bardin and Lipsett (54) demonstrated that in the hirsute female 74% of T is derived from glandular secretion and the blood production rates of T and androstenedione are almost always significantly increased in PCOD (52, 527,861). Higher mean levels of plasma T are generally noted in patients with hirsutism who also have menstrual disturbances such as amenorrhea (462,883,976). Although the mean concentrations of T and androstenedione are significantly elevated in hirsute women, only 50% of hirsute women demonstrate elevated androstenedione levels while plasma T is increased in 60% (3). Despite the increased production rates of these androgens in hirsutism, this paradoxical result is partially explained by the concomitantly increased extrahepatic metabolic clearance rate (MCR) of T in hirsute women due to a decreased level of TeBG (testosterone-estradiol-binding globulin) or also called sex-hormone-binding globulin (SHBG) (550). The determination of the free-testosterone index appears to be a more accurate reflection of the testosterone production (775). The steroidogenic pathways leading to testosterone (as well as glucocorticoids) are depicted in Fig. 6-5.

Acute variations of plasma testosterone may be quite significant with 15-minute, 4-hour and 24-hour variations ranging between 10–100 ng/dl in a series of hirsute females studied by Ismail et al. (409). The magnitude of variation differs from one patient to another. These investigators correctly view with caution any interpretation of data based on single determinations of plasma T (409). This also applies to acute suppression and stimulation studies, which makes making interpretation of such results difficult.

Twelve patients with PCOD and ovarian enlargement were studied by Southren et al. (861). The mean plasma T was 154 ng/dl (normal women, mean = 54 ng/dl), and the mean plasma androstenedione was 227 ng/dl (normal women, mean = 144 ng/dl). PCOD patients had a mean MCR of T of 1067 l/day or double that of normal women (584 l/day), and similar to that of normal men. The mean MCR of androstenedione was similar to that of normal women, at 2570 and 2399 l/day, respectively. The mean production rate (PR) of T in patients with PCOD was 1.67 mg/day, while that of normal women was 0.32 mg/day. The mean production rate of androstenedione in PCOD patients was 6.0 mg/day, while that of normal women was 3.2 mg/day (861). A two-fold increase in the percentage of free testosterone (223,861) and reduced binding of T was found in patients with PCOD as compared to normal women subjects as shown in Table 6-2 (861).

The mean production rate of T in this group of patients with PCOD was about five times that of normal women. Only 14% of the T could be accounted for by conversion from androstenedione (861). Bardin and Lipsett (54) noted that 26% of the plasma T was derived from androstenedione in PCOD, while Horton and Neisler

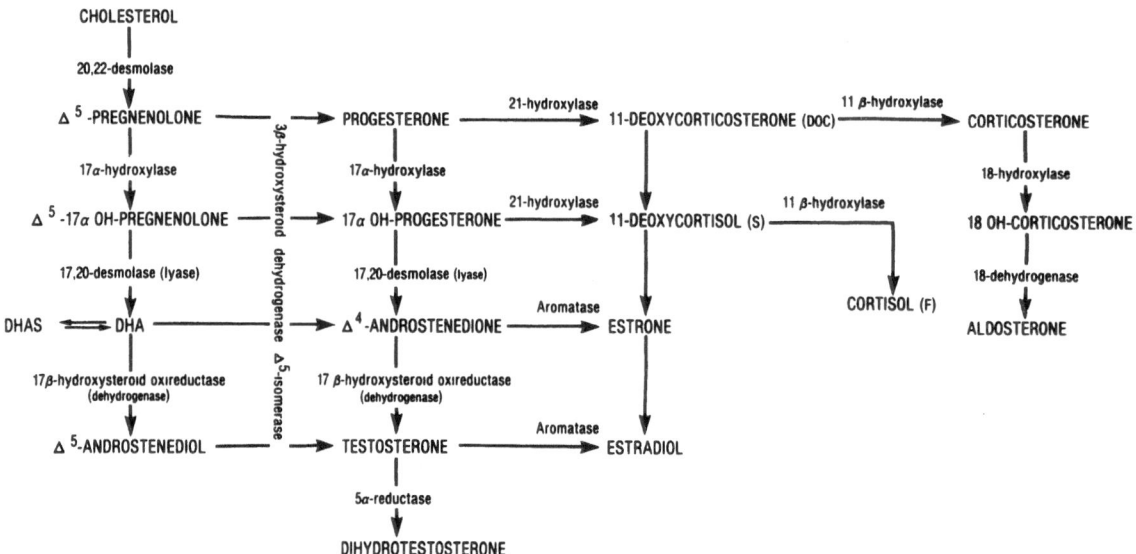

Fig. 6-5. Steroid pathways leading to androgens, estrogens, cortisol and aldosterone.

TABLE 6-2

GROUP	N	MEAN % BINDING OF T (SD)
PCOD	9	88.29 ± 4.15
Normal women	14	93.44 ± 0.89
Normal men	23	89.88 ± 0.99

(393) reported that 33% of the plasma T came from androstenedione. Thus the major portion of T in PCOD arises either from direct glandular secretion or by interconversion from a precursor other than androstenedione. Patients with PCOD have a greater ovarian overproduction of androstenedione than T, and an MCR of T which is greater than that of normal women (700 l/day) and almost similar to that of normal men (1250 l/day) (54). Chronic exposure to testosterone in women may cause a decrease in the percentage binding of T (861). The increased MCR and PR of T in PCOD may be enhanced by exceeding the saturation of the binding capacity of T (54).

Horton and Neisler (393) studied eight patients with PCOD. Seven of the eight patients had elevated levels of plasma T and androstenedione. Mean plasma T was 210 ng/dl, while that of androstenedione was 380 ng/dl. The MCR of androstenedione was normal at 2060 l/day, while the production rate was elevated to 7.8 mg/day (393). The conversion ratio of androstenedione to T was normal in PCOD as in normal women (18.5% vs. 15.0% in normal women). However, as previously noted, of the total plasma testosterone in PCOD, 33% was derived from androstenedione (393). The contribution of androstenedione to T in normal women has been reported as 50–60% (54,111), while in congenital adrenal hyperplasia, female children with the 21-hydroxylase deficiency have 76% of their T arise via conversion from androstenedione (394). The role of DHA and DHAS is minimal in PCOD because of the low conversion rate of DHA to T (395). These data therefore suggest that increased plasma T in PCOD arises as direct glandular secretion.

The adrenal glands have frequently been implicated as a significant source of hyperandrogenemia since exogenous glucocorticoid administration often lowers plasma and urinary androgens in hirsute women and patients with PCOD, presumably by selectively suppressing adrenal androgens (52,130,393,485,570).

DHT has also been reported to be suppressed in hirsute women with DXM administration (630). An adrenal contribution to the androgen excess in hirsute women and patients with PCOD has been suggested by ACTH stimulation studies of adrenal androgen production (330,346,432, 538,681), while others have proposed a combined adrenal and ovarian source of hyperandrogenemia (330,346,360,432,502,527). Previous studies by Bardin et al. (52) as well as Kirschner and Jacobs (466) have demonstrated that administration of exogenous corticoids to hirsute females may suppress the T production rate by 50%. The study by Horton and Neisler (393) of baseline and suppression levels of several plasma androgens in five patients with PCOD who were treated with 7.5 mg of prednisone for 30 days revealed suppression of plasma T and androstenedione levels to normal (393). See Table 6-3.

Rosenfield et al. (774) found no significant difference in the mean suppression of the total plasma T concentration of nine hirsute amenorrheic women with PCOD when compared to normal women, during treatment with 2 mg DXM for 2 days. The decrease in plasma T in both groups was almost similar to the reported 25% fall of plasma T reported by Bardin et al. (52) during DXM treatment to normal women. Hypersecretion of androgens from the ovaries of these nine patients with PCOD was proposed by Rosenfield et al. (774) in view of DXM failure to suppress the androgens to normal levels. Adequacy of adrenal suppression was documented by the normal fall of corticoids, DHA and DHAS following the DXM administration. Contradictory data has been reported by Abraham et al. (2), who studied 59 hirsute patients without specific data relating to the presence or absence of PCOD. Basal serum DHAS was elevated in 76% of his patients. A different dosage regimen of DXM, 0.5–1.0 mg four times daily, was employed for 7–14 days. Adequacy of adrenal suppression was considered if plasma corti-

TABLE 6-3

	MEAN PLASMA ANDROSTENEDIONE (NG/DL)	MEAN PLASMA TESTOSTERONE (NG/DL)
Baseline	365	223
Suppression	140	65

sol and serum DHAS were reduced below 4 μg/dl and 40 μg/dl, respectively. DXM treatment for 14 days was considered necessary for adequate adrenal suppression (2). Only 15% had an ovarian source of hyperandrogenism, while 38% had a combined adrenal and ovarian source, and 47% had an adrenal source. Thus Abraham et al. (2) considered 85% to have an adrenal component responsible for the hirsutism.

The effects of DXM and ACTH in nine patients with PCOD were reported by Lachelin et al. (502). Basal plasma levels of DHA, pregnenolone (Pe), 17-hydroxypregnenolone (17OHPe), progesterone (P), cortisol, delta^5-androstenediol, prolactin and urinary 17-KS were not significantly different in normal women as opposed to those with PCOD. Endogenous ACTH-circadian rhythms of cortisol, DHA, delta^5-androstenediol, Pe, and 17OHPe were quantitatively and qualitatively similar in PCOD and normal women. Plasma ACTH and urinary free cortisol levels have also been found to be within normal limits in a study by Lobo et al. (530). Lachelin et al. (502) did note, however, differences in other baseline parameters of PCOD subjects such as a 50% reduction of TeBG, and increased levels of mean free T, total T, androstenedione, and 17OHP. Following administration of 3.0 mg DXM for 24 hours, the suppression of plasma T, androstenedione and 17OHP was less pronounced in patients with PCOD than in normal women during the early follicular phase of the cycle. The elevated levels of androstenedione, T and 17OHP, and their failure to decrease to a normal range after a brief course of dexamethasone suppression, may be an indication of increased ovarian secretion of these steroids (502). Under physiological conditions the adrenal contribution to the circulating levels of C_{19} steroids and their C_{21} precursors in PCOD may not be different from that of normal women (502). The responses to small pulses of 200 μg/1.5 m^2 of ACTH to determine adrenal sensitivity also appeared similar in both groups of patients. However, an infusion of 20 μg/2 hours of ACTH revealed a significant difference in the PCOD group with an increased adrenal response (capacity) of DHA, 17OHPe, P and 17OHP. A significantly smaller increase was noted for delta^5-androstenediol, androstenedione and T in patients with PCOD (502). This may be interpreted as a mild compensated adre-

nal defect in 21- or 11β-hydroxylase deficiency in PCOD wherein the maintenance of normal cortisol secretion may occur at the expense of increased production of adrenal androgens. Other possibilities include (1) an increased MCR of delta^5-androstenediol, androstenedione and T in PCOD or (2) a relative deficiency of 3β-ol-dehydrogenase delta^5-isomerase activity necessary for the conversion of DHA to androstenedione. The selective hyperresponse of certain adrenal steroids in PCOD under sustained adrenal stimulation may, however, be secondary to the effect of increased ovarian androgen production (825) rather than a classical enzyme block. The evidence to support this view is based on in vitro studies of Sharma et al. (825) with bovine adrenal homogenates demonstrating that androstenedione can competitively inhibit 11β-hydroxylation of 11-deoxycorticosterone to corticosterone. Lesser inhibition may occur with DHA, DHAS and T, but not with P or 17OHP.

Some hirsute women have hyperresponsiveness of urinary 17-KS to ACTH, implying an adrenal component to their hyperandrogenism (527,528). Other than congenital adrenal hyperplasia, it is not clear how frequent ACTH-dependent hypersecretion is among hirsute women, and PCOD in particular. Givens et al. (330) studied hirsute females with amenorrhea, 12 of 20 of whom had enlarged ovaries suggestive of PCOD. Their responses were compared to normal cycling women as to their diurnal rhythms, overnight 1.0 mg DXM suppression, an ACTH stimulation study consisting of 0.5 units intravenously, and their response to a combination of 2.0 mg norethindrone and 0.1 mg mestranol for three weeks. Givens et al. noted that 5 of 12 of hirsute women had an exaggerated diurnal variation of androstenedione synchronous with cortisol, with 9 having an exaggerated androstenedione response to ACTH. Most of his subjects also had an exaggerated response of 17OHP, and a high 17OHP/cortisol ratio, suggesting a mild compensated 21- and/or 11β-hydroxylase activity defect. Hyperresponsiveness of plasma T was present in only 2 of 17 hirsute women. The degree of plasma androgen suppression of the combination estrogen-progestin was greater than that of the overnight DXM suppression. Presumptive evidence of ACTH-dependency of at least a portion of the androstenedione secretion in women who had an exaggerated diurnal swing of androstenedione was strengthened by an exaggerated response of androstenedione to physiological ACTH stimulation (0.5 units intravenously), without a concomitant increase in plasma T. This is similar to the data seen in prepubertal females with congenital adrenal hyperplasia who have minimal direct secretion of T but excessive androstenedione present (394). The data of Givens et al. (330) indicate approximately 50% of the hirsute women studied have ACTH-dependent hypersecretion of androstenedione, while only 12% have ACTH-dependent hypersecretion of T. Thus T secretion in most hirsute women including PCOD is usually ACTH independent and likely to be of ovarian origin (330).

Two of the cases of Givens et al. (330) with enlarged ovaries had an abnormally low response of cortisol and 17OHP to ACTH and may have had an uncompensated block in cortisol synthesis, possibly on the basis of deficient C_{21} 3β-hydroxysteroid dehydrogenase (3β-HSD) delta^5 isomerase enzymes which convert 17OHPe to 17OHP. Since hypersecretion of androstenedione was intact, $C_{19}3\beta$-HSD-delta^5 isomerase enzymes appeared adequate to account for the conversion of DHA to androstenedione. There is evidence for separate and specific 3β-HSD and delta^5 isomerase enzymes for the conversion of delta^5-C_{21} and C_{19} substrates (1009). These two cases differ from the one reported by Axelrod et al. (33), who had concurrent C_{19}- and $C_{21}3\beta$-HSD deficiency. Dexamethasone failed to influence the elevated androstenedione levels or T levels after an overnight suppression in approximately 50% of the hirsute patients studied by Givens et al. (330), suggesting concurrent ACTH-independent (i.e., ovarian) hypersecretion of androgens. This was further suggested by the estrogen-progestin suppression data which indicate more marked suppression of androstenedione and T than with DXM. Givens et al. suggest that an interplay between ovarian and adrenal factors may occur in PCOD, resulting in a combined ovarian and adrenal form of hyperandrogenism in 47% of their hirsute patients. Forty-seven percent also had ACTH-independent hyperandrogenemia, while only 6% had pure ACTH-dependent hyperandrogenemia (330). Although demonstrating a greater source of combined adrenal-ovarian source of hyperandrogenism than that noted by Kirschner and Jacobs (466), Givens et al. are in general agreement with the latter in that most hirsute women have either an ovarian or a combined ovarian and adrenal source of hyperandrogenism. Hyperresponsiveness of androstenedione and T to ACTH may be due to induced enzyme insufficiency in the adrenals by an abnormal androgen-estrogen milieu (330). Givens et al. also speculate that DHA from the adrenals may be converted to androstenedione by the ovaries.

Gibson et al. (314) studied 15 hyperandrogenic women, 7 of whom had clinical evidence of PCOD with elevated serum LH and normal FSH levels. Nine nonhirsute women controls were also studied before and after a bolus of 25 units ACTH intravenously (314). Abnormalities in circulating levels of adrenal steroids occurred in the majority of hyperandrogenic women tested. Basal levels of DHA were elevated in 3 of the 15 patients, while basal 17OHPe and 17OHP was elevated in 2 patients each. Basal pregnenolone levels were elevated in 5 of the 15 subjects. These hormonal elevations suggest an adrenal basis for the hyperandrogenism. Further abnormalities were noted following ACTH stimulation, suggesting partial deficiency of 3β-hydroxysteroid dehydrogenase (3β-HSD), delta^5 isomerase and 11β-hydroxylase activities. These included an increased ratio of 17OHPe/17OHP in 5 patients and an increased ratio of 11-deoxycortisol(S)/cortisol in 5 other patients. An additional 6 patients had an elevated DHA/cortisol ratio also suggesting a partial 3β-HSD deficiency (314). The exaggerated response of androgen precursors of adrenal origin with ACTH stimulation was associated with an inconsistent or minimal rise of T, similar to the results of others (236,330). Unlike the findings of Givens et al. (330), however, androstenedione did not rise significantly following ACTH. Those women who had an elevated ratio of 11-deoxycortisol(S)/cortisol had a normal basal level of S and no evidence of hypertension or fluid retention. Two of the 15 patients studied by Gibson et al. (314) had a mild hyperresponse of 17OHP following ACTH, suggestive perhaps of a very mild form of 21-hydroxylase deficiency. Although DHA normally accounts for only 10% of T production (395, 464), its increase following ACTH may suggest its role as a precursor for other potent C_{19} androgens, or it may exert its effect directly on target organs, such as skin, by local conversion to more potent androgens. It must be recalled that DHAS and DHA may be increased in hyperprolactinemic states (120,952) and perhaps in obesity (255), and that the adrenal abnormalities may be the result rather than the cause of the above states.

In adult women, partial 3β-ol-hydroxysteroid dehydrogenase (3β-HSD) deficiency has been implicated as a cause of hyperandrogenism associated with PCOD (330,342). In vitro studies of the ovaries, adrenals and testes demonstrate the occurrence of this enzymatic deficiency in some patients (33,799). A relative deficiency of 3β-HSD may be demonstrated as an alteration of the ratio of delta⁵ to delta⁴ steroids (1009). Elevation of serum DHAS may perhaps be a marker of an adrenal component to the hyperandrogenism of PCOD (2,37). Variable frequencies of elevation of DHAS have been described (2,37,203,218,442,540,736). Lobo et al. noted that 60% of women with hirsutism and oligomenorrhea had increased serum DHAS levels in the presence of normal delta⁴ androgens such as T and androstenedione (544). Twenty-four women with hirsutism, oligomenorrhea, absence of clinically enlarged ovaries and an elevated serum DHAS > 280 µg/dl were selected for the study of possible 3β-HSD deficiencies (538). The mean serum LH level in the hirsute group was higher (21 ± 8 S.E.) than that of a control group, and FSH levels were normal (mean 7 ± 3 S.E.). All but 2 of the 24 patients in this study had an elevated serum delta⁵-androstenediol with the elevated DHAS. Serum androstenedione was elevated in only 4 of the 24 patients, T was elevated in 5, while serum 17OHP was elevated in only one patient. In 9 of 24 hirsute patients, the immediate precursor of DHAS, i.e., 17α-hydroxypregnenolone (17OHPe) was significantly elevated (mean > 500 ng/dl) while normal and 15 other hirsute women had a mean value of 130 ng/dl. The basal serum 17OHPe/17OHP and delta⁵-androstenediol/T ratios were increased in 4 and 18 of the 24 hirsute patients, respectively, when compared to controls. The basal DHAS/androstenedione ratio, however, did not differ in the two groups and was a poor marker for the possible presence of 3β-HSD deficiency (538). Nine of the 24 patients underwent DXM – ACTH testing. A 1.0 mg DXM dose was given the evening before and an intravenous bolus of

250 µg of synthetic ACTH administered the next morning. The various steroids were measured at 0, 1 hour and 3 hours following intravenous ACTH. The maximal DHAS and delta⁵-androstenediol responses were achieved at 3 hours. As a group, the nine hirsute patients had a significantly higher 17OHPe/17OHP, DHAS/androstenedione, and delta⁵-androstenediol/T ratio than the six controls. The DHAS/androstenedione ratio was elevated in eight of the nine subjects tested (538). The data demonstrate that a subtle incomplete 3β-HSD deficiency may exist in some hirsute oligomenorrheic women who have baseline elevation of serum DHAS, as well as delta⁵-androstenediol and 17OHPe. The 3β-HSD deficiency is more firmly defined if elevated delta⁵/delta⁴ ratios occur following a DXM – ACTH study.

Both the ovaries and adrenals may possibly be similarly affected by 3β-HSD deficiency (514, 771). A reduced 3β-HSD activity may theoretically be induced by excessive androgens, much like that suggested for the 11-hydroxylase system (825). Its incidence may not be infrequent. The group selected in the previous study were those specifically chosen with elevated DHAS levels, but only nine were studied with DXM and ACTH. Only three of these nine women demonstrated abnormal delta⁵/delta⁴ ratios in all three ratio pairs tested following DXM – ACTH and probably qualify as having a subtle 3β-HSD defect (538). Clinically, the degree of hirsutism and the absence of clitoromegaly in this group of women did not differ from those with PCOD or those described with incomplete 21-hydroxylase deficiency, which may mimic PCOD (541). Basal and post-ACTH levels of 17OHP may serve as a marker for incomplete 21-hydroxylase deficiency (541), and in the latter study of five patients, the 3β-HSD activity was normal. The clinical hirsutism noted by Lobo and Goebelsmann (538) was probably due to the unbound elevated T, despite normal T serum values. In addition, serum delta⁵-androstenediol may be mildly androgenic. A major portion of the latter has been assumed to be of adrenal origin, but some delta⁵-androstenediol may perhaps also arise from the ovary (464, 771). A very subtle decrease in the response of cortisol to ACTH was noted when compared to controls (538), similar to that noted in patients with incomplete 21-hydroxylase deficiency (541). Treatment of patients with incomplete

3β-HSD deficiency consists of 0.5 mg dexamethasone administered daily at bedtime. The patients' androgens usually suppress well with this dosage with normal resumption of menses (538).

The true frequency of 3β-HSD deficiency in women with clinical PCOD is relatively small (538). Lobo et al. (540) have shown that one-third of women with PCOD have elevated levels of DHAS, and speculate that the adrenal may trigger the PCOD in some patients. Alternatively, it is also possible that ovarian derived T and androstenedione could result in similar findings. Once ovarian involvement occurs via LH stimulatory effects, the rise in unbound T, and perhaps delta[5]-androstenediol, leads to hirsutism, while the rise in unbound E_2 followed by increased LH production leads to IGS, chronic anovulation and androgen excess.

Serum DHAS may be used as an initial screen in identifying those with a possible significant adrenal component (2,37,442,486,540,1040). In the study by Ayers (37) of 38 normoprolactinemic patients with proven PCOD, 20 had levels of serum DHAS greater than 400 $\mu g/dl$. The normal DHAS group were heavier and tended to obesity at menarche. The age of onset of menarche did not differ in the two groups. Amenorrhea was present in 78% of the normal DHAS group. The high DHAS group had a 30% incidence of amenorrhea and more hirsutism than the normal DHAS group. Serum PRL was somewhat higher in the high DHAS group than in the normal DHAS group, although serum PRL was still in the normal range. The serum LH/FSH, E_2 and T were not different in the two groups. Higher basal serum P and 17OHP levels were noted in the high DHAS group (37).

Concurrent delta[5]-3β-hydroxysteroid deficiency (3β-HSD) in both polycystic ovarian and adrenal tissue has been reported (33). Gyory et al. (378) have also found evidence of such a deficiency in ovarian tissues of some patients with PCOD. Further suggestive evidence of a delta[5]-3β-hydroxysteroid dehydrogenase (3β-ol-dehydrogenase) deficiency in some hirsute amenorrheic women has been described by Lorber et al. (547), who noted elevated basal plasma levels of pregnenolone (Pe) and 17α-hydroxypregnenolone (17OHPe) associated with hyperresponsiveness to hCG. These investigators suggested that the latter steroids are derived both from the adrenals and the ovaries. Lobo and Goebelsmann (538) have suggested incomplete 21-hydroxylase and 3β-ol-dehydrogenase deficiencies in some hirsute women with PCOD, and also propose a concurrent abnormality of adrenal and ovarian tissues in these patients. The anomalous presence of adrenal enzymes in the ovaries (adrenal rests) has been suggested by other groups of investigators (1,592,770).

A prolonged ACTH test employing 500 μg synthetic ACTH intramuscularly twice a day for four days was employed to 15 patients with laparoscopic demonstration of PCOD and normal control women (442). The patients with PCOD were divided into two groups based on their LH response to LHRH before and at 44 and 92 hours after the administration of estradiol benzoate (443). Group A PCOD patients responded similarly to controls in the early follicular phase of the cycle, with an amplification of LH release at 44 hours and a greater amplification at 92 hours. Group B PCOD patients demonstrated an exaggerated response to LHRH before estrogen administration and an amplification of the LH response to LHRH at 44 hours, with a reduced response at 92 hours (443). Group B differed from Group A in demonstrating higher basal androgen and estrone values than those in Group A. Furthermore, Group B failed to ovulate in response to clomiphene therapy 100 mg daily for 5 days. Group A and B patients with PCOD were shorter than control subjects. Group B patients had significantly higher levels of DHAS, 17OHP and E_1 levels with lower TeBG values than those of Group A or controls (442). The elevated DHAS levels were not associated with hyperprolactinemia, although instances of hyperprolactinemia may be associated with elevated DHAS values (444). After the prolonged ACTH test the serum cortisol values were slightly lower in Group B patients with PCOD than those in Group A and normal controls. Serum E_2 values were lower in both groups after ACTH administration. A higher DHAS response was noted following ACTH in Group B. ACTH enhancement of serum E_1 was noted in both groups of PCOD. Elevated DHAS/cortisol, 17OHP/cortisol and E_1/E_2 ratios were also noted in Group B. A significant increase in the already elevated LH value in Group B was noted following ACTH (this finding had never been previously described in the literature). Two days after ACTH injection

Group A showed a greater increase in LH than the controls. FSH levels did not change significantly during the test in Group B, while a suppression of FSH was noted at the completion of the test in Group A and control subjects (442). Basal PRL levels were not significantly different in the three groups, but mean values tended to decrease after 2–4 days in all groups. One patient in Group B had a grossly abnormal 17OHP response to ACTH, while three subjects in each PCOD group had an increased 17OHP response similar to the ACTH-induced hyperresponsiveness of 17OHP noted by Givens et al. (330) and Lachelin et al. (502). Findings similar to Givens and Lachelin were also noted with increased DHAS/cortisol and 17OHP/cortisol ratios for Group B following prolonged ACTH stimulation (442). The data of Kandeel et al. (442) suggest that the increased 17OHP/cortisol ratio found in Group B PCOD indicates a temporary but compensated block in biosynthesis of cortisol due to a relative deficiency of 21- or 11β-hydroxylase. An association between PCOD and adrenal hyperplasia has been reported (76,299,552,731). Another possibility is that there may be a relative lack of 3β-HSD enzyme activity in some patients with PCOD in view of the elevated serum DHAS before and after ACTH. Givens et al. describe two patients who had impaired serum 17OHP and cortisol responses to ACTH, while an increased DHA response to ACTH was reported in the patients of Lachelin et al. (502). The probable presence of combined ovarian as well as an adrenal abnormality in PCOD is suggested by the elevated 17OHP and the response of 17OHP to ACTH in Group B, in association with a normal response of androgens to ACTH (442). This is also suggested by Givens et al. (330) and Lachelin et al. (502) by the fact that higher than normal androstenedione, T and 17OHP levels were seen in PCOD patients after an overnight DXM suppression study. An interplay between the adrenals and the ovaries in PCOD is again suggested (346,657,825). It is also possible that a primary ovarian disorder with increased androgen production may occasionally lead to inhibition of 11β-hydroxylase in the adrenals.

Hirsute patients with enzymatic defects such as 3β-HSD and 11β-hydroxylase or 21-hydroxylase deficiencies generally have an adrenal source of androgen excess. They may also be associated with inappropriate gonadotropin secretion (IGS) as with PCOD (532). Additional studies suggesting an adrenal source of hyperandrogenemia are data demonstrating ACTH-hyperresponsiveness of androgens and suppression with DXM. Some patients with adrenal excess of androgens, such as those with elevated serum DHAS and DHA may be hirsute despite absence of elevation of serum T (532). Delta^5-androstenediol production is increased two-fold in hirsute women (464) and it binds to TeBG almost as readily as T (18). Patients with 3β-HSD deficiency have an increase of free delta^5-androstenediol, and this reflects conversion from DHA and DHAS, and may partially account for the hirsutism of women with elevated DHAS and normal serum T levels (532). In patients with adrenal enzyme deficiences, Lobo and Goebelsmann (532) found elevated values of unbound T, delta^5-androstenediol and E$_2$, in association with a decreased TeBG lower than those of patients with PCOD. Patients with adrenal enzymatic defects also had elevated levels of unbound serum E$_2$ (532). A positive correlation was noted betweeen the level of unbound E$_2$ and the serum E$_2$. A positive correlation was also noted between the level of unbound E$_2$ and serum LH concentration as well as the LH/FSH ratio. This is consistent with the view that E$_2$ is at least in part responsible for the inappropriate gonadotropin secretion (IGS). The circulating E$_1$ or androgen levels did not correlate with serum LH (733) or the LH/FSH ratio (532). Other causal factors which may contribute to IGS may be reduced dopaminergic modulation of LH or the effect of β-endorphin on the amplitude and frequency of LH discharge (766).

Previous data of Bardin and Lipsett (54) demonstrated that hirsute women with normal-sized ovaries and no significant menstrual dysfunction ("idiopathic hirsutism") have lesser degrees of androgen production than hirsute women with enlarged polycystic ovaries. "Idiopathic hirsutism" may possibly be considered one end of the spectrum of systemic androgen ovarian production. The ovarian and adrenal vein catheterization data of Kirschner et al. (463) suggest that most hirsute women with no clinically enlarged ovaries have an ovarian source of hyperandrogenism. One may have to reexamine and expand the spectrum of PCOD to include androgen-producing normal sized ovaries with no or minimal histologic changes (325,463). Cases of androgen suppression by exogenous corticoids in hirsute women may represent an early stage of PCOD, while those who fail to suppress with DXM are in a more advanced stage of the disease (463). This implies that when ovarian changes are found in PCOD they may be secondary to the effects of increased circulating androgens. Some evidence supports this concept: (1) thickening and capsular fibrosis has been induced in animals given exogenous androgens (781,807); (2) polycystic ovarian changes have been described in non-ovarian causes of hyperandrogenism such as congenital adrenal hyperplasia (76,299,552,731); (3) testosterone secreting adenomas have been associated with ovarian stromal hyperplasia (974); and (4) estrogens as well as progestins may reverse sclerocystic ovarian changes (301,997).

LH-stimulated thecal production of androgens (230) may potentiate the initial androgen production whether it is ovarian or adrenal (203). This occurs because the increased androstenedione leads to increased E_1 by peripheral conversion which subsequently may increase LH. A relative deficiency of FSH reduces conversion of intra-ovarian androgens to E_2 (231). This not only leads to an increased circulating androgen level but also to a lower E_2/T ratio reducing TeBG production. Longcope and Williams (546) suggest that the rate-limiting factor in this cycle may depend on the peripheral conversion of E_1 to E_2, which counterbalances the effect of the androgens on TeBG production.

As previously noted, short-term diagnostic suppression for testing plasma T is generally useless in predicting long-term results (2,235). They do not enable the investigator to predict either the source of androgen (236) or the clinical response. Adrenal glucocorticoids like DXM can suppress adrenal androgens but may also suppress ovarian T and androstenedione production (466). A serious argument, however, against the study of Kirschner and Jacobs (466) is their assumption that cortisol and androgens are secreted at parallel rates by the adrenal. This was questioned in a later publication by Huq et al. (403), who demonstrated that the ratio of adrenal vein levels of androstenedione and cortisol are not constant. A similar view challenging the conclusions of Kirschner and associates (463,466) has been published by Rosenfield (772). Abraham (5) and Kim et al. (459) have demonstrated that 2 mg DXM/day for 1-2

menstrual cycles does not suppress E_1, E_2, P or LH levels. Kirschner et al. (463) used the criterion of 50% suppressibility of plasma testosterone and androstenedione following DXM to indicate an adrenal source of androgens. It may be that their criterion for the determining DXM suppressibility was inadequate (463), since prolonged adrenal suppression for at least 1-2 weeks may be necessary for adequate interpretation (2,579). Many studies have utilized short duration of glucocorticoid suppression tests, which may explain discrepancies in the literature in the evaluation of the source of hyperandrogenism (130,158,235,432,805,882). Similarly, it is clear that further studies defining the effect of glucocorticoids on ovarian steroidogenesis are necessary.

Evidence for excessive adrenal secretion due to mild 21- or 11β-hydroxylase deficiency has been gathered from clinical studies of hirsute women by Newmark et al. (681). Enzymatic defects had been previously noted by Axelrod et al. (33) in a patient with PCOD resulting in concurrent 3β-ol dehydrogenase deficiency (3β-HSD) in the adrenal and ovaries. Mild abnormalities of steroidogenesis may not be apparent unless tested under conditions of maximal glandular stimulation (513,681). Thus Newmark et al. (681) found normal basal excretion but exaggerated urinary tetrahydro-11-deoxycortisol and pregnanetriol excretion during ACTH administration, suggesting mild 21- and 11β-hydroxylase deficiencies. Similarly Lee and Gareis (513) found normal basal 17OHP levels in heterozygote parents of children with congenital adrenal hyperplasia (CAH) who had an abnormal increase in 17OHP following ACTH testing.

The finding of enhanced pregnanetriol following ACTH stimulation (681) may not necessarily reflect 21-hydroxylase deficiency in hyperandrogenic women, rather it may suggest mild 3β-HSD deficiency in the conversion of 17OHPe to 17OHP (314). This may also occur in PCOD (33), and abnormal function of the enzyme may reflect a combined ovarian and adrenal hyperfunction. As already indicated, selective catheterization data of adrenal and ovarian veins (681) suggest that the adrenals rarely are the major site of origin of excessive amounts of androgens (463).

Established evidence indicates that the ovary does not contain 11β-hydroxylase. Maschler et al. (591,592), however, incubated mitochondria from polycystic ovaries of five patients and demonstrated 11β-hydroxylase activity with C_{21}-deoxy substrates (17OHPe and 17OHP), but not with C_{21}-hydroxy compounds. (The adrenal 11β-hydroxylase has preferential activity of C_{21}-hydroxylated precursors such as 11-deoxycortisol). This is a unique report demonstrating biosynthetic 11β-hydroxylase potential of typical adrenal cells in polycystic ovaries, and accounts for the origin of the pregnanetriolone found in the urine of some patients with PCOD. Pregnanetriolone is a urinary steroid metabolite which is not normally detected in human urine except in large amounts in the 21-hydroxylase deficiency of congenital adrenal hyperplasia, in certain instances of Cushing's syndrome and virilizing adrenal tumors, and in some patients with PCOD (262,834,923). In PCOD there may be a dormant ovarian 11β-C_{21}-deoxysteroid hydroxylase which is selectively activated prior to or during adolescence or which may be present due to derangements in the embryonic development of the ovary. It may be possible that in certain instances of PCOD, penetration of primordial coelomic epithelial cells may have occurred early in the sixth week of gestation from the prospective adrenocortical site into the gonadal ridge. Nebel et al. (673) found primitive cells resembling the early coelomic epithelial cells in patients with PCOD, which may perhaps be the site of the abnormal 11β-hydroxylase.

An attempt to select the appropriate hyperandrogenic patient who is suitable for glucocorticoid suppressive therapy was reported by Steinberger et al. (882). These authors compared the results of an 1 mg acute DXM suppression test the night before a 250 μg ACTH test intravenously, to the eventual outcome of a 7.5 mg course of prednisolone therapy daily for 2–3 months to hirsute women. These results were compared to a group of normal women. The mean suppression of T after DXM was 30% with a return to presuppression values following ACTH. All the patients whose elevated T levels were suppressed, regardless of degree, responded to prednisolone therapy with essentially a normalization of T levels. On the other hand, those whose plasma T levels remained unaltered following DXM responded poorly to chronic prednisolone therapy. Some patients, however, with poor suppression following DXM (<10% suppression of plasma T) nevertheless

responded to 2–3 months of prednisolone therapy. The non-responders to DXM or prednisolone had a higher mean LH and LH/FSH ratio (2.9–4.1), suggesting that the elevated T may have been LH-dependent (882). These were also the patients whose plasma T remained greater than 40 ng/dl during 2–3 months of prednisolone administration. Chronic prednisolone therapy resulted in an approximate 50% reduction of T except in the group that failed to suppress following DXM. Since the validity of DXM or glucocorticoid suppression tests to differentiate between an adrenal from ovarian source of hyperandrogenism has been questioned (81,418,463), the origin of the androgens may sometimes be clinically academic (882). The beneficial effect of glucocorticoids has been variable in the literature, but appears to be related to the adequacy of suppression of elevated androgen levels (882). Although glucocorticoid therapy may reduce the plasma levels of 17β-hydroxyandrogens, it does not increase the TeBG (18).

While short courses of high doses of prednisolone do not alter responsiveness of LH to LHRH, chronic administration of prednisolone diminishes the LH response to LHRH (787) and causes disordered menstruation. A reduction of plasma LH as well as the mid-cycle LH peak with reduced plasma E_2 was noted by Cortes-Gallegos et al. (171) following administration of 6 mg/day of paramethasone to five ovulatory women. No effect on plasma P was noted by the latter group, suggesting that ovulation still occurred despite a probable direct effect on ovarian E_2 biosynthesis. Normal female subjects received 25 mg triamcinolone acetatonide intramuscularly on day 1 or 2 of their cycle, and variable suppression of plasma estrogens were noted associated with loss of the mid-cycle gonadotropin surge and deficient or absent rise in plasma progestins (184). This occurred in the presence of normal plasma or elevated plasma LH, suggesting a possible ovarian resistance to stimulation of gonadotropins. The response to LHRH was impaired, suggesting possible hypothalamic suppression by the glucocorticoid as well (184).

The fact that plasma ACTH levels are normal in PCOD patients (139,530) suggests the presence of a possible putative factor, adrenal androgen-stimulating hormone.

Short-term administration of estrogen for 10

days to five patients with PCOD (3 mg diethyl-stilbestrol) was insufficient to differentiate between an ovarian and adrenal source of hyperandrogenemia (186). Daily hormonal analyses of LH, T, and androstenedione fluctuated widely in the basal state and during treatment. The authors wisely stress the importance of multiple sampling before any meaningful data can be assessed as to the efficacy of suppressive therapy (186).

Givens et al. (332) studied seven patients with PCOD using a combination regimen of 2.0 mg norethindrone and 0.1 mg mestranol for 17–21 days. All seven patients had elevated LH/FSH ratios (mean = 3.7) with elevated mean plasma androstenedione and T levels of 515 ng/dl and 93 ng/dl, respectively. Urinary 17-KS were normal. Treatment with the combination drug regimen reduced the mean plasma androstenedione level 58% and the mean T level 65%. All PCOD patients achieved normal plasma androgen levels during treatment (332). Similar findings have also been described by Ettinger et al. (235) and Gordon et al. (350). Gordon et al. (350) suppressed the serum LH level 50% to normal, and the plasma T values 60% to normal, with a treatment regimen of 40 mg medroxyprogesterone acetate orally daily for 4–6 weeks to patients with PCOD. Correlations between androstenedione, T and LH during suppression and recovery revealed good correlation between LH and the two androgens. The mean levels of LH and FSH after 13–16 days of treatment were 6.3 mIU/ml, and 2.7 mIU/ml, respectively, a drop of 70% for LH and 58% for FSH. At this time, the mean levels of plasma androstenedione and T were 216 and 33 ng/dl, respectively (332). Goldzieher et al. (345) have shown that LH is suppressed more readily than FSH (71% vs. 31%) in normal women receiving long-term (>7 years) treatment with the same dose of oral contraceptive. The data of Givens et al. (332) suggest that the hyperandrogenism of PCOD is LH-dependent and that the most resistant patient to therapy was the one with lowest pretreatment LH level. Additional studies must be done to see if there is any correlation between low LH levels and resistance to combination estrogen–progestin treatment. It is of interest that the abnormally high LH/FSH ratio noted during pretreatment was unchanged at the end of the treatment period. Thus the inappropriate gonadotropin secretion (IGS) of PCOD

persists even during suppression of both LH and FSH. This also is an argument against a role of the high androgens levels in the pathogenesis of the IGS in PCOD, and points to a possible primary hypothalamic-pituitary abnormality (332). In view of the presence of a refractory period of suppression which may last up to 10 days and which is followed by suppression of plasma androstenedione and T concentrations, an evaluation of the degree of suppressibility of androstenedione and T by potent combination-type oral contraceptives should consist of at least three weeks of therapy with androgen measurements during the last week of drug administration.

In another study two women with PCOD were given ethinyl estradiol orally in a dosage of 0.1–0.25 mg daily for a period of 16–23 days (467). One of the two patients with PCOD had no suppression of LH, androstenedione or T following 16 days of 0.25 mg estinyl estradiol treatment, while the other patient receiving 0.2 mg daily had a drop in LH from 35 to 10 mIU/ml, associated with a suppression of plasma T from 139 to 57 ng/dl and a suppression of androstenedione from 490 to 75 ng/dl. Five of seven hirsute patients had no significant suppression of plasma LH with estrogen therapy. It is apparent, however, that estrogens uniformly decrease the MCR of T since the TeBG increases with estrogen therapy. Values of plasma T may not always correlate with the plasma T production rate. The usefulness of estrogens in diagnostic suppression studies of hirsute women must be questioned (467). Serum DHAS and ACTH has been reported to be decreased during oral contraception treatment by Madden et al. (562). Wild et al. (979) noted that combination oral contraceptive therapy for one cycle of 21 days (2 mg norethindrone and 0.1 mg mestranol) to 15 hirsute women with probable PCOD reduces adrenal androgen activity by (1) a reduction of the magnitude of the diurnal change in plasma androstenedione synchronous with cortisol, (2) a reduction of plasma androstenedione response to exogenous ACTH and (3) a mean 28% reduction in the concentration of plasma DHAS below pretreatment levels. DHAS is primarily an adrenal androgen and a valid marker of adrenal androgen production (544). Plasma DHAS may decrease in postmenopausal women due to reduced adrenal androgen production (584). Combination sex-steroid therapy may reduce DHAS in normal women and affect adrenal steroid production, turnover, or both (64). It must be concluded that combination estrogen–progestin therapy not only suppresses LH-dependent ovarian hyperandrogenism, but also exerts suppressive effects on adrenal androgen production. The mechanism for this is not clear. The use of this modality of testing for identifying a specific ovarian source of hyperandrogenism appears inadequate. It is of interest that adrenal neoplasms have been described sensitive to estrogen suppression (341).

Estrogens may inhibit the enzyme complex delta^5-3β-hydroxysteroid dehydrogenase (3β-HSD) isomerase in human testes and adrenal glands (854,1007,1009). Yates and Deshpande (1009) demonstrated an in vitro inhibitory effect of E_1 and E_2 on 3β-HSD from the human adrenal. Similarly, the effects of estrogens on the adrenal cortex have been documented experimentally and on postmenopausal and ovariectomized women (4,346). Contradictory data have been reported by Anderson and Yen (22), who performed basal ACTH infusion studies in four ovariectomized women before and after administration of 50 μg ethinyl estradiol orally for 5–6 weeks. An acute infusion of E_2, 50 μg/hour, was also given for 2 hours prior to the chronic dose of estrogens for 4–6 weeks (22). Both high-dose estrogen regimens had no effect on 3β-HSD activity in the four ovariectomized women, nor were changes in DHAS levels noted. ACTH stimulation did not alter the delta^5/delta^4 pairs. It appears that in vivo experiments do not support the notion that estrogens influence adrenal function directly (22). Similar conclusions were drawn by Mahajan et al. (567), who found no effect of a 3-week course of 200 μg of ethinyl estradiol to eight ovariectomized women on plasma DHAS, DHA, T or androstenedione levels. Long-term studies of the effects of estrogens on adrenocortical androgens are necessary to resolve this question.

HCG administration in the presence of DXM suppression may not stimulate ovaries which may already be maximally stimulated by endogenous LH. Approximately 50% of patients with proven PCOD show no increased plasma T following hCG-DXM testing. Ettinger et al. (235) as well as Abraham et al. (2,3) have found hCG stimulation studies in patients with hirsutism

and PCOD to be of no practical value. Furthermore, hCG administration may stimulate secretion of androgens from adrenal tumors (19, 334,974). Although some investigators have found dynamic testing with ACTH, DXM and hCG (158,915) and estrogen suppression studies to be of value in differentiating between and ovarian and adrenal sources of androgen excess (72,705,805), the conclusion of most workers is that these studies are of little diagnostic value.

Clomiphene testing may also not be useful in hyperandrogenemic states, in that possible adrenal stimulatory effects may occur (327).

Combined Ovarian and Adrenal Venous Catheterizaton Data. An increased adrenal production of DHA and androstenedione has been reported in adrenal vein catheterization data of hirsute women (966). In a study of 20 patients with PCOD, Stahl et al. (872) utilized selective adrenal and ovarian venous catheterization data to investigate the source of increased androgens. They noted that previous suppression and stimulation studies with DXM and hCG to be of little value in predicting clinical response to glucocorticoids, clomiphene or wedge resection. Their data revealed that no patient demonstrated excess androgens of ovarian origin alone and that no morbidity was present with their technique (872). Nine had combined ovarian and adrenal T hypersecretion, eight were shown to have increased T from the adrenals and three were felt to have increased T on the basis of peripheral conversion. These results differed from those of Kirschner and Jacobs (466), who noted 9 of 13 hirsute patients to have ovarian androgen hypersecretion while four had a combined adrenal and ovarian disturbance. The four patients with a combined ovarian and adrenal source of hyperandrogenemia had a 50% decrease in plasma T and androstenedione after 4 mg of oral dexamethasone administration for five days. In addition, in three of nine patients whose origin of androgen production was "ovarian," a similar decrease in the plasma androgen concentrations was also noted (466). No readily discernible clinical or chemical features characterized the latter group. Although none of the 13 patients had enlarged ovaries, all had elevated blood production rates of testosterone. In another study, Kirschner el al. (463) investigated 44 hirsute females with elevated T production rates (41 with normal sized ovaries) by studying the gradients of T, androstenedione and cortisol of adrenal and venous effluents obtained by catheterization (a gradient is defined as the effluent blood concentration divided by the peripheral vein concentration). The major source of T in 42 of the 44 women was ovarian, i.e., either direct ovarian secretion of T or ovarian secretion of androstenedione which was peripherally converted to T. The mean T gradient observed in ovarian veins was 7.2 times the peripheral blood levels, in contrast to a mean adrenal gradient of 2.6 times. Androstenedione gradients averaged 20 times the peripheral blood levels in ovarian versus 6 times in adrenal vein samples. Nineteen of the 20 women who demonstrated at least a 50% suppression of plasma T and androstenedione after 4–5 days of 2–4 mg DXM daily had an ovarian vein effluent of T and androstenedione higher than that of their adrenal veins. This was similar to the group that failed to suppress plasma androgens after DXM (463). The latter group had mean higher plasma concentrations and blood production rates of T and androstenedione, as well as a higher free T concentration. This study suggests that the ovaries are the site of excessive androgen production in most women with unexplained hirsutism and normal sized ovaries, and that the use of indirect glucocorticoid suppression studies are not accurate in assigning an adrenal etiology to the site of the excessive androgen production. The authors claim that glucocorticoid suppression of ovarian steroidogenesis of androgens does not alter serum LH, and thus the mechanism of corticoid action does not appear to occur via hypothalamic–pituitary suppression (466). In vitro studies by Janata and Starka (418) have demonstrated that glucocorticoids suppress androgen production from polycystic ovaries, and thus a direct ovarian effect of corticoids on ovarian androgen production is possible (463). The fact that DXM may exert a direct effect on ovarian androgen synthesis cannot be excluded (418, 463) and its usefulness in testing the origin of the hyperandrogenemia must be questioned (236,463,466,976).

Increased amounts of T and particularly androstenedione have been demonstrated from ovarian catheterization data of patients with PCOD by Rivarola et al (753). These investiga-

TABLE 6-4

MEAN VALUE ± S.D. (NG/DL), PERIPHERAL BLOOD		
T	Androstenedione	DHA
NL 49 ± 13	181 ± 59	502 ± 88
PCOD 115 ± 60	473 ± 243	2108 ± 2860
(range	(range.	(range·
73–216)	216–908)	390–10,050)

tors determined the concentrations of T, androstenedione, and DHA in ovarian and peripheral venous blood of four normal women and 10 patients with PCOD as shown in Table 6-4 (753).

The mean ovarian venous plasma T value of normal women was found to be 130 ng/dl while the mean androstenedione value was 1627 ng/dl (753).

The enzyme 17β-hydroxysteroid oxidoreductase (17β-HOR) catalyzes the interconversion of androstenedione and T. The relative amounts of androstenedione and T from ovarian venous blood was obtained from 10 women undergoing ovarian wedge resection, and ovarian tissue was obtained and analyzed for 17-ketoreductase and 17β-dehydrogenase activities. The in vitro studies indicated no difference in 17-ketoreductase and 17β-dehydrogenase activites in PCOD and normal ovarian tissues. The major source of secreted T in PCOD may arise, however, from DHA conversion to delta⁵-androstenediol and then to T (723).

Concentrations of T and androstenedione were elevated in ovarian venous blood and present in greater concentration than in peripheral blood of all patients with PCOD. Only five of eight subjects studied had an increase of DHA in ovarian venous blood greater than that of peripheral blood. The mean and range of ovarian vein plasma concentration of T was 732 (216–1516 ng/dl), while that of androstenedione was 10,400 (739–20,085 ng/dl) (753). Pittaway et al. (723) found that elevated androstenedione levels were the most common finding of ovarian venous blood in women with PCOD, while increased T was present in approximately half of the patients.

In another report of three patients with PCOD (Table 6-5), the mean androgen levels in ovarian and peripheral venous blood were as follows (820):

TABLE 6-5

	OVARIAN V. (NG/DL)	PER. V. (NG/DL)
Androstenedione	8433	approx 400
DHA	approx 1650	approx. 480
T	294	approx. 45
DHT	approx 40	approx. 20

An increased gradient was found for androstenedione, DHA and T. A small gradient of DHT may be present in PCOD. This may be a reflection of the increased T concentration and presumably of the presence of some 5α-reductase activity in the ovary (820).

Laatikainen et al. (500) studied ovarian and peripheral venous blood samples of seven normal subjects in the follicular phase of the cycle and six patients with PCOD. In normal women the ratio between ovarian and peripheral venous plasma concentrations was highest for estradiol, followed by androstenedione, DHA and 17OHP. Pregnenolone was also demonstrated in the ovarian venous blood of normal subjects as a small gradient for DHT (500). Ovarian venous blood of six patients with PCOD demonstrated marked elevation of androstenedione and testosterone. Lesser elevations were noted for DHA, DHT and androsterone. Three of the six patients with PCOD had an elevated ovarian blood concentration of 17OHP. No difference between control subjects and those with PCOD was noted in the DHAS concentration of ovarian and peripheral blood. The absence of a higher concentration of DHAS in ovarian venous blood as compared to peripheral blood, even in hyperandrogenic states, indicates that the ovaries play little if any role in the elevation of DHAS in hyperandrogenic states. Ovarian venous levels of E_2 were similar in the PCOD and control groups.

Lloyd et al. (527) found an average ovarian–peripheral venous T difference of 25 ng/dl in two patients with PCOD. The ovarian venous T concentrations were 299 and 355 ng/dl, respectively.

Kirschner and Jacobs (466) state that their catheterization technique of both adrenal and ovarian veins was performed without any undue difficulty. The authors also state that dilution of effluent samples may occur due to admixture from collateral blood flow in both adrenal and gonadal vessels. Similarly, a single effluent sample collected within a 5- to 10-minute period may not be relevant in view of the episodic and diurnal pattern of adrenal secretion. They do suggest, however, that cortisol concentrations be measured together with the adrenal androgens so that a proportionate ratio may be calculated (466). Others have established that difficulties may be encountered in catheterizing the right adrenal vein (873). On the other hand, apparent reliable catheterization data have been reported in subsequent studies by other investigators (84,682,747). There has been sufficient concern, however, regarding the tendency of the catheter to obstruct against the vein wall during aspiration of adrenal venous blood (806). Unlike the report of Stahl et al. (872), Wentz et al. (970) claim that bilateral catheterization techniques appear to be more difficult than previous reports indicate. First, anatomic variation in venous size and drainage make catheterization and bilateral sampling difficult, with less than 80% of patients having adequate bilateral venous sampling. Second, adrenal secretion appears to be both episodic and parallel, necessitating both simultaneous catheterization and serial sampling for adequate diagnosis. The stress of the procedure itself may provoke an increased adrenal output. Third, since ovarian secretion is not parallel and since increased hormone output occurs in the ovary containing the dominant follicle or corpus luteum, distinguishing ovarian dysfunction may be difficult to interpret. Finally, in view of the fact that this is a time-consuming procedure, patient discomfort must be considered. In a report by Bayliss et al. (62) a 5% complication rate was noted in 359 venous catheterization cases including thrombosis of the adrenal and iliac veins, extravasation of the contrast medium and hematoma formation in or around the adrenal gland. In the study of Wentz et al. (970), 2 of 22 patients suffered adrenal hemorrhage as a result of the catheterization. Another concern which may be pertinent to younger patients is the time of radiation exposure in subjects of reproductive age. Wentz et al. (970) strongly recommend its abandonment in the routine evaluation of hirsute women, and this has been also stated by Maroulis (579), who prefers its use mainly in the evaluation of an adrenal or ovarian tumor.

Measurements of urinary 17-KS, the suppressibility of peripheral plasma androgens with DXM, and stimulation of plasma androgens with hCG correlate poorly with selective catheterization data (250).

The uncertainties inherent in diagnostic stimulation and suppression studies to localize the source of increased androgen in PCOD have been stressed by Goldzieher (341) and others (235,250). To place all the above data in proper perspective, it may be helpful to consider the following:

1. Short-term administration studies with DXM or other corticosteroid may be relatively useless unless administered for at least 14 days, or definite criteria presented of adequate adrenal suppression. This would include demonstration of a reduction of serum cortisol below 4 μg/dl, or DHAS below 40 μg/dl. It may yield some information regarding adrenocortical resistance to suppression. More uniform data of the combined DXM–ACTH test in PCOD is indicated with detailed clinical correlation. A direct effect of glucocorticoids on ovarian androgens cannot be excluded in hyperandrogenic subjects. Similarly, glucocorticoids may suppress LH secretion (171), while certain hirsute females may demonstrate a DXM-induced rise in LH (330).
2. Administration of estrogen as an androgen-suppressive regimen must be performed for a least three weeks before any meaningful information may be assessed. Contradictory data on the effects of estrogen on adrenal steroidogenesis makes one cautious in relying on this testing modality. The addition of a progestin to the estrogen may make interpretation even more difficult, particularly in view of different effects of various progestins on the TeBG.
3. Human chorionic gonadotropin (hCG) stimulation studies of the ovaries have been of little value in differentiating between an adrenal from an ovarian source of hyperandrogenism. In addition, the fact that adrenal tumors frequently respond to hCG, makes this modality useless and misleading.
4. Although ACTH testing has occasionally been of some value in demonstrating sub-

clinical adrenal enzymatic defects, its role is limited. Physiological intravenous ACTH tests may be of more value, but are not practical or always useful.

5. Bilateral catheterization data are of most direct interest, but possible sampling difficulties and occasional medical complications makes this procedure more of a research-oriented tool, but quite valuable in the diagnostic evaluation of a patient suspected of harboring an adrenal or gonadal tumor. Controversy exists regarding the observations of Kirschner et al. (463). It is clear that although a number of patients with PCOD and/or hirsutism may have a major source of androgens arising from the ovaries, many patients may well have a combined adrenal and ovarian source of hyperandrogenism. It is not unlikely that instances of adrenal hyperandrogenism may be the trigger in some patients which provides the hormonal milieu for the development of a subsequent functional ovarian defect and finally an abnormality that manifests itself as PCOD. It is possible that different enzymatic deficiencies seen in hyperandrogenic women including PCOD may be secondary to elevated circulating androgen levels. Another possibility has been the proposed existence of a pituitary factor which selectively stimulates adrenal androgen production. Its possible existence does indeed present a challenge, and further investigation of this putative factor may perhaps be rewarding.
6. A more specific test for an ovarian source of hyperandrogenism may be the use of LHRH analogues (137).

Testosterone Binding Globulin, Androgens and Obesity in the Pathogenesis of PCOD

Low levels of TeBG (SHBG) may occur in obese women (398,483,695,727,773). Suppression of TeBG in obese patients is likely to increase the levels of free testosterone in the plasma. The lowering of TeBG in obese women may explain the higher incidence of menstrual disturbances in such patients (763). Weight reduction in obese women has been associated with an increased TeBG level (695,1040) and improvement of menstrual function (319,336). These observations suggest that reduced hepatic synthesis of TeBG may be associated with obesity. As previously stated, plasma androgens are usually elevated and consequently TeBG suppressed in hirsute females. In a study of 57 undefined hirsute patients by Mathur et al. (593), a reduction of TeBG was noted in the obese group as opposed to the non-obese group. The two groups were comparable in their plasma androgen and E_2 levels but differed with a further reduction of TeBG in the obese group. This suggests that in hirsute females obesity is associated with a further reduction of TeBG through a mechanism independent of androgens.

In another study by Plymate et al. (727), obese and non-obese patients with oligo- or anovulation were studied and divided into two groups, depending on their ideal body weight. Although the authors label these patients as having PCOD, no clinical data substantiating the diagnosis was presented. No differences were noted in both groups as measured by serum FSH, T or E_2. However, serum LH levels in the obese group were almost double that of the normal weight group. TeBG was significantly lower in the obese patients compared to the normal weight patients. TeBG correlated negatively with body weight, suggesting that obesity has an influence on TeBG independent of hormonal status. When TeBG is lowered the increase in free (unbound) T may inhibit follicular maturation, thereby enhancing the sequence of events seen in PCOD. The increase in free T which is associated with increased body fat may be also associated with increased peripheral conversion of androgens into estrogens (39,203,742). This, in turn, increases LH secretion and suppresses FSH secretion, resulting in the increased LH/FSH ratio characteristic of PCOD. Since not all obese women have PCOD, the change in TeBG is obviously not the primary factor in causing the disease. However, it may be an additional factor, among others, in the development of PCOD in the obese patient. The frequent prepubertal onset of obesity in patients with PCOD is of particular interest and may indeed play a role in the pathogenesis of the disease (1011).

In both spontaneous and experimental obesity, an increased cortisol production rate has been noted accompanied by an increased cortisol secretion rate (304). Normal values for total and free plasma T have been found in obese women with normal menstrual cycles (398). A progressive increase in the delta[5] and delta[4] adrenal steroids is noted in the development of normal children (217,512). Genazzani et al. (313) demonstrated that obese prepubertal children and those at Tanner stage P1 of puberty, have adrenal delta[5] and delta[4] levels higher than those found in normal children at the same stage of sexual maturation. A significant rise of plasma Pe is found in obese girls as early as 7–9 years of age while E_2 levels are depressed. Similarly, plasma DHA, P and PRL levels are higher in obese girls than non-obese children. The possible existence of a pituitary hormone other than ACTH and PRL which stimulates the adrenal zona-reticularis may be responsible for this prepubertal adrenal hyperactivity in the obese child (22). This factor has been called adrenal androgen-stimulating hormone (AASH).

Hosseinian et al. (398) studied the extent to which oligomenorrhea and obesity may be manifestations of high androgen levels independent of hirsutism. Most patients with obesity, oligomenorrhea and/or hirsutism had clinical evidence of PCOD. Obese women with oligomenorrhea had plasma and free T increases greater than those women with hirsutism alone without obesity or oligomenorrhea. The authors noted that free androgen levels were frequently elevated with minimal or no hirsutism in obese oligomenorrheic women (398). Other investigators have had similar findings of elevated plasma androgens in PCOD without hirsutism (468, 773). Obese hirsute women also had higher plasma-free androgens than non-obese women with the same degree of hirsutism. The authors suggest that obesity is an important variable in the expression of androgen action (398,773). One-third of the women with high free androgen levels were not hirsute. In non-obese oligomenorrheic women the degree of hirsutism correlated with free T levels, while no significant correlation was noted in the obese hirsute subjects. Oligomenorrhea alone was not associated with plasma-free androgen or binding protein levels, suggesting that this was a result of the androgen excess. Obesity alone was not associated with abnormal androgen levels. The authors conclude that obesity is either a response to high androgen levels of certain oligomenorrheic women or an incidental finding which blunts the expression of androgen effect on hair follicles (398,773). This may occur as a result of conversion of androgens to estrogens in fat tissue, or the subcutaneous fat may remove some of the androgen before it reaches the hair follicle. It is not inconceivable that slight hyperandrogenism even in the absence of hirsutism may stimulate appetite and lead to obesity. The hyperinsulinism of obesity in PCOD may be related to increased levels of β-endorphin (321). In addition, data of Burghen et al. (106) suggest that perhaps androgens may be responsible for causing moderate insulin resistance in some patients with PCOD. Regardless, obese oligomenorrheic women must be suspected of having elevated androgen production even in the absence of hirsutism (398).

Extragonadal extrahepatic aromatization of androstenedione to E_1 is increased with obesity, aging and liver disease. A direct correlation with obesity and the fractional conversion of androstenedione to E_1 has been demonstrated in pre- and postmenopausal females (226,556). Thus extraglandular estrogen formation occurs in adipose tissue where aromatase activity has been demonstrated (688). Aromatase activity appears in both adipocytes and stromal cells prepared from human adipose tissue (8,716). Ackerman et al. (8) found the major portion (87%) of the aromatase activity of human adipose tissue to reside in the stromal cells rather than the adipocytes. Estradiol was also synthesized significantly in addition to E_1. With increasing obesity, there is not only an increase in the number of adipocytes but its probable precursors, the stromal cells. It is likely that estrogens produced in the stromal cells have paracrine function in adipose tissue. Roncari and Van (765) have reported that E_2 stimulates replication of human adipocytes in culture. In the female, approximately 1.3% of androstenedione is converted to E_1 and only 0.15% of T is converted to E_2. Because of the increased ovarian production of androstenedione in PCOD there is a relative increase in the E_1/E_2 ratio when compared to normal ovulatory women. The increased estrogen concentrations in PCOD increases pituitary LH secretion which perpetuates the vicious cycle of PCOD. A primary ovarian cause of PCOD is discounted by Yen et al. (1015), since no obvious enzymatic deficiency is present if gonadotropin stimulation is administered or a wedge resection performed. Yen (1011) notes that obesity is frequently present at puberty associated with menarchal hair growth. Pubertal onset of obesity or its occurrence postpubertally

may be one of the mechanisms responsible for the onset of PCOD (61), since extraglandular aromatization of androgens increases with increasing body weight (226,556,844).

Bates and Whitworth (61) addressed the question as to whether the signs of androgen excess in PCOD are the consequence of exogenous or independent of exogenous obesity. They compared plasma androgen concentrations in obese anovulatory infertile women, with plasma androgen concentrations, from infertile women of normal body weight with nonendocrine causes of infertility (61). The 18 obese infertile women with anovulation had no specific diagnostic tests to suggest PCOD other than a mean elevated LH/FSH ratio of 3.0 and plasma androstenedione and T levels of 352 and 66 ng/dl, respectively. Control subjects had mean androstenedione and T levels of 173 and 41 ng/dl, respectively. Following a weight loss of greater than 15% of their body weight, 10 of 13 of the obese infertile patients became spontaneously pregnant. A measurement of plasma androgens in seven of these women revealed a decrease in the mean pre-weight loss level of androstenedione from 295 to 179 ng/dl prior to conception. Similarly, the plasma T decreased from 75 to 39 ng/dl. The authors conclude that weight loss to within 125% of ideal body weight (IBW) is a primary method of treatment of obese women with PCOD and suggest that obesity plays an important role in the genesis of PCOD (61). Other reports also confirm reduction of free T (695) and T (336) with weight loss in obese subjects.

Eight hirsute oligomenorrheic women of varying weights were studied by Givens et al. (321). Four of eight had elevated LH/FSH ratios and two had proven PCOD. Mean plasma β-endorphin and β-lipotropin were significantly elevated (15- and 5-fold, respectively) in the hirsute patients above the mean values of age-matched non-obese subjects with normal endocrine function. Significant correlation between body weight and β-endorphin and β-lipotropin was noted (321). Individual androgen levels and the degree of hirsutism were not significantly correlated with either β-endorphin or β-lipotropin, although plasma levels may not reflect the secretion rate of various androgens which may be distributed into fat and/or as a result of altered metabolic clearance rates of these androgens. A possible mechanism whereby pituitary

β-endorphin may influence body weight appears to be stimulation of hyperinsulinemia (68).

Patients with PCOD have a reduction of TeBG with a consistent increased MCR of T and free T in plasma. Although individual sensitivity in the response of the skin occurs in some hirsute women, it is clear that the major factor in the hirsutism is an increase of 17β-hydroxyandrogens in the plasma (18). An increased plasma ratio of 17β-hydroxyandrogen/TeBG is found almost uniformly in hirsute women (18). The activity or "utilization" of testosterone 5α-reductase activity in pubic skin samples of hirsute women with normal menstrual cycles were similar to that of patients with PCOD (499). Both groups converted T to DHT and 3α- and 3β-androstanediols to 3–4 times the levels seen in normal women, and equal to the activity which is present in normal men. In contrast, women with an adrenal source of hirsutism had only a minimal increase in the testosterone 5α-reductase activity of the skin (499).

Clinical Features of Polycystic Ovarian Disease

7

The original description of the syndrome which bears the names of Stein and Leventhal (880) emphasized the association of amenorrhea, hirsuitism and sterility with enlarged polycystic ovaries. They established specific criteria for the diagnosis of their syndrome that included bilaterally enlarged ovaries, normal urinary 17-ketosteroid excretion and absence of virilization. These criteria were established as a basis for their selection of patients for bilateral ovarian wedge resection (521,876,878,879). Using the classic description of patients originally described in 1935, Stein (874), in 1964, reported only 108 patients who conformed to the original description. In this strictly defined group he was able to report a 95% return to ovulatory cycles and an 85% conception rate following bilateral ovarian wedge resection. Subsequent reports by numerous investigators have emphasized that enlarged ovaries are not necessarily present, nor is infertility or anovulation always present (347,349,852,905,909,945). Similarly not all patients are hirsute (347,349,423,737,852, 895,905,909) and the original observation that most women with Stein-Leventhal syndrome have hypoplastic breasts has not been noted by others. Most have normal sized breasts or "unusually well developed" breasts (324,423).

From a practical viewpoint the eponymic syndrome of Stein and Leventhal has been replaced by an emergence of a spectrum of a diffuse syndrome of overlapping disorders of ovarian and adrenal dysfunction. The fact that hypothalamic dysfunction may also be present in this syndrome complex makes differentiation of a specific etiology virtually impossible. The clinical syndrome, however, has come to be known as polycystic ovarian disease (PCOD) on the basis of the frequent presence of multiple subcapsular follicular cysts 2–6 mm in diameter and a thickened ovarian capsule. The multifollicular cysts and frequently associated thickened ovarian capsule is undoubtedly an ovarian response to a multiplicity of entities associated with inappropriate gonadotropin secretion and/or hyperandrogenemia.

In view of the broad clinical spectrum of PCOD a reevaluation of signs and symptoms which may lead one to consider the presence or association of PCOD will follow. Numerous excellent reviews by Goldzieher (341,347), Yen (1011,1013), Givens (324), and others (206, 430,852,905,) have shed light on many aspects of this enigmatic state.

Although hyperthecosis, namely, the presence of nests of luteinized theca cells in hyperplastic ovarian stroma, appears to be one end of a spectrum of what has been described as PCOD (858), histologically most cases of hyperthecosis have less polyfollicular elements and a greater tendency to virilization with its concomitant biochemical findings. In view of this, the clinical signs of hyperthecosis will be discussed separately in Chapter 9.

It must be emphasized that no matter what term is applied to this disease complex, the histopathological expression of polyfollicular ovaries in various stages of growth and atresia is a sign and not a disease (324).

Clinical Signs and Symptoms

The major presentations of patients with PCOD are (1) hirsutism, (2) menstrual dysfunction and (3) infertility. These are the reasons most of these patients seek medical advice. Most women have normal onset of menarche, although oligomenorrhea may be significant and persistent from the beginning. Infrequently, primary amenorrhea may be present in PCOD (115, 647,1015). Four of 98 patients reported by Yen et al. (1015) had primary amenorrhea. A careful history which may be elicited from parents indicates that frequently one may detect some degree of hirsutism and obesity *prior* to the onset of menarche (1011). In most instances hirsutism is recognized following the onset of menarche, and increased body hair may be noted facially,

in the intermammary, periareolar and pubic areas as well as over the extremities.

Hirsutism implies the presence of terminal pigmented hair in areas of hair growth normally found in the male. With the exception of the eyelashes and eyebrows, most other terminal pigmented body hair growth is androgen dependent. Genetic factors are important in determining local sensitivity to androgens and accounts for the relative hirsutism of those of Mediterranean descent compared with those of Northern European ancestry (976).

In the hirsute female the primary abnormality is an increase in the androgen production rate (52,54,462). Progressive manifestations of hirsutism and menstrual dysfunction correlate with the testosterone production rates (Fig. 7-1) (462). Increased level of circulating androgens increase 5α-reductase activity of the skin (598). Genetic factors may modify the effects of increased androgens in that some women with increased androgen levels may not be hirsute (54, 206). A possible potentiation of the effects of T

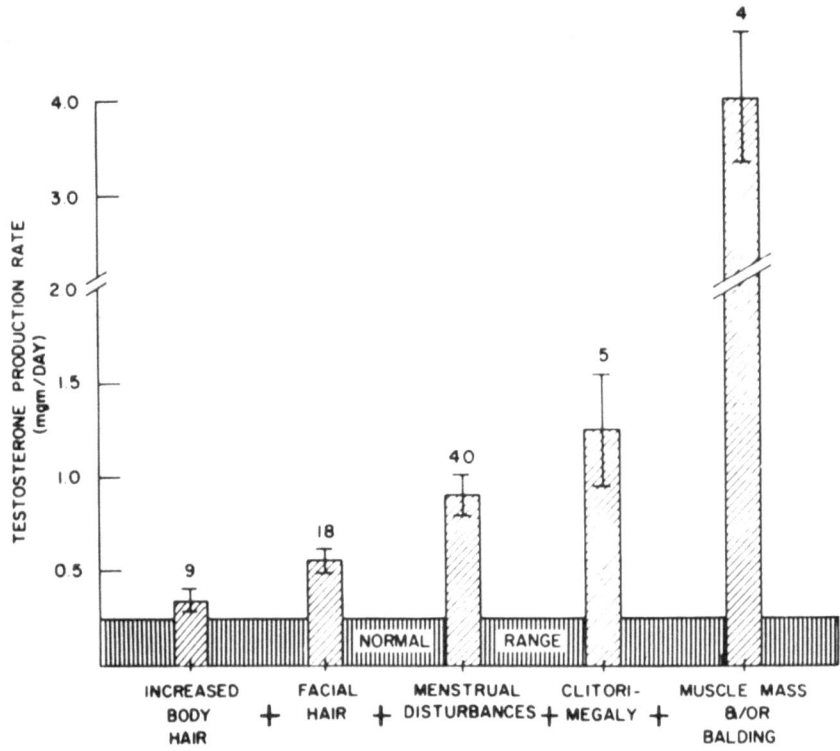

Fig. 7-1. Testosterone production rates ($\pm$ SE) in women with progressive hirsutism and virilization. The number of patients examined in each category is noted above the respective bar (Reproduced with permission from Kirschner MA, Zucker IR, Jespersen DL. Ovarian and adrenal vein catheterization studies in women with idiopathic hirsutism. In: James VHT, Serio M, Giusti G, eds. The Endocrine Function of the Human Ovary. New York: Academic Press Inc, 1976:443–456.) (462).

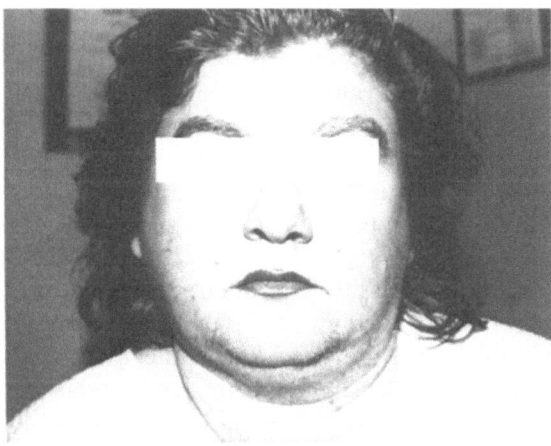

Fig. 7-2. Coarse terminal facial hair in a 44-year old woman with generalized hirsutism.

of the pilosebaceous apparatus causing the transition of villous hair (small, lightly colored and cosmetically insignificant hair) to the terminal type hair which is large, coarse and strongly pigmented (Figs. 7-2 and 7-3) (499). Once terminal hair has developed due to chronic androgen excess, only small amounts of androgens are necessary to maintain full growth (409). Significant hirsutism will, however, be associated with the growth of terminal coarse hair on the face, intermammary and linea alba regions associated with a male pattern pubic hair distribution (Fig. 7-4) (909). Increased oiliness of facial skin, seborrhea and acne may also be present (Fig. 7-5). In the more advanced stage of hyperandrogenemia, severe resistant cystic acne may develop on the face and upper back. A male escutcheon is usually associated with a moderately signifi-

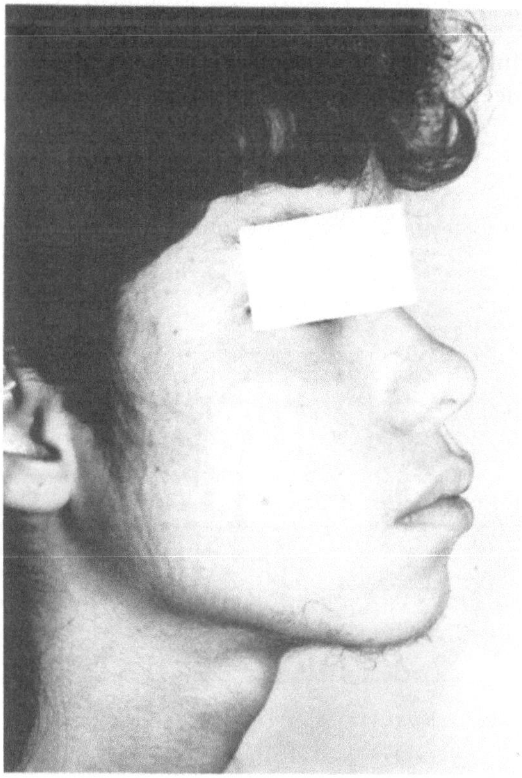

on hair growth may be a reduced E_2/T ratio (931).

Hirsutism is often a difficult symptom to evaluate in view of the constitutional predisposition to develop increased facial, periareolar and suprapubic hair. Androgens influence the growth

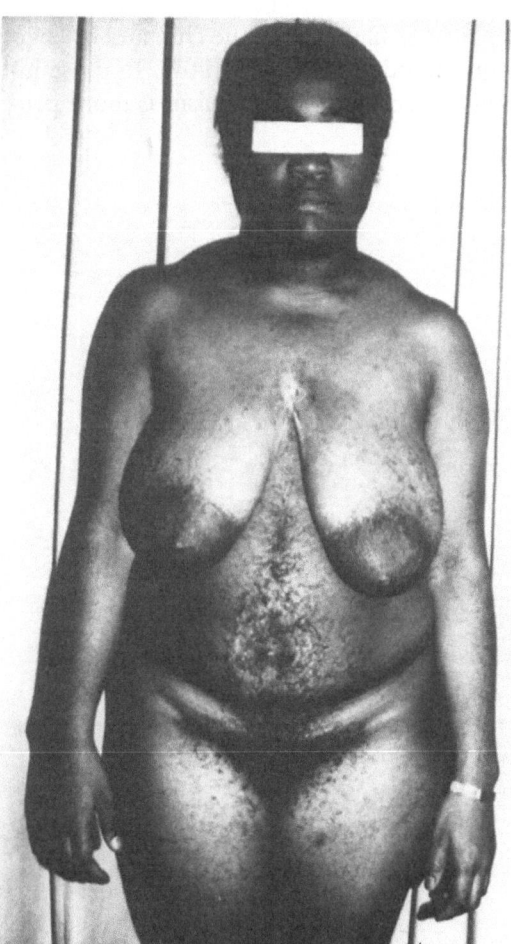

Fig. 7-4. Moderately severe hirsutism and male pattern pubic hair distribution. Note significant amount of breast development which is present in many patients with PCOD.

Fig. 7-3. Facial hirsutism and acne in a 20-year-old female with PCOD.

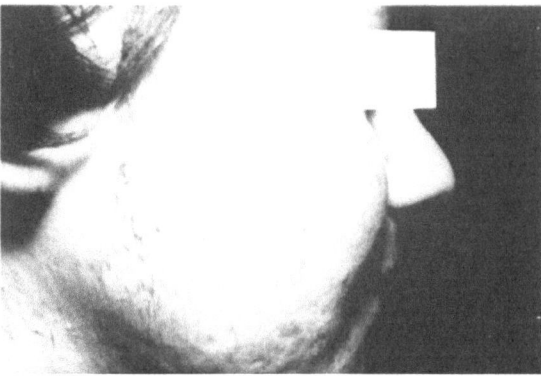

Fig. 7-5. A 21-year-old female with facial hirsutism, oiliness of the skin and cystic acne.

cant hyperandrogenemia. Racial factors must be taken into account in the evaluation of hirsutism as being abnormal or normal. A study of Causasian women between the ages of 15 and 44 years demonstrated that 33% had hair on the upper lip, 9% had hair on the chin and 6% had hair on the sides of the face (907). In those instances where hyperandrogenism is more pro-

nounced, temporal scalp hair loss may be bothersome and is usually associated with more severe and generalized hirsutism. A diffuse pattern of scalp hair loss may also be present with a pronounced midcephalic distribution (Figs. 7-6 and 7-7). A familial history of hirsutism makes PCOD a likely possibility in the individual patient (324).

Although obesity is frequent in PCOD, the most distressing symptoms to the teenager is the hirsutism, and not necessarily the menstrual dysfunction. Facial hirsutism may present as coarse long hair over the sides of face, chin, as well as neck. For the teenager hirsutism may involve considerable emotional anguish and psychosexual adjustments. The fact that irregular menses may or not have been present since onset of menarche may occasionally be further compounded by the fact that a number of these teenagers have been placed on oral contraceptive-type drugs to "regulate their periods." This frequently causes a delay in alerting the physician to the significance of the irregular menses.

Mild hirsutism with no significant menstrual dysfunction may be one end of the spectrum of systemic androgen ovarian production. This implies that the ovarian changes found in PCOD are secondary to the effects of increased circulating androgens. Some evidence supports this concept: (1) thickening and capsular fibrosis has

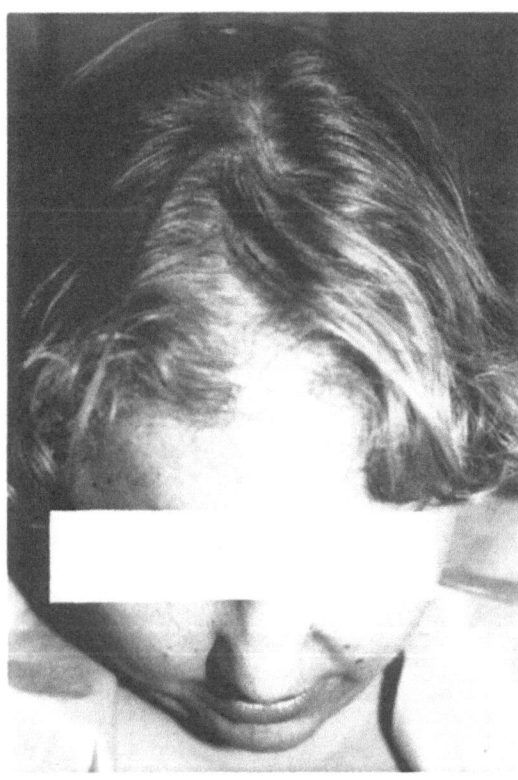

Fig. 7-6. Severe degree of mid-cephalic hair loss in a 25-year-old female with PCOD.

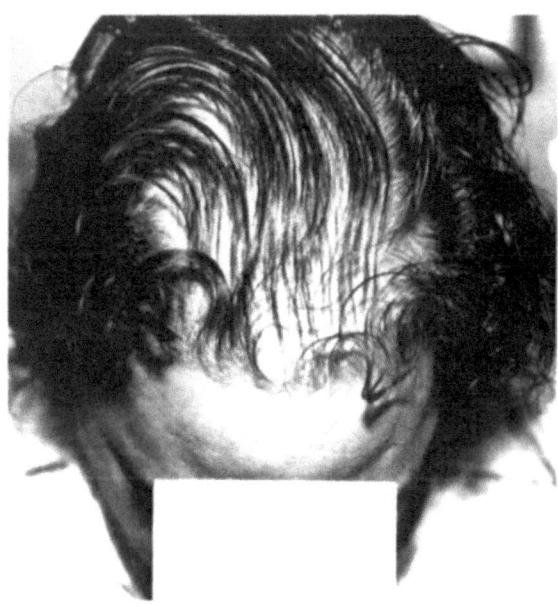

Fig. 7-7. Marked diffuse scalp hair loss in a 43-year-old woman with PCOD

been induced in animals given exogenous androgens (781,807); (2) in non-ovarian causes of hyperandrogenism such as congenital adrenal hyperplasia (76), polycystic ovarian changes have been described; (3) testosterone-secreting adrenal adenomas have been associated with ovarian stromal hyperplasia (974); and (4) estrogens may reverse sclerocystic ovarian changes (301).

By stimulating thecal production of androgens (230) an elevated LH level may potentiate the initial androgen production whether it was predominantly ovarian or adrenal in etiology (203). This occurs because the increased androstenedione is converted peripherally to E_1, which may increase LH. A relative deficiency of FSH reduces conversion of intra-ovarian androgens to E_2 (231). This leads to an increased circulating androgen level but also to a lower E_2/T ratio reducing TeBG production. Longcope and Williams (546) suggest that the rate-limiting factor in this cycle may depend on the peripheral conversion of E_1 to E_2, which counterbalances the effect of the androgens on TeBG production.

In an analysis of 98 cases of PCOD, Yen et al. (1011,1015) noted the following suggestive clinical findings which implied endocrine aberrations occurring before and during puberty, and prior to the establishment of cyclicity of the hypothalamic–pituitary–ovarian axis:

1. Mean age at menarche (12.3 years) was close to the mean of 12.9 years found in the general population (279). Although it is rare, primary amenorrhea may occur (115,1015). Four of 98 patients with PCOD had primary amenorrhea in Yen et al.'s series (1015).
2. The onset of clinically discernible excessive hair growth may be noted before or around the time of menarche. Parents may give a reliable history of this if questioned carefully.
3. Continuation of postmenarchal menstrual irregularity is present in most instances. Seventy of 88 patients had irregular menses following onset of menarche (1015).
4. Obesity prior to onset of menarche is common with "heaviness" being described in 90 of 98 cases (1015).

In the United States, menarche occurs at a mean age of 12.7–12.9 years with a standard deviation of just over one year (278). At menarche the breasts and pubic hair have reached Tanner stage IV (586) and linear growth rate is slowing. Patients with PCOD may present with a normal onset menarche, but the flow and frequency of cycles may be abnormal. Less frequently onset of menarche may be delayed. Although some girls continue to have regular cyclic menses they may or may not be associated with significant premenstrual symptoms of pelvic discomfort, bloating or breast engorgement. Some have erratic menstrual intervals of varying lengths and in most instances the oligomenorrhea will respond to a progestational agent resulting in withdrawal bleeding. In some instances the oligomenorrhea gradually proceeds to intervals of prolonged amenorrhea. To further add to the variability of menstrual abnormalities, dysfunctional uterine bleeding may be present with a mean incidence of 29% (347). Table 7-1 lists the reported frequencies of menstrual dysfunction in PCOD. It must be stressed again that regular menses may be present as well as signs of ovulation (Table 7-1) (286,347,349, 423,737,756,852,895,905,909), and that their presence does not exclude the presence of polycystic ovaries.

In the comprehensive review by Goldzieher and Axelrod (347) of 1079 published cases of surgically proven polycystic disease, the mean incidence of amenorrhea was 51%, hirsutism 69%, infertility 74%, "functional" bleeding 29%, obesity 41%, cyclic menses 12%, and corpus luteum evidence of ovulation in 22% (Table 7-1). A number of smaller series that followed this review demonstrated similar findings (349,423,737,852,895,905,909,945). The mean incidence of 21% of virilization reported by Goldzieher and Green (349) may reflect a higher incidence of associated stromal disease or other diseases such as the various types of congenital (or adult-onset) adrenogenital syndromes. In most instances of PCOD, enlargement of the clitoris is unusual and its presence warrants careful investigation for the presence of possible adrenal or ovarian tumors (Fig. 7-8).

It is also apparent from Table 7-1, that normal sized ovaries are present in approximately 20–40% of patients (349,852,905). Palpation of the ovaries in obese women is at best difficult and additional information regarding ovarian size may have to be obtained by ultrasonography of the pelvis. However, as stated earlier, enlargement of the ovaries is not always present

TABLE 7-1. Clinical Features of Patients with Polycystic Ovarian Disease.

Author	Ref.	No.	Infertility	Obesity	Hirsutism	% OF PATIENTS Oligo & amenorrhea	Dysfunctional bleeding	Cyclic menses	Ovulation	Corpus luteum	Spont. pregnancy
Goldzieher and Green	349	39	76	49	62	92	0	8	14		
Goldzieher and Axelrod	347	1079	74 (35–94)	41 (16–49)	69 (17–83)	51 (15–77)	29 (6–65)	12 (7–28)		22 (0–77)	18
Taymor et al	905	40	100	43	58	58	12	10	20	25	
Jeffcoate	423	46	32	50	57	100			11		
Smith et al.	852	127		54	47	65		35			
↑ tunica		68		65	79	72		28			
nl tunica		59		42	8	58		42			
Raj et al	737	101	55	37	86	89	7	7			
Type I		67	64	31	82	91	4	6			
Type II		34	35	44	100	85	12	9			
Tacchi	895	78	32	32	64	92		4			
Thompson and Taymor	909	101	55	37	86	89	7	7	15		
Futterweit and Mechanick	286	93	19	46	92	78	12	10			3

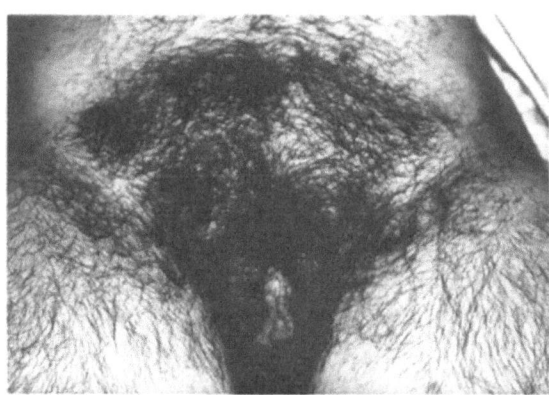

Fig. 7-8. Marked increase in pubic and peripubic hair associated with minimal clitoromegaly in a 27-year-old obese female with PCOD. Diagnostic studies did not indicate the presence of an adrenal or ovarian tumor.

in polycystic ovaries and instances of unilateral enlargement have also rarely been reported (206,945).

Galactorrhea may be present in PCOD (509, 912,998). Its exact frequency is as yet not defined, but it is our experience that it is present in 13% of patients with PCOD (286). The patient may or may not be aware of this sign, but careful examination of the breasts should be performed routinely to look for its presence. The significance of galactorrhea in association with hyperprolactinemia in these patients will be discussed in Chapter 8.

Flier has noted that 5% of hyperandrogenic women have acanthosis nigricans (AN) (121). This is a brown velvety, sometimes verrucous discoloration of the skin most often seen around the nape of the neck and axillae (Figs. 7-9, 7-10, 7-11). It is present in a number of endocrine disturbances including PCOD, hyperthecosis and pituitary tumors. Its significance lies in the fact that in these patients AN may be a marker of insulin resistance and that they may fall into a category described by Kahn et al. (440) as having type A or type B (903) insulin resistance. (See later section of this chapter on AN and Insulin Resistance.)

Careful follow-up examination of patients with PCOD is necessary to look for possible complications or associations such as endome-

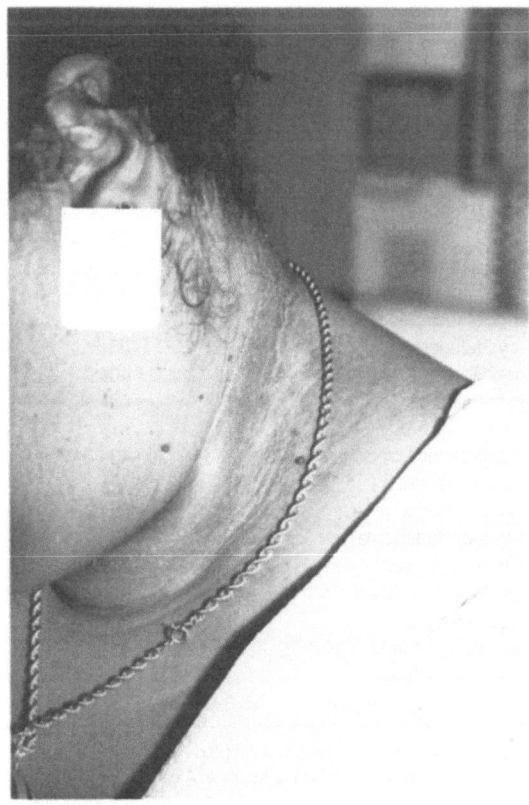

Fig. 7-9. Patient with PCOD and acanthosis nigricans

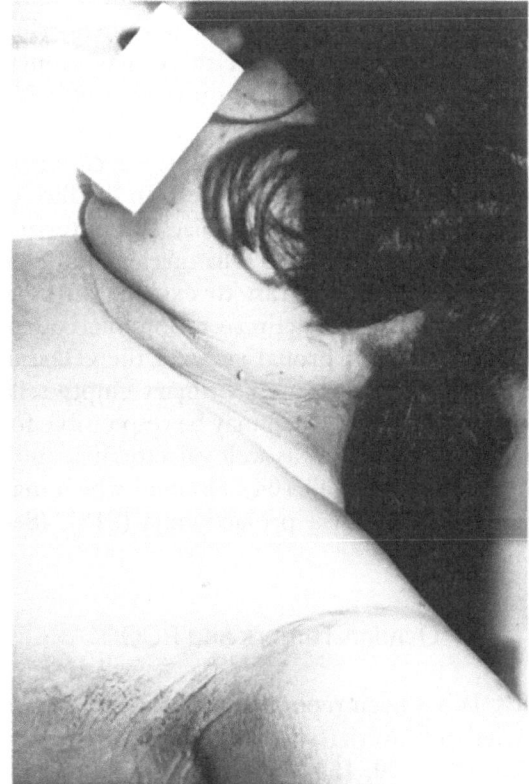

Fig. 7-10. Patient with PCOD and acanthosis nigricans

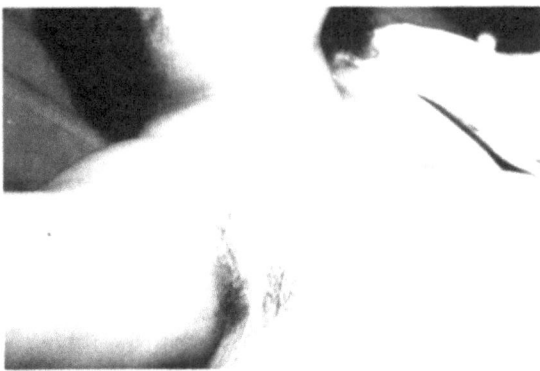

Fig. 7-11. Patient with PCOD and acanthosis nigricans.

trial carcinoma, ovarian tumors, and pituitary tumors. (See later sections of this chapter, and Chapter 8 on hyperprolactinemia.)

Any rapid development of progressive hirsutism, scalp hair loss, amenorrhea, with or without galactorrhea, deepening of voice and onset of clitoromegaly or a palpable new mass on pelvic examination requires explanation for its cause. The fact that a higher incidence of ovarian tumors is present in PCOD (287) should make interval ultrasonography every two years or so mandatory, particularly in the face of a rapidly developing virilizing syndrome or adnexal mass. Similarly, a patient with prolonged amenorrhea and galactorrhea, whether there may or may not have been a previous history of protracted treatment with a combination of an estrogen–progestin drug, should have serial serum prolactin measurements performed. In the face of significant hyperprolactinemia, computerized tomography (CT) of the sella turcica should be performed with contrast to exclude an associated pituitary-prolactin secreting microadenoma (284,290). Coronal views of the CT scan (937) may demonstrate a primary empty sella syndrome (PESS) which may be responsible for hyperprolactinemia, as well galactorrhea and/or amenorrhea (100,104,288), and which may also co-exist with a prolactinoma (213). (See Chapter 8.)

Ovarian Tumors and PCOD

PCOD has been reported in association with a variety of ovarian neoplasms (16,38,80,125, 126, 128, 159, 169, 180, 237, 287, 329, 333, 358,404,406,601,654,880,1041). The incidence of ovarian tumors which have been re-

ported in patients with polycystic ovaries has ranged from 4.6 – 17.0% (38,404). Of the many types of ovarian neoplasms associated with PCOD (Table 7-2) the most commonly found are dermoid cysts (38,159,287,404,406,654). Ovarian dermoids constitute 24 of the 69 cases of ovarian tumors reported with polycystic ovaries (35%) (287). Bilateral dermoid cysts of the ovaries in association with polycystic ovaries is extremely rare, and only two cases have been reported (287,406). Insulin resistance was noted in both instances, while AN was described in the patient of Imperato-McGinley et al. (406). Stromal luteinization was absent in the dermoid cysts and in the surrounding polycystic ovarian tissue in both patients (287,406).

TABLE 7-2. Polycystic Ovaries and Coexisting Ovarian Tumors.

	NUMBER OF PATIENTS	REFERENCES
Dermoids	24	38,159,287, 404,406,654
Arrhenoblastomas	8	16,38,80,125, 128,180, 1041
Thecomas	5	237,329,333, 404
Papillary fibromas and papillomas	5	38
Cystic granulosa cell tumors	4	38,126
Adrenal rest tumors (lipid cell)	4	38,404,1041
Hilar cell tumors	4	38,169,358
Papillary cystadenomas	3	38,880
Pseudomucinous cystadenomas	2	38
Adenofibromas	2	404
Dysgerminoma	1	404
Serous cystadenocarcinoma	1	404
Bilateral mucinous cystadenoma	1	654
Serous cystadenoma	1	654
Hemorrhagic cyst	1	654
Mesonephroma (clear cell tumor)	1	38
Interstitial cell tumor	1	481
Gynandroblastoma	1	601
TOTAL	69	

No tumor classification in this table attempted

From Futterweit W, Scher J, Nunez AE, et al A case of bilateral dermoid cysts, insulin resistance and polycystic ovarian disease association of ovarian tumors with polycystic ovaries with a review of the literature Mt Sinai J Med 1983, 50 251 – 255 (287)

Endometrial Cancer and PCOD

There is evidence suggesting a relationship between estrogen use by menopausal women and an increased incidence of endometrial cancer (824,848,849,969,1038). A relationship between chronic estrogen therapy and endometrial abnormalities in hypogonadal subjects with gonadal dysgenesis has also been reported (777). Patients with estrogen-secreting ovarian tumors and women with PCOD are also at high risk for development of uterine cancer (212, 411,575). In PCOD the excessive production of androstenedione leads to increased levels of estrone via peripheral aromatization (844). It appears that estrone is the strongest stimulator of endometrial hyperplasia of all the estrogens (843). Obesity is another predisposing factor in the development of uterine cancer via increased peripheral conversion of androstenedione to estrone. The transfer constant of conversion of plasma androstenedione to estrone is greater in obese than in non-obese women (227,755,844). A causal relationship between endogenous estrogen production and endometrial carcinoma has been provided by the studies of MacDonald and Siiteri (557,843,844). Schindler et al. (796) noted that adipose tissue of patients with endometrial cancer convert androstenedione to estrone nearly four times as fast as those women without uterine cancer.

An epidemiological study of 1000 women with endometrial carcinoma confimed the primary association of obesity in such patients. Wynder et al. (1005) suggested that the risk of developing endometrial cancer in obese women is increased 3 to 9 times depending on the severity of the obesity. Most extraglandular estrogen formation occurs in adipocytes since aromatase activity is present in such tissue. The extent of conversion of plasma androstenedione to estrone is significantly correlated with excessive body weight in postmenopausal as well as in young ovulatory and anovulatory women (226). MacDonald et al. (556) found no difference in the conversion of plasma androstenedione to estrone in postmenopausal women with endometrial carcinoma than in those without endometrial disease when both groups were paired by age and degree of obesity. However, women with endometrial cancer had 1.5 times more excessive body weight than did women without uterine neoplasia (556). Aging and hepatic disease also predispose women to an increased risk of endometrial carcinoma.

Fechner and Kaufman (254) described four cases of well differentiated adenocarcinoma of the endometrium and reviewed previous reports of the endometrial lesion in patients with PCOD. Most of the uterine cancers have been well differentiated adenocarcinomas or adenocanthomas with only few instances of more aggressive tumors. The ages at time of diagnosis of these endometrial carcinomas in women with PCOD have ranged from 16–40 years of age (254). In some instances an initial diagnosis of endometrial hyperplasia preceded the diagnosis of adenocarcinoma. Some reports note the spectrum of hyperplasia to include such terms as cystic glandular hyperplasia, polypous hyperplasia, adenomatous hyperplasia and atypical adenomatous hyperplasia (135). Fechner and Kaufman (254) as well as Grattarola (356) have stressed that the histologic distinction between atypical adenomatous hyperplasia and well-differentiated adenocarcinoma is not sharp (254, 356). The relatively benign prognosis of well-differentiated adenocarcinoma of the endometrium in PCOD has been stressed (254), with metastases occurring rarely in these patients under the age of 40 years. A combined study of 57 cases of PCOD and associated endometrial carcinoma (254,411,414,607,993) with a review of the literature (254) revealed that only four were poorly differentiated carcinomas.

In 1949, Speert (866) reported 14 cases of endometrial carcinoma in women under the age of 40 years and found that 8 had associated sclerocystic ovaries. The association of endometrial carcinoma and PCOD was also described by Jackson and Dockerty (411) and Sommers et al. (860). Dockerty and Mussey (212) noted that 20% of women under the age of 40 who developed carcinoma of the endometrium had clinical evidence of PCOD. In a study by Chamlian and Taylor (135) of 97 young women with endometrial hyperplasia, 14% developed endometrial carcinoma in a 14-year follow-up and 25% of these patients had PCOD. Conservative therapy of patients with endometrial carcinoma and PCOD has been advocated by some, including the use of hydroxyprogesterone caproate (225). Others, however, are of the opinion that these patients should be treated as any other such neoplasm whether PCOD is present or not (414).

Adenocarcinoma of the endometrium is usually a disease of post-menopausal women with less than 25% of cases occurring during child-bearing age. In 1957, however, Jackson and Dockerty (411) reported 45 cases of PCOD, 17 of whom had carcinoma of the endometrium. Additional studies also demonstrated an association of PCOD and endometrial cancer (254,414,607,993), with the ages of the patients ranging from 16–40 years. Frequent screening of patients with polycystic ovaries is necessary for early detection of the lesion. Although conservative therapy with progestins may be of some value in reducing the risk of progression of the disease, it appears to offer little in promoting fertility in these women with endometrial hyperplasia (135).

McDonald et al. (607) reviewed 72 cases of concomitant ovarian disease and endometrial cancer at the Mayo Clinic from 1905 through 1975, and noted that the associated disorders were functioning ovarian tumors in 44 patients (mostly theca cell tumors) and polycystic ovaries in 28 patients. While there was no patient with an associated functioning ovarian tumor younger than 46 years of age, only 2 of the 28 cases of PCOD were older that 40 years. Although the vast majority of patients were seen for abnormal uterine bleeding (86%), those with postmenopausal bleeding all had associated functioning ovarian tumors. Ten of the 72 patients complained of lower abdominal pains and swelling. Hypertension was noted in 32% of patients with PCOD and in 66% of those with functioning ovarian tumors. Twenty-five percent of both groups also had associated diabetes mellitus, while 79% of patients with associated PCOD were obese. In the 28 cases of PCOD, ovarian pathology revealed bilateral enlargement with thickened tunica albuginea, multiple subcapsular follicular cysts, cortical and stromal fibrosis and numerous primordial ova. The survival rate in both groups was 86% at 10 years, and suggested that the prognosis of the endometrial cancer in most instances where a coexisting endogenous estrogenic stimulus is present is more favorable than endometrial carcinoma alone (607). Four of the 72 patients had breast cancer preceding, concurring with, or after diagnosis of their endometrial cancer.

A recent study by Coulam et al. (174) of a cohort of 1270 patients with chronic anovulation syndrome at the Mayo Clinic from 1935–1980 revealed associated neoplasms in 74 patients. Thirty patients had neoplasia diagnosed before and concurrent with the chronic anovulation syndrome and 44 subsequently developed neoplasms. Fourteen instances of concurrently diagnosed endometrial carcinomas were noted, which is an incidence of 1.1%. Comparison to the expected number of incidence rates of neoplasm revealed that the only site of increased risk for development of a malignancy was the endometrium. The relative risk for the development of endometrial carcinoma after the diagnosis of chronic anovulation syndrome was made was 3.1. There was not a statistically high risk for the development of breast cancer in this group of patients. The concept of a chronic anovulation syndrome being a spontaneous biologic experiment of unopposed estrogen production appears to be of some interest in relating a possible cause and effect of estrogens in the development of endometrial cancer (174). The incidence of 1.1% of such patients having endometrial carcinoma is much lower than the 37% reported by Jackson and Dockerty (411). The difference appears to be one of patient selection bias, since the latter study was performed on surgical specimens, where a diagnosis of endometrial carcinoma was made because of symptoms suggestive of such a neoplasm.

Acanthosis Nigricans and Insulin Resistance in PCOD

Givens et al. (333) in 1974 described the association of acanthosis nigrican (AN), hirsutism and insulin resistance. Kahn et al. (440) in 1976 reported women with this triad in whom the insulin resistance resulted via decreased numbers of insulin receptors (type A receptor defect). The type B patients with AN, autoimmune disease and insulin resistance) have decreased affinity of the receptor to insulin due to the presence of antireceptor antibodies (440). A post-receptor defect as reported by Bar et al. (47) necessitates total insulin binding as being unaltered. Clinical studies have demonstrated a positive correlation between hyperandrogenism and hyperinsulinism in patients with PCOD (106). Furthermore, gonadotropin suppression with oral contraceptives has been reported to be occasionally effective in modifying excess androgen production and reducing AN in certain patients where AN is associated with PCOD (333).

AN is characterized by brown symmetric, hyerpigmented, verrucous, or fine papillomatosis, and hyperkeratotic thickening of the skin. Gentle stroking of the skin may elicit a soft velvety texture. It most often affects the nape of the neck, axillas and groin. AN may be diagnosed by punch biopsy of the skin which usually shows characteristic papillomatous, hyperkeratotic formations (333). Although it may be associated with visceral malignancies, it also occurs in metabolic and endocrine disorders including obesity and diseases of the thyroid, pituitary and adrenal glands (103,121). AN may also be associated with an uncommon group of disorders characterized by target resistance to insulin (265,266). The type A syndrome of insulin resistance is characterized by hyperandrogenism with a clinical onset near the time of puberty (440). Hyperthecosis and polycystic ovaries have been reported in some cases (121,406). Some are symptomatic diabetic patients and others have a normal glucose tolerance, but in all cases there are high endogenous insulin levels and resistance to endogenous insulin (440). A normal range of fasting plasma insulin is up to $15-20\ \mu U/ml$, and insulin resistant patients have a high level of basal insulin. Instances of insulin resistance may be due to a deficiency in the number of insulin receptors that their cells express (46,440), or to an abnormality of early steps beyond (post-) receptor binding (47).

Approximately 5% of hyperandrogenic women have AN (121), and these women have resistance to endogenous insulin despite a normal glucose tolerance. Although insulin resistance may be correlated with hyperandrogenism (106), it is not a direct cause for the insulin resistance, nor does bilateral oophorectomy correct this defect.

A striking elevation of plasma insulin to exogenous glucose provides evidence that the pancreatic β-cell is functioning.

Insulin resistance can result from (1) an abnormal secretory product of the β-cell, (2) insulin antagonists (pre-receptor causes), and (3) tissue insensitivity to insulin action (an abnormality at the receptor or post-receptor level) (517). Insulin resistance may also occur in the presence of excess growth hormone or glucocorticoids.

A 17-year old premenarchal female with marked reduction of the clearance of plasma insulin was studied by Ferraninni et al. (259). Excessive post-hepatic delivery of insulin was noted. She also demonstrated fasting hyperinsulinemia with glucose intolerance, primary amenorrhea, hirsutism and PCOD. AN, glucose intolerance and onset of menses occurred following wedge resection of the ovaries. The results, however, were not sustained one year following the surgery. Pre-operatively there was a hyperresponse of plasma insulin to glucose from 170 to more that 1000 $\mu U/ml$. Post-operatively a glucose tolerance test caused the basal plasma insulin to rise from 37 to maximum of 412 $\mu U/ml$ at 60 minutes. Fasting euglycemia was maintained at the expense of a 20-fold increase of the plasma insulin level. Since anti-receptor antibodies were absent and insulin binding was near normal, it was inferred that the insulin resistance was in part due to a post-receptor defect. Insulin degradation was severely depressed in the absence of organ failure of the liver or kidney. Impaired insulin degradation was demonstrated in this patient with severe insulin resistance and a normal number of insulin receptors were found (259). A recent study by Minaker et al. (641) also demonstrated three patients with AN and reduced insulin clearance.

Elevated circulating β-endorphin and β-lipotropin levels have been found in hirsute patients including some with PCOD (321). A direct correlation has been found with increased body weight. A significant correlation between body weight and elevation of β-endorphin and β-lipotropin has been reported, while no correlation between androgen levels and β-endorphin or lipotropin levels has been noted. Since β-endorphin stimulates insulin secretion it may play a role in the hyperinsulinism of obesity. The relationship of β-endorphin or β-lipotropin in hyperandrogenism is not clear. Obsesity has been reported to be associated with a rise in DHA secretion from the adrenal (255).

Six non-obese patients with aplastic anemia who were treated with the synthetic androgen oxymetholone have been reported (994). All had normal blood glucose levels but demonstrated abnormal glucose tolerance associated with increased plasma insulin response to glucose. Thus insulin resistance developed in this group of patients with aplastic anemia treated with a synthetic androgen.

Because insulin resistance may be clinically

silent and AN is often not observed, the incidence of type A syndrome is unknown. Severe but clinically silent insulin resistance with AN was reported in two siblings (a 30-year-old hirsute infertile woman with PCOD and her 26-year-old brother) (264). Large thickened hands suggestive of acromegaly were present in both patients in association with normal growth hormone and elevated basal plasma insulin levels. A long history of episodic extremity muscle cramps was described and a type A insulin resistance with reduced concentration of insulin receptors on circulating monocytes was found in both patients. A genetic basis for this syndrome appears probable. Perhaps the hyperinsulinism may account for acral hypertrophy via an effect on somatomedins (264).

One of the original patients of Kahn et al. (440), was restudied with fibroblast cultures (439). She demonstrated a primary defect in insulin receptors, possibly a genetic abnormality. Decreased receptor affinity was noted and this was different from previously reported patients, where a decrease in the number of receptors was noted. An alteration of receptor structure with decreased receptor affinity may lead to insulin resistance and secondary hyperinsulinism, and a decrease in the number of receptors by the process of "down-regulation."

Obesity is a frequent occurrence in PCOD and may be associated with subclinical insulin resistance and exaggerated hyperinsulinemia to a glucose tolerance test. Fasting hyperinsulinemia was found in 10 of 14 patients with PCOD (most were obese), and this correlated with their body weight (996). Fasting hyperglycemia was not found in any of 25 PCOD patients studied. Mean peak serum insulin response following a glucose tolerance test was approximately $200 \mu U/ml$ with no correlation to body weight noted. Despite normal serum cholesterol and triglyceride levels in this group, the high density lipoprotein cholesterol (HDL-cholesterol) did not exceed 50 mg/dl in any patient (996).

A comparison of the response of 16 obese patients with PCOD and 16 with simple obesity matched for age and weight revealed higher basal insulin levels and higher glucose stimulated insulin levels in the PCOD group (710).

Although the basal C-peptide levels were similar in obese patients with PCOD to that of control obese subjects, the C-peptide response to an oral glucose load was also significantly higher in the obese PCOD patients. This suggests that the secretion rate of the β-cell in PCOD is stimulated to a greater extent following glucose administration than the subjects with simple obesity (710).

In a study to determine whether insulin resistance occurs in PCOD in the absence of obesity and AN, circulating levels of insulin in response to oral glucose administration were measured in 10 non-obese PCOD subjects without AN and in 10 normal women matched for height and weight (136). There was no statistical difference between patients with PCOD and the control subjects in the levels of FSH, growth hormone, PRL, cortisol, E_1 and E_2. The 10 non-obese PCOD subjects had a mean percent ideal body weight of 104.4%, which was not significantly different from the control group (101.3%). The mean basal insulin level in the PCOD patients was $18.7 \pm 2.9 \mu U/ml$, which was significantly higher than that of the normal control group ($11.0 \pm 0.8 \mu U/ml$). The mean rise of circulating insulin to 100 g of oral glucose was much greater in PCOD than in normal subjects (Fig. 7-12) (136). The mean peak insulin level achieved in PCOD patients following the glucose load was $158 \pm 23 \mu U/ml$ while that in normal subjects was $57 \pm 10 \mu U/ml$. The blood glucose response following the glucose administration did not differ between the two groups. A highly significant correlation was found between serum T and androstenedione concentrations and basal insulin levels, as well as the sums of the increased insulin concentrations during the oral glucose tolerance test. Serum DHA, DHAS, cortisol, E_1 and E_2 levels did not correlate with insulin secretion. These observations of Chang et al. (136) suggest that hyperandrogenism may perhaps be responsible for the insulin resistance in PCOD. It appears that a significant degree of insulin resistance exists in PCOD which is not related to obesity or AN.

Although extreme insulin resistance and AN has usually been associated with hirsutism, PCOD, and elevated plasma T values (type A syndrome due to a genetic reduction in the number of insulin receptors), a recent report by Taylor et al. (903) found a similar clinical picture in a hirsute, fertile, 25-year-old woman with secondary amenorrhea, enlarged ovaries and absence of clitoromegaly having the type B syndrome. They demonstrated that type B syndrome may be associated with androgen excess

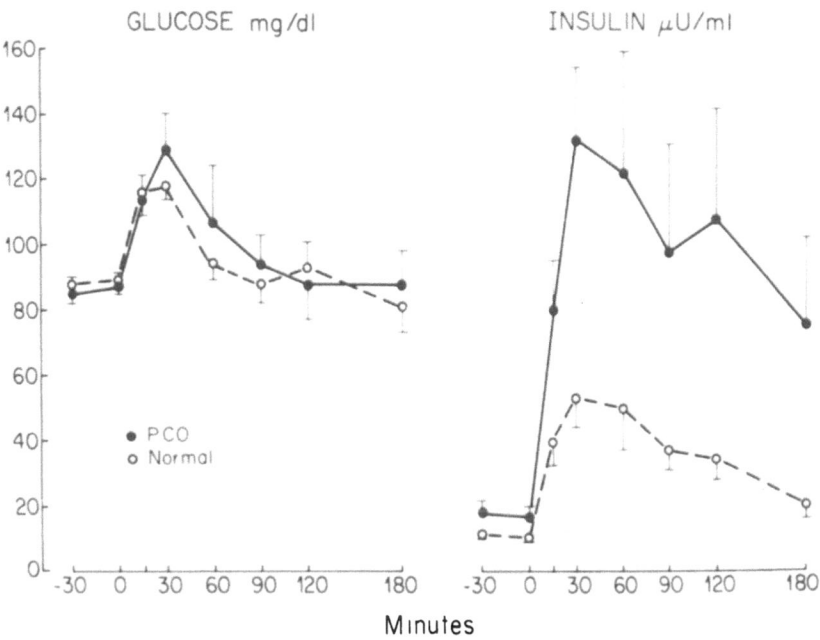

Fig. 7-12. Circulating levels of glucose and insulin in PCOD and normal control subjects in response to oral glucose administration (Reproduced from Chang RJ, Nakamura RM, Judd HL, et al Insulin resistance in nonobese patients with polycystic ovarian disease. J Clin Endocrinol Metab 1983, 57:356–359) (136)

as well, and this represented a modification of their earlier findings (440). It appears that post-menopausal females with type B syndrome do not characteristically develop signs of hyperandrogenism in association with the insulin resistance which has plasma autoantibodies directed against the receptor for insulin. On the other hand, four of their five type B patients under the age of 45 years, had elevated levels of plasma T ranging from 88–1033 ng/dl. The younger patients tended to have markedly elevated plasma T concentrations. Levels of E_2 and gonadotropins were usually in the normal range in these patients (903). Selective venous catheterization showed increased T from both ovaries in the one patient studied. Estrogen suppression treatment for two months caused a decline in the peripheral T value from 1000 ng/dl to less than 100 ng/dl. The authors state that in the syndromes of extreme insulin resistance, masculinization is commonly present in both types of syndromes with the AN and hyperinsulinism. Their hypothesis is that hyperinsulinemia per se may play a role in the production of hyperandrogenemia, rather than the proposal of Burghen et al. (106), who suggested that andro-gens may be responsible for causing moderate insulin resistance. It has been hypothesized that insulin itself may stimulate ovarian hyperandrogenism since the degree of hyperinsulinemia is frequently correlated with the severity of the hyperandrogenism (106). Whether insulin and growth factors may modulate gonadal sensitivity to gonadotropin stimulation has not as yet been clinically documented.

Barbieri et al. (50) studied the in vitro effects of insulin on porcine thecal steroidogenesis. Insulin alone had no stimulatory effect on andros-tenedione accumulation, but insulin plus LH resulted in significantly greater accumulation of androstenedione and progesterone as compared with LH alone in the cultures of dispersed theca cells. This suggests that insulin may be a regulatory protein for thecal steroidogenesis, although the mechanism is not clear. It is possible that in cultured theca cells, insulin is a regulator of LH receptor induction.

A direct causative effect of androgen production in PCOD and type A insulin resistance must be viewed with caution since insulin resistance may persist despite normalization of androgen production and reduction of AN (47).

Hyperprolactinemia and Polycystic Ovarian Disease

8

Hyperprolactinemia is a frequent concomitant of infertility, hypogonadism, and may be found in 27% of patients with PCOD. The isolation of prolactin and the development of a sensitive radioimmunoassay for its measurement has enabled the clinician to identify those clinical states that may be associated with hyperprolactinemia, and offers an option of medical treatment which may be useful in the treatment of the underlying pathological disturbance. It must be stressed that hyperprolactinemia is the most common hypothalamic–pituitary disorder in the human and an understanding of the pathophysiological effects of hyperprolactinemia is clearly important in the evaluation and management of such patients who may present with galactorrhea and/or menstrual abnormalities. Excellent reviews of PRL secretion and physiology have been reported (27,240,275,415,967).

The purpose of this discussion is to analyze the pathophysiology of hyperprolactinemia and its effects on the hypothalamus, ovaries and adrenal cortex, as well as its possible etiology and role in PCOD.

Causes of Hyperprolactinemia

Hyperprolactinemia may be found in a number of clinical conditions as indicated in Table 8-1.

Von Werder et al. (959) suggest that hyperprolactinemia may be caused by one of three mechanisms:

1. Autonomous PRL secretion by a pituitary adenoma

2. Reduced DA effect on the pituitary lactotrope
   (a) Reduced hypothalamic secretion of DA due to space-occupying lesions.
   (b) Reduced hypothalamic secretion of DA due to disturbed neurohormone transport (e.g., pituitary stalk compression or suprasellar extension of a pituitary adenoma).
   (c) DA receptor blocking drugs which antagonize DA at the lactotrope level.
3. Lactotrope stimulation which overrides physiologic inhibition (e.g., large doses of estrogens or hypothyroidism).

Pathophysiology of Hyperprolactinemia and the Hypothalamic–Pituitary–Ovarian Axis

The mechanism of altered reproductive functions in the hyperprolactinemic female is complex. At an early stage, follicular maturation may be suppressed leading to an inadequate corpus luteum (CL) associated with a short luteal phase, and subnormal P secretion (168, 815). With more pronounced hyperprolactinemia the preovulatory E_2 rise is lost and the length of the cycle is lengthened as a result of prolongation of the follicular phase. Anovulation results at this point but clomiphene and gonadotropin induction of pregnancy may still occur. Occasional patients may have spontaneous pregnancy despite moderately elevated PRL levels (667). However, pregnancy in hyperprolactinemia appears to be associated with a higher miscarriage rate. With further progres-

TABLE 8-1. Causes of Hyperprolactinemia (744,920)

1. Pituitary lesions
   (a) Prolactin-secreting pituitary tumors
   (b) Acromegaly
   (c) Combined growth hormone and prolactin secreting tumors
   (d) Cushing's disease
   (e) Nelson's syndrome
   (f) Primary empty sella syndrome
2. Hypothalamic lesions, (craniopharyngioma, surgical stalk section, sarcoidosis, histiocytosis X, leukemia, primary or metastatic tumors)
3. Primary hypothyroidism
4. Chronic renal failure (20%)
5. Polycystic ovarian disease
6. Irritative chest wall lesions (trauma, herpes zoster, thoracic burns, post-thoracotomy)
7. Pharmacological
   (a) Reserpine, alpha-methyldopa
   (b) Haloperidol, chlorpromazine (CPZ), metoclopramide (MCP)
   (c) Cimetidine
   (d) Tricyclic antidepressants
   (e) Opiates (e g , morphine, methadone)
   (f) Estrogens
   (g) Verapamil
8. Idiopathic hyperprolactinemia (presumed decrease of PIF or increase of prolactin releasing factor (PRF); an occult radiologically undetectable microadenoma of the pituitary may be present)
9. Ectopic production of prolactin
10. Physiologic
    (a) Pregnancy
    (b) Breast stimulation
    (c) Nursing mothers

sion of the hyperprolactinemia the hypothalamus demonstrates a decreased episodic and pulsatile LH pattern despite normal levels of LH and FSH, and stimulation with LHRH may result in a normal or exaggerated LH and FSH release. It is of interest that the normal levels of LH and FSH encountered in patients with hyperprolactinemia is inappropriate in view of the frequently found reduced serum E_2 levels (240). Failure to respond to LHRH, however, makes it unlikely that bromocriptine will be effective in restoring gonadal function, since a lack of LH response to LHRH usually occurs in large macroadenomas with considerable loss of gonadotrope function. In patients with pituitary microadenomas the administration of bromocriptine increases the LH frequency and amplitude (660).

Administration of LHRH to hyperprolactinemic patients frequently causes a normal or exaggerated response of serum LH (23,25,337, 475,503,648,867). High levels of PRL do not inhibit the E_2 rise following LHRH administration (28,472,503). Thus prolactin does not appear to act at the gonadotrope level to desensitize the pituitary gland to the action of LHRH. A hypothalamic action of hyperprolactinemia, however, may result in loss of the nocturnal increase of PRL and loss of pulsatile LH release as well as acyclic gonadotropin secretion (90,94, 628,798).

Lachelin et al. (503) studied the character of the hypothalamic–pituitary–ovarian axis in two groups of hyperprolactinemic patients in different stages of their disease: (1) Group I with an initial diagnosis of idiopathic hyperprolactinemia and/or probably microadenoma who later developed radiologic evidence of pituitary microadenoma in 9 of the 13 patients, and (2) Group II which consisted of five patients with surgically proven pituitary microadenomata with similar mean PRL levels as Group I (100 ng/ml). Serial intravenous pulses of TRH (200 μg) and LHRH (10 μg) were given alternately at hourly intervals for three doses each for a total period of 6 hours, and results compared to seven normal women in the early follicular phase of the menstrual cycle. Of interest was the augmented pituitary FSH response to LHRH in Group I > Group II > controls, while the LH response to LHRH was similar in Group I and controls but reduced in the subjects with surgically proven pituitary tumors. This indicated a significant reduction of the LH/FSH ratio during pulses of LHRH stimulation. The mean basal E_2 levels were reduced in both hyperprolactinemic groups, but an ovarian response of LHRH was observed to be similar in Group I and controls, and slightly reduced in Group II. Although the TSH response to TRH was normal in all three groups the serum PRL response was reduced or absent in Group I and absent in Group II.

The following conclusions were drawn from the above study (503): (1) basal LH and FSH levels of hyperprolactinemic subjects early in the course of a pituitary microadenoma overlap those of normal women in the early follicular phase of the menstrual cycle; (2) a progressive decline of pituitary LH sensitivity and response to LHRH was noted from Group I to Group II patients despite comparable basal LH secretion; (3) while the basal FSH level was similar to that found in the controls, the functional capacity of FSH to LHRH was increased in Group I > Group II, resulting in a significant reduction of the LH/FSH ratio, which may be in keeping with the associated reduction of serum E_2 of the hyperprolactinemic patients and consistent with the fact that there may be preferential inhibition of FSH by E_2 (1023,1027) — in the presence of hyperprolactinemia FSH synthesis and storage is favored by the gonadotrope; (4) the presence of a response of endogenous E_2 to LHRH in the hyperprolactinemic subjects (Group I > Group II) suggests that the ovarian response to stimulation (endogenous or exogenous) may not be appreciably impaired. Lachelin et al. (503) suggest that an alteration of the norepinephrine (NE) to DA ratio in the hypothalamus may be responsible for the diminished pulsatile LH release and acyclic gonadotropin secretion in hyperprolactinemia. An alteration of the lactotrope–dopamine system may lead to hyperprolactinemia and possible pituitary adenoma formation. The latter may possibly arise via a relative DA deficiency at the adenoma–lactotrope DA receptor, or an anomalous arterial supply to an area of the pituitary leading to reduced DA delivery (919).

A direct suppressive effect of prolactin on ovarian steroid secretion, however, may be one of the causes of hypogonadism associated with hyperprolactinemia. Acute effects of PRL inhibit the hCG-stimulated release of P and E_2 in ovarian perfusion studies (199). Hyperprolactinemia may also exert an inhibitory effect on the induction of ovulation by gonadotropins (1008). Prolactin may act directly at the gonadal site in the presence of specific binding sites. Prolactin receptors in the gonads have been demonstrated in experimental animals (751,962) and in human ovaries (70,728). In the period of postpartum lactation and ovulation, E_2 and P secretion are inhibited even though gonadotropin levels are relatively high. It appears that refractoriness to gonadotropins is the mechanism responsible for postpartum amenorrhea (764, 1034). In vitro studies of human granulosa cells by McNatty et al. (626) show a dose-dependent inhibition of progesterone by prolactin. This may be responsible for the deficient luteal phase which may occur in hyperprolactinemic women.

McNatty (617) attempted to study the relationship between circulating PRL levels at time of ovariectomy and the endocrine micro-environment and development of antral follicles in the excised ovaries of a variety of gynecological patients. Prolactin, FSH and E_2 were measured in peripheral plasma and in antral fluid of excised follicles collected at varying stages of the menstrual cycle. Granulosa cells of each follicle greater than 4 mm also were isolated and quantitated. There was no difference in the peripheral hormone levels of FSH and E_2, the mean number of follicles per ovary as well as their mean diameter, in women with hyperprolactinemia and those with normal prolactin levels. However, women whose serum PRL exceeded 100 ng/ml during surgery had antral fluid PRL levels that were significantly higher than those of follicles recovered from women whose serum PRL was less than 100 ng/ml (28–39 ng/ml, and 14–16 ng/ml, respectively). In addition, no FSH was detectable in the follicles of women with serum PRL over 100 ng/ml. Parenthetically, the highest levels of antral fluid FSH were found in subjects with the lowest serum PRL, and this also correlated with increased concentration of antral E_2. An approximate four-fold increase of E_2 was noted in the antral follicles of women with serum prolactin under 50 ng/ml. It was further shown that when serum FSH was absent in follicles of women whose serum PRL exceeded 100 ng/ml, most follicles more than 4 mm in diameter had less than 50% of their maximal granulosa cell number per follicle size. The study of McNatty (617) indicates that elevated levels of serum PRL are associated with a reduced level of ovarian follicular activity and reduction of aromatase activity. The major criticisms of the above study are that most patients may have had a rise in serum PRL due to surgical trauma, the hyperprolactinemia was probably transient and no prior clinical endocrine information was available.

Conjugated estrogen administered (20 mg i.v.) to normal women at days 7–9 of the menstrual cycle causes an initial decrease of LH at 8 hours followed by a rebound LH peak 48 hours after injection (1010). Patients with hypothalamic amenorrhea have an LH increase only half that of normal women, while patients with the amenorrhea–galactorrhea syndrome do not have an LH surge following an estrogen provocation test (25,337). The latter group of patients usually have reduced serum E_2 and their hypothalamic receptors are usually not responsive to clomiphene (387,914). Thus hypothalamic rather than pituitary dysfunction may occur in patients with amenorrhea–galactorrhea. The impaired positive feedback of the hypothalamic–pituitary unit to estrogen may be partially responsible for anovulation and amenorrhea in patients with hyperprolactinemia. Additional evidence for hypothalamic dysfunction in women with galactorrhea–amenorrhea syndrome is suggested by loss of sleep-related rise in PRL secretion (94,572), attenuation of pulsatile release of gonadotropins and a reduction of the LH/FSH ratio (90,94,503) due to inhibition of LHRH release, and frequent failure of chlorpromazine to cause an increased PRL secretion (572).

The short-loop feedback of hyperprolactinemia increases hypothalamic DA. L-dopa is converted to DA in the CNS and pituitary gland by the enzyme dopa-decarboxylase. The frequent failure of patients with prolactin-secreting pituitary tumors to suppress on L-dopa-testing represents the presence of already maximal tuberoinfundibular DA turnover in such patients which cannot be increased further by L-dopa administration (643). The persistence of a short-loop negative feedback mechanism may cause blunted PRL responses to TRH of the remaining lactotropes following successful surgical removal of a prolactinoma (930).

Evans et al. (240) have concluded that a hypothalamic abnormality in hyperprolactinemia may result in hypogonadism via one of three causes:

1. Prolactin-enhanced hypothalamic dopaminergic tone resulting in the inhibition of LHRH release.
2. Increased β-endorphins in some patients with hyperprolactinemia may exert an effect on increasing PRL release by reducing hypothalamic dopaminergic tone. (This relationship to hypogonadism in hyperprolactinemia is not as well understood as #1.)
3. Suppression of positive feedback to E_2 in hyperprolactinemia results in acyclic gonadotropin release and anovulation (25,337).

The large body of evidence establishing the importance of dopamine (DA) in inhibiting prolactin secretion by the pituitary has been well reviewed elsewhere (73,520,674). Dopamine does not account entirely for the hypothalamic inhibition of prolactin, and the identity of the additional prolactin inhibitory factor is unknown (520). A stimulatory mechanism for prolactin release by the pituitary gland has been supported by the finding of prolactin-releasing activity in purified fractions of hypothalamic extracts. A profusion of substances have been reported to cause prolactin increases by a direct action on the pituitary gland. These include TRH (178), vasoactive intestinal peptide (VIP), serotonin, β-endorphin, LHRH, vasopressin, estradiol and others (520). Leong et al. (520) speculate that estradiol may regulate prolactin secretion to some extent, and act as a prototype of a class of hormones which have been coined "prolactin responsiveness factors." The foundation for such changes in prolactin responsiveness is a study by Raymond et al. (740) who demonstrated that prior incubation of cultured pituitary cells with estradiol caused a decrease in prolactin responsiveness to DA in addition to a marked increase in PRL responsiveness to TRH. Small amounts of TRH in combination with estradiol treatment were sufficient to cause significant PRL increases in the presence of inhibitory amounts of dopamine. By comparison, acute treatment with estradiol given alone causes a modest increase in PRL release (386, 520), and similarly TRH has no effect on PRL release in the presence of dopamine. The effect of estradiol may therefore be viewed as a "prolactin responsiveness factor" with little or no direct influence on prolactin release but which has significant effects on the pituitary by altering PRL responsiveness to hypothalamic releasing and inhibitory factors. It may act by altering PRL responsiveness to DA and, more importantly, increasing PRL responsiveness to TRH (520). This effect of estradiol may be mediated by its conversion to 2-hydroxyestradiol, a catecholestrogen in the pituitary gland.

Diffuse prolactin cell hyperplasia may be induced by estrogen administration. This process is reversible, but in time, a nonreversible state with adenomatous histologic changes may occur (282). Diffuse prolactin cell hyperplasia has rarely been convincingly demonstrated as the lesion responsible for hyperprolactinemia in humans. Preliminary evidence documenting this association was presented by McKeel and Jacobs (611) in five hyperprolactinemic patients who were initially suspected of harboring pituitary adenomas. Subsequently, 9 of a series of 33 patients who underwent transsphenoidal pituitary surgery for hyperprolactinemic syndromes at Barnes Hospital were found to have prolactin cell hyperplasia (887). McKeel et al. (610) further demonstrated that prolactin cell hyperplasia occurred in 25% of the hypophyses of 300 autopsied males and females aged 16 weeks to 101 years who died in hospitals. The lesion was clinically silent, even though 57% of affected persons had known associated causes of hyperprolactinemia. Serum prolactin measurements were not available, however, for the latter series of patients.

Prolactin cell hyperplasia does not appear to be uncommon in hyperprolactinemic states. Its occurrence in primary hypothyroidism has also been reported (887). Indeed, hyperprolactinemia may occur in primary hypothyroidism, and the associated galactorrhea is also corrected with thyroid replacement therapy (291,920). Stoffer et al. (887) suggest the following pathological criteria for the diagnosis of pituitary cell hyperplasia: (1) lack of obvious demonstration of pituitary adenoma, (2) diffuse proliferation of immunoreactive prolactin cells, (3) a diffusely abnormal reticulum pattern suggesting cellular overgrowth and fusion of adjacent acini, (4) an admixture of cytologically normal secretory cells of nonprolactin functional types, and (5) focal rather than diffuse intracytoplasmic distribution of immunoreactive prolactin sites.

In female Long-Evans rats the development of prolactin cell adenomas with advancing age is preceded by hyperplasia of prolactin cells (488). Experimental evidence of hypothalamic damage of dopaminergic neurons has been described in rats with spontaneous prolactin-secreting tumors as well as in young rats with prolactinomas induced by prolonged estrogen treatment (790).

There is in vitro evidence of a direct effect of estrogens on the pituitary gland (524) with an enhanced release of PRL and TSH. In the chronic anovulation syndrome the estrogen pool is augmented by increased synthesis from androgen conversion (557). The fact that not all of these patients have hyperprolactinemia reflects different individual sensitivity to estrogens. In the human pituitary, numerous prolactin cells have been described in the nontumorous portions of the pituitary glands which contain prolactin-secreting adenomas (489). This may suggest that in some cases, prolactin cell adenomas may be associated with and pre-

ceded by prolactin-cell hyperplasia. However, a study by Sherman et al. (837) of 35 cases of pituitary prolactinomas revealed no evidence of concomitant prolactin-cell hyperplasia. Nine to 30% of the adult population have clinically silent pituitary microadenomas at autopsy (644). Sherman et al. (837) state that at least half are potentially prolactin-secreting tumors and may be enhanced by estrogen. Conflicting epidemiologic studies exist regarding the role of oral contraceptives and the development of pituitary prolactin-secreting tumors (176,644,724,745, 906,989). It is not unlikely that the possibility exists that oral contraceptives, and estrogens in particular, may cause the expression of a previously silent pituitary microadenoma (837). It is of interest that 8 of 14 patients with pituitary tumors associated with PCOD had a history of post-pill amenorrhea (284).

Induction of ovulation with clomiphene or gonadotropin in hyperprolactinemic states is generally   unsuccessful   (90,267,665,1008, 1026), although ovulation induction with gonadotropins has been reported by Archer and Josimovich (28) in some of the latter patients with galactorrhea–amenorrhea. A significant reduction of serum PRL in four of five hyperprolactinemic patients with PCOD was noted following treatment with 100 mg spironolactone daily for three months (640).

The serum T and androstenedione levels are usually normal in hyperprolactinemic women (60,67,120,203,338,503,706,817), while the TeBG binding capacity in both men and women with prolactinomas is significantly decreased (338,949). As a result the free testosterone is increased in patients with prolactinomas (949). The mean free T in normal women is 1.05 (range 0.6–1.4), while women with prolactinomas have a free T concentration of 2.0% (range 1.2–2.8) (949). Hirsutism is occasionally present in hyperprolactinemic women (284, 290,818), and DHA and/or DHAS may be increased   (60,120,133,338,425,444,536,542, 951,952). Glickman et al. (338) also observed normal total T concentrations in hyperprolactinemic subjects with a two-fold increase of plasma free T, a one-third reduction in TeBG, a significant reduction in plasma DHT with a normal free DHT, and a moderate increase in DHAS. These androgenic abnormalities resemble those of most hirsute women except for the absence of DHT elevation (3), which may result from a PRL-induced decrease in 5α-reductase activity. A normal responsiveness of T to hCG stimulation was noted while the response of DHT was decreased (565,566). On the other hand, recent data by Vermeulen et al. (949) demonstrate no defect in the conversion of T to DHT in male patients with prolactinomas. The cause of the low TeBG in hyperprolactinemia is elusive. The modest increased androgens in elevated PRL states do not appear to be the cause. PRL receptors have also been found on liver (730), and theoretically an elevated PRL level could directly suppress TeBG. Pituitary surgery or bromocriptine may be associated with a fall in serum DHA and/or DHAS and an increase of the TeBG. Prolactin receptors have been identified on adrenocortical cells (690,730), and an effect of hyperprolactinemia on adrenal androgen production has been suggested (60,120, 317,338,444,542,559,951,952). The possible enhanced adrenal androgen biosynthesis may result in a further increased extraglandular conversion of androgens to estrogens. Parenthetically, the adrenal gland has the highest PRL-binding activity of all tissues of the body (840).

Conflicting data have appeared concerning the possible role of hyperprolactinemia on adrenocortical androgen production and DHAS in particular. It is clear that DHAS is secreted solely by the adrenal cortex since no gradient has been observed between ovarian and peripheral venous levels of DHAS in normal women (684). Ten women with amenorrhea and hyperprolactinemia were studied by Bassi et al. (60). All hyperprolactinemic patients showed an increase of plasma DHAS, and free DHA was increased in 4 of 10 subjects. Normoprolactinemic women with amenorrhea and normal control subjects showed no increase of plasma DHAS or free DHA. The increase in free DHA in some hyperprolactinemic patients may be the result of conversion from DHAS (768). As previously suggested one of the possible mechanisms of increased plasma DHAS in hyperprolactinemic subjects may be a specific prolactin action on synthesis and secretion of steroid sulfates by the adrenal cortex (60). Similarly, plasma androstenedione, T and cortisol were similar in hyperprolactinemic subjects, normoprolactinemic patients with amenorrhea, and controls. Three hyperprolactinemic patients treated successfully with bromocriptine for

26–90 days demonstrated a reduction of plasma DHAS, although not quite to normal levels (>275 μg/dl). No increase in plasma growth hormone or ACTH has been demonstrated in hyperprolactinemic patients with galactorrhea and amenorrhea (914). Elevated plasma DHAS levels were also noted in all 10 hyperprolactinemic amenorrheic subjects studied by Giusti et al. (318).

Mean plasma DHA and DHAS concentrations were found to be elevated in another study of 19 men and women with prolactinomas by Vermeulen and Ando (951). Two of three postmenopausal women with prolactinomas had elevated DHAS levels. Plasma DHA was also significantly increased in these two groups compared to normal controls, while plasma DHA was normal in seven male subjects with prolactinomas and an intact pituitary–adrenal axis. Treatment with bromocriptine for six weeks caused a significant decrease in plasma DHAS and DHA concentrations in patients with prolactinomas, although treatment with 40 mg/day of hydrocortisone for several weeks caused a decline in serum DHA and DHAS despite the elevated prolactin levels. Thus intact ACTH is necessary for the effects of PRL on the adrenal cortex. Unlike normal subjects who had a rapid increase in plasma DHA and no response of DHAS following 0.25 mg Synacthen i.v., four subjects with prolactinomas demonstrated a rapid increase in both plasma DHA and DHAS, indicating a higher androgen reserve capacity. Sulpiride treatment (100 mg/day for one month) caused plasma PRL levels to range between 132–159 ng/ml in three normal postmenopausal women with an associated rise in plasma DHAS and DHA. Plasma DHA and DHAS decreases during pregnancy despite the hyperprolactinemia because pregnancy is associated with an increased MCR of DHAS (303). An increased blood production rate of DHAS with a normal MCR was noted in two patients with prolactinomas. This excluded the possibility that the elevation of plasma DHAS was due to a reduced MCR in patients with prolactinomas (951). Postmenopausal women treated chronically with phenothiazines or butyrophenones also demonstrated elevated DHAS levels associated with the drug-induced hyperprolactinemia. No effect of increased plasma PRL was noted on serum androstenedione (60,952). This is in keeping with a possible modulating effect of prolactin on the adrenal delta^5-3β-ol-dehydrogenase activity (338,444,951), or a direct effect of PRL on adrenal sulfate synthesis (60). A direct effect of prolactin on the adrenal cortex has been shown by animal experiments demonstrating an inhibition of 5α-reductase activity (374, 992). The lack of effect of TRH or short-term (10-day) sulpiride treatment on DHAS may indicate that prolonged hyperprolactinemia is necessary before PRL exerts an adrenocortical effect. In summary, prolonged chronic stimulation of PRL is necessary for the adrenal cortex stimulating effect to be manifest, and this requires the presence of an intact pituitary–adrenal axis (951).

Twenty-one women with hyperprolactinemia with a mean plasma PRL of 191 ng/ml (range, 36–991 ng/ml) were studied (338) and compared to normal female controls in the follicular phase of the menstrual cycle. Plasma DHAS values in the 26 controls were 153 μg/dl, while in the hyperprolactinemic group the mean DHAS level was moderately higher at 272 μg/dl ($P < 0.125$). However, only 4 of 21 (19%) hyperprolactinemic subjects had elevated levels of plasma DHAS. Six of 15 hyperprolactinemic patients with elevated plasma free testosterone levels did not demonstrate a correlation with elevated plasma DHAS levels. Both the hirsute and nonhirsute hyperprolactinemic subjects had higher DHAS levels than control subjects (338). ACTH testing following overnight DXM suppression revealed no differences in the response of DHA, DHAS, cortisol or 17α-hydroxypregnenolone. These data are similar to the findings of Carter et al. (120). It is difficult to assess rapid changes in plasma DHAS by ACTH stimulation studies of the adrenal cortex in that DHAS has a long half-life with a low MCR and large pool (542). Hyperresponsiveness of DHAS to ACTH in hyperprolactinemia has, however, been noted by others (444,951). ACTH administration for four consecutive days by Kandeel et al. (444) caused a greater increase in serum DHAS in hyperprolactinemic subjects than in normal controls (338), while DXM suppressibility of both DHAS and free T was normal in hyperprolactinemic women (338,951). This again suggests that the effect of PRL on adrenal adrogens is ACTH-dependent.

A combination of 21 women with idiopathic hyperprolactinemia and pituitary adenomas presenting as amenorrhea–galactorrhea were studied by Lobo et al. (542). The mean plasma PRL in this group was 257 ng/ml while the mean DHAS was 254 μg/dl. The mean DHAS value was significantly higher than that of 11 normoprolactinemic amenorrheic women and 41 normal controls. Administration of bromocriptine to the hyperprolactinemic subjects for three weeks resulted in a 32% decline in basal plasma DHAS levels. A reduction of adrenal androgens following bromocriptine has been noted by several groups (60,120,133,317,444, 951).

Other studies have also demonstrated elevated androgens associated with hyperprolactinemia. Carter et al. (120) noted a correlation between the serum PRL and DHAS levels in 35 hyperprolactinemic women, most of whom presented with amenorrhea and galactorrhea following cessation of oral contraceptives. Similar findings have been reported by Jones et al. (425). Seven of 14 hyperprolactinemic women studied by Kandeel et al. (444) also had elevated serum DHAS. In a study by Lobo and Kletzky (536) of 28 women with amenorrhea, galactorrhea and hyperprolactinemia (mean serum PRL, 204 ng/ml), without hirsutism and with no evidence of pituitary macroadenomas or PCOD, significant mean elevation of serum DHAS as well as androstenedione was noted when compared to controls. This was associated with an increase of the free T and free delta^5-androstenediol. The total T was slightly lower than the control subjects. A positive correlation was found between serum PRL levels and the percentage of unbound T as well as increased ratios of total T and DHT to unbound T and DHT in the hyperprolactinemic subjects ($P < 0.05$) (536). The latter evidence, suggestive of a reduced 5α-reductase activity in hyperprolactinemia, may explain the rarity of severe hirsutism in such subjects since DHT may be necessary for the expression of androgen action. The reported association of hirsutism and hyperprolactinemia (819) appears to be relatively uncommon (536). After two months of treatment with bromocriptine and the return of serum PRL to normal levels, the elevated DHAS and androstenedione returned to normal levels. Normalization of TeBG may only occur after three months of bromocriptine therapy (949). DHAS and androstenedione are weak androgens and would not be expected to decrease TeBG-binding capacity. It is possible that in hyperprolactinemia a direct effect of prolactin on the liver may result in a decreased TeBG-binding capacity (536). ACTH-testing did not elicit any obvious defects of 3β-ol, 17β-hydroxysteroid dehydrogenase, or 17-20-desmolase enzymatic activities (536).

Unlike the previously mentioned finding of reduced 5α-reductase activity in hyperprolactinemia (536), Giusti et al. (317) found elevated levels of serum DHT in hyperprolactinemic subjects in the presence of normal levels of T and androstenedione. The rise in circulating DHT may perhaps occur as a result of increased peripheral conversion of delta[5] androgens in hyperprolactinemia (758), or as a result of serum prolactin on 5α-reductase activity.

Contradictory data on the effects of hyperprolactinemia on the adrenal cortex have been reported by other groups. Studies have shown an overlap in serum DHA values in hyperprolactinemic and control subjects (60,149,503). Sera of 13 patients (5 men and 8 women) with pituitary tumors and marked hyperprolactinemia (mean, 198 ng/ml) were compared to normal controls (706), and no difference was noted between the two groups in values for cortisol, androstenedione, DHA and DHAS. This was interpreted as a negative evidence for a correlation between hyperprolactinemia and adrenal adrogen secretion (149,706).

The lack of correlation between plasma prolactin and DHAS was also noted by Metcalf et al. (638). Only one of 12 subjects with hyperprolactinemia had an elevated DHAS level, and reduction of serum prolactin was not accompanied by significant decrease of plasma DHAS concentration. The authors conclude that it is difficult to establish with certainty that PRL influences adrenal androgen secretion in man.

Buvat et al. (110) studied 23 women with PCOD. Although serum DHA, DHAS and androstenedione levels were higher in the 10 patients with modest hyperprolactinemia, the statistical difference was not significant when compared to the nonhyperprolactinemic group. As a group the DHAS was elevated in patients with PCOD, suggesting an adrenal source of hyperandrogenism associated with the ovarian hyperandrogenism in PCOD. The data of Buvat et al. (110), however, does not support the role of hyperprolactinemia in the elevated adrenal androgen secretion in PCOD. In vitro studies of steroid secretion of normal women and those

with polycystic ovaries have failed to demonstrate ovarian DHAS secretion (986).

In a study by Belisle and Menard (67) normal levels of DHA and DHAS were found in 10 subjects suspected of having prolactinomas with hyperprolactinemia, galactorrhea and amenorrhea. The range of plasma prolactin was 56–108 ng/ml. The MCR of DHA and DHAS was unchanged from normal controls, as was the production rate (67). Normal androstenedione and T levels were found in all hyperprolactinemic subjects similar to the data of others (120). Tolis (919) was unable to detect elevated serum DHAS, DHA or T in prolactinoma patients or a reduction of DHA or DHAS with bromocriptine. It appears that perhaps the degree of hyperprolactinemia as well as duration may be of importance in determining the effect of hyperprolactinemia on the adrenal cortex. Six of seven non-PCOD hyperprolactinemic women with galactorrhea and amenorrhea with mean serum PRL levels of 178 ng/ml also had no increase in serum DHAS (239). Drucker and David (215) observed marked heterogeneity of serum DHAS in normal subjects, and noted no significant association between hyperprolactinemia and elevated DHAS values. The presence of possible DHAS subgroups in control subjects makes it difficult to assess any correlation between hyperprolactinemic and control subjects.

One must conclude from the above studies that the role of prolactin on the adrenal cortex is far from clear. The reasons for elevated adrenal androgens in some hyperprolactinemic subjects and not in others may be related to different pathophysiological circumstances which lead to the hyperprolactinemia. It may well be that the elevation in adrenal androgens may be coincidental. Further investigation in this area should lead to a resolution of this question.

Hyperprolactinemia in PCOD

Hyperprolactinemia in PCOD is not uncommon (15, 79, 110, 164, 165, 197, 218, 228, 246, 248, 284, 286, 290, 332, 352, 417, 443, 553, 640, 715, 818, 911, 912, 913, 935, 976, 997) with an approximate reported frequency of 20–40% (164, 197, 218, 228, 246, 286, 341, 443, 715, 976, 997, 998). Combined data from series of patients with PCOD comprising 394 cases re-

TABLE 8-2. Combined Data of 394 Cases of Polycystic Ovaries with Hyperprolactinemia.

INVESTIGATOR	REF.	NO. OF PATIENTS	NO. OF PATIENTS WITH HYPERPROLACTINEMIA
Duignan	218	21	4
Kandeel et al	443	17	5
Jaffee et al	417	12	5
Givens	322	30	6
Alger et al	15	9	3
Del Pozo & Falaschi	197	47	12
White & Ginsburg	976	96	26
Wortsman et al	997	21	6
Buvat et al.	110	23	10
Corenblum & Taylor	164	25	13
Futterweit & Mechanick	286	93	16
		Total = 394	106 (26 9%)

vealed an incidence of 26.9% with associated hyperprolactinemia (Table 8-2).

Hyperprolactinemia in PCOD may occur as a result of stimulatory effects of estrogens on pituitary lactotropes. Hyperresponsiveness to TRH is frequently noted in patients with PCOD since PCOD is characterized by estrogen excess (164,165,197,715) and TRH hyperresponsiveness is more pronounced in hyperprolactinemic subjects with PCOD. This compares to the blunted response to TRH and the dopaminergic antagonist haloperidol found in patients with hyperprolactinemic amenorrhea–galactorrhea. PCOD patients hyperrespond to TRH regardless of baseline serum PRL level, more than control subjects. Hyperresponsiveness to haloperidol also occurs in hyperprolactinemic subjects with PCOD and may be due to a priming effect of estrogens (197).

Falaschi et al. (247) evaluated the pituitary PRL response to nomifensine (a dopamine reuptake-inhibitor) and domperidone (a peripheral DA-receptor blocker). Patients with PCOD had a significant reduction of serum PRL with nomifensine, while their response to domperidone was excessive as compared to normal control subjects. Patients with prolactinomas failed to respond to domperidone. The studies of Falaschi lend support to the notion that PCOD may demonstrate hyperprolactinemia as a consequence of estrogen priming (197). Of interest is that E_1 is incapable of stimulating PRL secretion in normal cycling women, whereas E_2 has an immediate effect (445). Recent data indicate that identical serum PRL responses to nomifensine and carbidopa plus L-dopa (both are central

dopaminergic stimulatory agents) occur in patients with prolactinomas and in hyperprolactinemic subjects without radiological evidence of pituitary tumors (178). This suggests the existence of a common defect in dopaminergic inhibition of PRL secretion in hyperprolactinemic states of tumorous and unknown etiologies. It may well be that most patients with hyperprolactinemia may harbor a small microadenoma or may have pituitary lactotrope hyperplasia (178).

Dopamine infusion significantly suppresses LH in patients with PCOD, and this occurs in both normoprolactinemic and hyperprolactinemic subjects with PCOD (715). The decrease in LH following DA infusion in patients with PCOD correlates with basal LH levels. Abnormal prolactin and LH secretion in PCOD may reflect altered dopaminergic control and allows a rationale for the use of the dopamine agonist bromocriptine in the treatment of patients with PCOD (164,197,248,914). No correlations have been found between basal serum PRL levels, T and androstenedione production or MCR (715). Recent data indicate synchronized pulsatile release of PRL and LH in normal cycling and hypogonadal women, suggesting that the ovarian steroidogenic environment may modulate pulse frequency and amplitude of both LH and PRL (134).

The clinical frequency of hyperprolactinemia in PCOD perhaps may be related to the hyperestrogenemia which in turn, may be associated with lactotrope hyperplasia and possible adenoma formation (282,284,290,386,412,413, 488,524,610,837,906,956). It is becoming more apparent that estrogens may also play a role in stimulating growth of pre-existing pituitary tumors (837). Diffuse lactotrope hyperplasia has been noted in one patient with hyperprolactinemic PCOD who underwent pituitary biopsy (164).

The association of hyperprolactinemia with PCOD may be due to the following mechanisms: 1) abnormal central neurotransmission, particularly in the dopaminergic control of PRL release (15,183,733,759); 2) increased lactotrope activity produced by an abnormal steroidal milieu resulting in unopposed action of estrogens (197,246); 3) a distinct clinical entity of hyperprolactinemic PCOD. In a study by Corenblum and Taylor (164,165), 13 of 25 patients with PCOD had elevation of serum prolactin in at least two of three measurements. Clinically, hyperprolactinemic patients with PCOD are similar to those without hyperprolactinemia (163). Twelve of the 13 patients with hyperprolactinemia had elevated serum LH/FSH ratios. The remaining 12 normoprolactinemic patients with PCOD had an abnormal LH/FSH ratio in 6 and a normal ratio in the other 6. Hyperresponsiveness to TRH testing was noted in the hyperprolactinemic group as well as the PCOD patients with normal serum PRL and an elevated serum LH/FSH ratio. A normal response to TRH similar to that seen in normal ovulatory subjects studied during the early follicular phase of the cycle was noted in those PCOD subjects with a normal LH/FSH level. Thirty-two women with CT visualization of a pituitary tumor and hyperprolactinemia did not demonstrate an increased serum prolactin response to TRH testing (164, 165).

It has been suggested that hyperprolactinemia may have an initiating or maintaining role in the chronic ovulation in PCOD (161,759), possibly by a direct effect on steroidogenesis and/or an enhanced adrenal androgen production which further increases extraglandular estrogen production. Treatment of patients with PCOD with bromocriptine may cause a return of ovulatory menstrual function (197,914). Bromocriptine may act not merely in suppressing PRL, but also may have a central dopaminergic action which may suppress LH and T (248), suggesting that PCOD may involve a relative decrease in central dopaminergic activity (183). This may result in a reduction of LHRH and thus LH. Further evidence that hyperprolactinemic patients with an elevated LH/FSH

ratio may have decreased central dopaminergic activity has been the report of Quigley et al. (733), demonstrating enhanced LH suppression following dopaminergic stimulation. It is possible, however, that the augmented extraglandular estrogen production enhances pituitary lactotropes and gonadotropes resulting in an overproduction of PRL and LH. Chronic estrogen administration has been shown to decrease hypothalamic dopamine (853). Furthermore, estrogen may inhibit the ultra-short feedback effect of PRL on inhibiting its own secretion (791). Consequently, prolactin cell hyperplasia may result from decreased central dopaminergic inhibition (183,733) and/or direct estrogen stimulation (488). Enhanced responsiveness to TRH may suggest underlying pituitary lactotrope hyperplasia. Animal and human models suggest that pituitary hyperplasia may indeed be the precursor of adenoma formation (166,488)

Cyclic LH discharge to estrogen is impaired in hyperprolactinemic patients. Bromocriptine itself or the suppression of hyperprolactinemia may restore cyclic LH discharge to intravenous estrogen, restoring positive feedback. With bromocriptine treatment serum LH and E_2 also increase while no rise in FSH is noted (23). Experimental evidence indicates that PRL may augment ovarian changes resulting in multiple cyst formation, which is prevented by bromocriptine therapy (161).

It is likely that the hyperprolactinemia in PCOD may result from 1) an abnormal hormonal milieu which consists of primarily an enhanced estrogen effect which stimulates the pituitary lactotrope (i.e., a secondary effect of PCOD), and/or 2) hypothalamic dysfunction resulting in decreased dopaminergic secretion or action which occurs in association with a fundamental series of pathophysiological events leading to PCOD.

Hyperprolactinemia and Pituitary Tumors in PCOD

The association of hyperprolactinemia with or without galactorrhea has been described in anovulatory states and secondary amenorrhea (90, 274,471,819,912). Galactorrhea and/or hyperprolactinemia have been described in some patients with polycystic ovarian disease without a demonstrable pituitary tumor (79,165,218,

246,417,443,509,819,912,976). Galactorrhea is a relatively infrequently reported symptom in patients with polycystic ovarian disease (228, 284,290,349,443,509,912,913,914,998). Its probable frequency in PCOD may range from 10–15%. Although hyperprolactinemia has been described in approximately 27% of patients with polycystic ovaries (Table 8-2), there is no single study defining the incidence of hyperprolactinemia in a large group of such patients.

The occasional clinical finding of hirsutism in association with hyperprolactinemia, galactorrhea and amenorrhea (819,914) as well as elevated levels of DHAS in some patients with PCOD suggests possible stimulation of adrenocortical androgen production (120,318,432, 573,640). Administration of bromocriptine frequently results in a decrease in serum DHAS, and normalization of serum prolactin levels, while serum testosterone and androstenedione levels are unchanged (120,817). Elevated levels of serum DHAS have also been found in patients with polycystic ovaries in whom prolactin determinations were not performed (203).

While most patients with polycystic ovarian disease have elevated serum LH levels (24,39, 74,203,473,539,742,1029), the majority of hyperprolactinemic subjects have normal or reduced levels of LH (244,914,976). This again stresses the wide clinical spectrum of PCOD. Patients with polycystic ovarian disease may include those with or without hyperprolactinemia or galactorrhea as well as many other varying manifestations. Those with galactorrhea and hyperprolactinemia may also manifest different endocrine abnormalities (i.e., decreased serum LH and estradiol levels) as a result of LHRH suppression, thus varying from the classic description of an elevated LH/FSH ratio in PCOD. As with other series of patients with "idiopathic" or "functional" galactorrhea associated with oligomenorrhea or amenorrhea, some PCOD patients when followed for a period of time may eventually demonstrate clinical evidence of pituitary adenoma (284,290). When a careful investigation is made, evidence of such adenomas in this subgroup may occasionally be manifest at the initial presentation (284,290). Similarly, patients with elevated DHAS levels may later be found to have polycystic ovaries on ultrasonography or by surgical confirmation.

Prospective and retrospective studies suggest that between 13% to 39% of the patients with secondary amenorrhea have hyperprolactinemia (90,274,833). Similarly, the association of amenorrhea, hyperprolactinemia and/or galactorrhea in patients with polycystic ovarian disease is not uncommon. Consequently, the presence of significant hyperprolactinemia in PCOD or a progressive rise in serum PRL in these patients should make one suspect the possible presence of a pituitary prolactin-secreting tumor or significant lactotrope hyperplasia. This may represent only a small group of anovulatory women with PCOD, but an important one with specific diagnostic and therapeutic implications (284,290).

Since the original description of the association of pituitary tumors with hyperprolactinemia in three patients with polycystic ovarian disease (290), 18 other instances of pituitary tumors in PCOD have been noted in the literature (7,49,77,310,381,487,497,504,797,822). Although no extensive survey of the incidence of this association of a large series of patients with PCOD has been reported, the finding of three additional patients over a three-year period prompted another report (284). The six combined cases in the two reports (284,290) had the following characteristics: 1) amenorrhea, 2) hyperprolactinemia with or without galactorrhea, 3) varying degrees of hirsutism without significant clitoromegaly, 4) failure to experience withdrawal bleeding after administration of progesterone, 5) failure of clomiphene citrate to induce ovulation or bleeding, 6) histopathologic and/or clinical evidence of PCOD preceding roentgenographic findings suggestive of an intrasellar tumor (284,290).

Reports have described pituitary tumors and PCOD in patients with Cushing's syndrome (77,487) and acromegaly (7). Lamotte el al. (504) reported a 28-year-old female with amenorrhea and galactorrhea of eight years duration who had orange-sized ovaries. Pituitary surgery was performed for visual symptoms and a macroadenoma was removed. Serum prolactin bioassay revealed markedly elevated levels of prolactin.

Kurisaka et al. (497) recently described two young women who developed elevated serum prolactin levels of 51 and 90 ng/ml with galactorrhea 1–4 years following wedge resection of polycystic ovaries. One patient had an associated benign dermoid cyst which was removed

TABLE 8-3. Clinical Summary of 14 Patients with Polycystic Ovarian Disease and Pituitary Tumors.

PATIENT NO.	REF.	AGE (YR)	PRESENTING COMPLAINTS	AGE AT MENARCHE (YR)	DURATION AMENORRHEA (YR)	DURATION GALACTORRHEA (YR)	PRE-OP PROLACTIN (NG/ML)	POST-OP PROLACTIN (NG/ML)	OVARIES & PARITY	HIRSUTISM	VISUAL LOSS	PITUITARY
1	284	23	Am	13	1	—	67–72	—	Clinical PCOD	+	—	CT-micro
2	284	25	Oligo-Gal(pp)	11	4	.25	39.2	—	WR(age 21)	+	—	CT-micro
3	284	31	Am-Gal	13	7	1	5–29	—	WR(age 16)	+	—	CT-micro, ES
4	290	36	Am-Gal	13	12	12	180	32	WR(age 26)	+	—	OR,8mm
5	290	30	Am-Gal(pp)	11	7	1	540	102	WR(age 25)	+	—	OR,8mm
6	290	28	Am	16	7	—	480	—	WR(age 20)	+	—	Polyt-micro
7	381	30	Am		2			9.0	PI-WR(age 28)		+	OR,supr
8	381	33	Am		13			194	WR(age 26)		+	OR,supr.
9	797	30	Am-Gal(pp)	13	12	12	51		WR			OR-no data
10	797	33	Am-Gal(pp)	13	5	8	61	9.0	PI-WR			OR-no data
11	797	27	Am-Gal(pp)	12	3	3	84		WR			OR-no data
12	797	28	Am-Gal(pp)	15	8	3	343		GI-WR			OR-no data
13	822	25	Am(pp)	12	1	—	7.0–25 6	"nl"	G5-spont ab	+		OR,micro
14	822	26	Am-Gal(pp)	13	3	9	30–42	9 6	Laparoscopy(age 23)	+		OR,micro

Abbreviations

Am — amenorrhea, Gal — galactorrhea, Oligo — oligomenorrhea, pp — postpill, GI — gravida I etc, PI — para I, supr — suprasellar extension, polyt — polytomography of sella, ES — empty sella, micro — microadenoma, OR — transsphenoidal surgery, WR — wedge resection

Reprinted with permission from the American College of Obstetricians and Gynecologists, from Futterweit W Pituitary tumors and polycystic ovarian disease Obstet Gynecol 1983, 62 S74–S79 (284)

at the time of surgery. Both were parous and presented because of the galactorrhea. Transsphenoidal microsurgery was performed on one patient because of a blunted PRL response to TRH and chlorpromazine stimulation testing, and an associated CT scan abnormality was noted in the sella turcica of the other patient. Pathology revealed multiple mucin-filled cysts interspersed in the pituitary adenoma tissue in both patients, with the adenomas measuring less than 1.0 cm. Immunoperoxidase preparation revealed the adenoma to be of the prolactin-secreting type. The cyst lining cells did not stain with the immunoperoxidase preparation and was consistent with Rathke's cleft epithelium. The latter is probably due to a failure in embryonal differentiation of the adenohypophysial anlage. The rare type of pituitary tumor which is composed of mixed tissue elements of Rathke's cleft cysts with prolactin-secreting adenoma has previously been termed "cystic prolactinoma" (714). The authors suggest that continuous estrogenic stimulation of receptors in the pituitary–prolactin secreting cells may be related to the development of prolactinomas in patients with polycystic ovarian disease. Indeed, Case 1 of the two patients described by Kurisaka et al. (497) was also unique in that she had an associated ovarian as well as a pituitary tumor with her polycystic ovary syndrome.

Geller et al. (310) described a patient with polycystic ovaries that had a 6 mm pituitary microadenoma at surgery. The serum prolactin level was not described in the report, but injection of 100 μg of LHRH revealed adequate responsiveness of the tumor. In an abstract by Baranowska et al. (49), three patients with proven PCOD and hyperprolactinemia had CT evidence of pituitary microadenomas. No specific data of prolactin levels were described in their report. Glickman et al. (338) commented on two women with focal erosion and enlargement of the sella turcica who had histologically confirmed polycystic ovaries 7–8 years prior to discovery of hyperprolactinemia (139 and 167 ng/ml, respectively). No documentation of the presence of a pituitary tumor in these two patients was reported and they were not included in the above series (284).

Table 8-3 (284) is a published summary of 14 patients with proven PCOD and pituitary tumors (290,381,797,822). The age at time of diagnosis of the pituitary tumor ranged from 23–36 years (mean = 29 years). Prior wedge resection of the ovaries was performed in 11 of the 14 patients studied; 4 were gravid and 2 had one child each. Eight patients presented with postpill amenorrhea, and galactorrhea was noted in 9 of the 14 subjects. The duration of amenorrhea and galactorrhea varied from 1– 13 years (mean = 6 years) and 0.25–12 years (mean = 5.5 years), respectively. In instances where the presence or absence of hirsutism was described, all eight patients had varying degrees of hirsutism without clitoromegaly. Ten of the 14 patients underwent transsphenoidal surgery. In two instances there were visual symptoms associates with suprasellar extension. Microadenomas were noted in eight other patients with histopathological evidence of chromophobe adenoma. Clinical CT confirmation of pituitary microadenomas was noted in four other instances, with one case demonstrating a pituitary tumor with an associated empty sella on metrizamide cisternography. Hyperprolactinemia was present in 11 of the 14 cases. The range of serum prolactin levels was 30– 540 ng/ml in patients who had operative evidence of pituitary tumors. In two instances the serum prolactin did not exceed 30 ng/ml. Following surgery, two of six patients had persistent hyperprolactinemia of 102 and 194 ng/ml, respectively.

Certain features about several of the patients described in Table 8-3 bear further mention. Case 1 developed hyperprolactinemia 15 months after an initial evaluation which was clinically consistent with PCOD (increased LH/ FSH ratio and elevated serum androstenedione). The serum DHAS level was slightly elevated with normal serum testosterone and prolactin levels. Subsequent amenorrhea responded briefly to prednisone therapy but later the amenorrhea persisted in association with hyperprolactinemia and CT evidence of a pituitary microadenoma. A normal rise of serum prolactin following TRH administration in Case 2 demonstrated the occasional unreliability of TRH testing in patients with prolactin-secreting microadenomas. Case 3 had surgically proven PCOD associated with a symptomatic premature menopause and the subsequent development of a pituitary microadenoma with an associated empty sella. Lack of suppression of the elevated serum LH level was noted following 5.0 mg conjugated estrogens daily for three weeks. There was insufficent data to prove the presence of an LH-secreting microadenoma in the latter patient. Although the majority of pituitary tumors associated with PCOD are prolactin-secreting tumors, Geller et al. (310) have suggested that some may harbor LH-secreting tumors. It is clear that the demonstration of hyperprolactinemia in patients with PCOD warrants careful exclusion of an associated pituitary adenoma. This should be done with careful thin section CT studies of the sella turcica. Further studies to define the incidence of pituitary tumors in PCOD appear indicated. It is possible that pituitary hyperplasia may precede CT demonstration of a pituitary adenoma in some patients with hyperprolactinemic PCOD. This may result in roentgenographic enlargement of the sella turcica, diffuse contrast enhancement on CT scanning without actual demonstration of a pituitary tumor.

Serious questions have arisen regarding interpretation of polytomography of the sella turcica in establishing a diagnosis of pituitary microadenomas (107,666,933). This must be stressed before meaningful analyses of polytomographic data in the literature is attempted. A study of 254 cases of PCOD by Tzingounis et al. (935) revealed abnormal radiographic findings in 22 subjects (8.7%). Of significance was that 3 of the 22 subjects with abnormal sella polytomograms had an enlarged sella turcica associated with elevation of serum prolactin ranging between 45–65 ng/ml. Galactorrhea was present in one patient with a serum prolactin level of 65 ng/ml. Roentgenographic abnormalities of the sella turcica were also noted in 3 of 8 patients with hyperprolactinemia in another series (998). In a case-control study, patients with chronic anovulation syndrome appear to have an increased risk of developing or harboring a pituitary tumor (175).

PCOD is not an infrequent disease and an incidence of 1.4% to 3.5% has been described (859,944). Some of the above evidence suggests that the association of PCOD and pituitary tumors is more than coincidental and that the pathophysiology in these instances may reside in an abnormality of hypothalamic-pituitary function. In 1956, Sommers and Wadman (859) performed necropsy studies of the pituitaries of seven females with PCOD and demonstrated unusual numbers of normal heavily granulated basophiles collected into hyperplastic nodules. Pituitary basophil hyperplasia was noted by comparing these patients to controls. The presence of hyperprolactinemia with or without galactorrhea in approximately 27% of patients with PCOD (15,110,164,197,218,228,246, 286,322,341,417,443,715,976,997,998) may be causally related to hyperestrogenemia, which in turn may be associated with lactotrope hyperplasia leading to possible adenoma formation (282,412,413,524,610,837,906,956). As previously mentioned, estrogens may play a role in the pathogenesis of some prolactin-secreting adenomas by stimulating growth of pre-existing pituitary lesions (837). Furthermore, it has been noted that diffuse lactotrope hyperplasia was found in a patient with hyperprolactinemic PCOD who underwent pituitary biopsy (165), as well as nine other patients who underwent transsphenoidal surgery for suspected prolactin-secreting pituitary tumors (887). The clinical frequency of hyperprolactinemia in PCOD may reflect an abnormality in dopaminergic tone. Quigley et al. (733) demonstrated that the elevated LH secretion in PCOD was promptly suppressed by dopamine infusion. Statistical enhanced LH sensitivity to dopamine was noted when the resulting LH decrement was compared with that of normal women during the early follicular phase of the menstrual cycle. Indeed the elevated LH secretion and high sensitivity to dopamine inhibition in patients with PCOD may reflect reduced endogenous dopamine inhibition of LHRH secretion resulting from the tonic feedback of chronically elevated estrogen levels (733). The adequacy of estrogen levels in PCOD is due to increased extraglandular conversion of androgens. As a result of an adequate estrogen pool, a normal response usually occurs to clomiphene citrate (742) with unimpaired negative and positive feedback responses to estrogen testing (39,510,742).

Normo- and hyperprolactinemic patients with PCOD (246,417,998) have demonstrated abnormalities following hypothalamic–pituitary testing. Jaffee et al. (417) demonstrated a chlorpromazine-induced paradoxical rise in growth hormone in six of seven normoprolactinemic and hyperprolactinemic subjects with PCOD as well as abnormalities in L-dopa responsiveness. Hyperresponsiveness of serum PRL to TRH (164,165,197,246) and an exaggerated response to dopamine blockade with haloperidol (197) may be due to enhanced sensitivity of pituitary lactotropes to estrogen priming (246).

In conclusion, the presence of hyperprolactinemia in approximately 27% of patients with PCOD may reflect hypothalamic–pituitary dysfunction leading to lactotrope hyperplasia and possible adenoma formation. Appropriate CT scanning of the sella should be performed to exclude the presence of a pituitary tumor. An enlarged sella may also represent pituitary hyperplasia and/or a primary empty sella syndrome which may be diagnosed with the newer CT scanning techniques.

9

Laboratory Diagnosis and Differential Diagnosis of Polycystic Ovarian Disease

Laboratory Diagnosis of PCOD

The introduction of radioimmunoassays in clinical medicine has opened new approaches in the understanding of disease processes and in diagnosis. Similarly, rapid advances in computerized tomography and ultrasonography have aided the physician in the diagnosis of patients who present with hirsutism, anovulatory states, amenorrhea, dysfunctional uterine bleeding, galactorrhea and a variety of other clinical signs which may suggest polycystic ovarian or other endocrine disease states. It is the purpose of this chapter to outline a laboratory approach and differential diagnosis of PCOD, which will be helpful in evaluating the endocrine factors responsible for the patient's complaints.

The absence of enlarged ovaries on clinical examination is of little importance in the diagnosis of PCOD. Since anovulation (monophasic basal body temperature and nonsecretory endometrium) with hirsutism is frequently the presentation of PCOD, the following laboratory parameters may be useful in the initial evaluation of the patient (Table 9-1). Adequacy of estrogenization should be demonstrated by a history of regular menses or withdrawal bleeding following five days of 10 mg medroxyprogesterone acetate orally. Injection of progesterone in oil is not recommended in that laboratory parameters such as plasma LH, FSH and possibly androgens may be altered for several weeks. Failure to achieve withdrawal bleeding after a progesterone challenge is infrequent in PCOD and a diagnostic approach in these patients will be discussed later in this section.

A pooled specimen of three blood specimens taken at 45–60-minute intervals is of importance in avoiding the initial "stress factor" which may raise plasma androstenedione or PRL. In addition, spontaneous fluctuations of androgens may be minimized and an average obtained (385). Multiple sampling for T and other androgens is necessary to avoid inaccurate results and interpretation. Large fluctuations of plasma T and androstenedione have been described (186,409), and the pooling of three blood specimens has been recommended by Goldzieher et al (344). The diurnal variation of the adrenal contribution to androstenedione may also be reduced by drawing the plasma samples after 10 A.M. The pulsatility of LH in PCOD is taken into account to some extent by multiple sampling, and a truer "average" reading obtained for plasma LH.

Although not present in all patients with polycystic ovaries, approximately 60–70% of patients demonstrate an increased LH/FSH ratio if tested frequently enough. The inappropriate gonadotropin secretion (IGS) is an important diagnostic consideration which indicates the probability of increased LH stimulation leading to ovarian hyperandrogenism and functional ovarian changes. An elevated LH/FSH may also be present in hyperthecosis, and inappropriate gonadotropin secretion may sometimes occur in adrenal sources of hyperandrogenism which may be associated with polycystic ovaries (Tables 9-2 and 9-3). The concomitant demonstration of increased plasma androgens and IGS makes it likely that the patient has PCOD, although an initial adrenal defect cannot be ex-

TABLE 9-1. Initial Laboratory Evaluation of Patients Suspected of Having PCOD.

1. Plasma LH/FSH
2. Testosterone
3. DHAS
4. PRL
5. Androstenedione
6. 17-OHP

cluded. In the absence of an elevated plasma T value a repeat determination is indicated with the addition of a free T determination (see Table 9-4.).

Hyperprolactinemia usually less than 50 ng/ml is present in 20–30% of patients with PCOD and may also occur in those with a significant adrenal contribution to the hyperandrogenism found in PCOD. Hyperprolactinemia in excess of 100–150 ng/ml necessitates exclusion of a prolactin-secreting pituitary tumor. Withdrawal bleeding following medroxyprogesterone acetate is less likely to occur in amenorrheic subjects with markedly elevated serum prolactin levels. Although most subjects with PCOD have either an increase in plasma T or androstenedione, some relatively nonhirsute patients may only present with an increased LH/FSH ratio greater than 2.5 and with borderline plasma DHAS and acne without obvious menstrual dysfunction as has been suggested by Marynick et al. (590).

Elevation of plasma 17OHP and 21-deoxycortisol is characteristic of the 21-hydroxylase deficiency noted in patients with congenital adrenocortical hyperplasia (490). This syndrome

TABLE 9-2. Diagnostic Possibilities which May Be Encountered by the Initial Laboratory Screening Tests for PCOD.

(a) ↑LH/FSH

PCOD
Ovarian hyperthecosis (335,971)
PCOD with significant adrenal component
    a. congenital adrenal hyperplasia (CAH)
    b. late-onset ("acquired") adrenal hyperplasia
Mid-cycle gonadotropin surge in women with PCOD.
Mid-cycle surge in normal women.

(b) ↑LH/FSH + ↑Testosterone and/or DHAS

    PCOD
    Ovarian hyperthecosis
    PCOD with significant adrenal component

TABLE 9-3. Diagnostic Possibilities which May Be Encountered in the Absence of Increased LH/FSH.

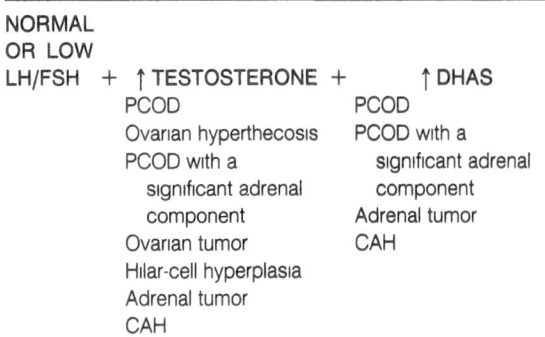

NORMAL OR LOW LH/FSH + ↑TESTOSTERONE +	↑DHAS
PCOD	PCOD
Ovarian hyperthecosis	PCOD with a significant adrenal component
PCOD with a significant adrenal component	Adrenal tumor
Ovarian tumor	CAH
Hilar-cell hyperplasia	
Adrenal tumor	
CAH	

is frequently associated with the development of polycystic ovarian changes. A 3–10-fold increase in plasma androstenedione was present in non-salt losers with CAH aged 15–41 years described by Rivarola et al. (754), while a variable increase of DHAS was present. Ten of the 51 patients (19.6%) with PCOD had androstenedione values which were in the normal range (<130 ng/dl) with the mean value for androstenedione for the entire PCOD group approximately 300 ng/dl (736). Although plasma androstenedione is frequently increased in PCOD, its contribution is both ovarian and adrenal. In most instances of PCOD, however, the increased androstenedione level in the blood reflects increased ovarian secretion of this androgen. Peripheral plasma T and androstenedione levels are both elevated in 58% of women with PCOD (324). Fifteen percent are reported to have normal plasma T in the presence of elevated plasma androstenedione, while 17% have normal androstenedione with an associated elevation of plasma T. Both androgens may be normal in 9% of patients with PCOD, but in these instances, plasma TeBG binding capacity is usually reduced, indicative of increased free T.

TABLE 9-4. Ancillary Studies of Patients Suspected of Having PCOD.

1. Plasma TeBG, free testosterone, % free T
2. E_2
3. E_1
4. DHT
5. Insulin (insulin resistance)
6. Cortrosyn® Test (if hyperandrogenemic)
7. LHRH test
8. TRH test (if hyperprolactinemic)

A combination of normal or reduced gonadotropins and elevated plasma androgens such as T as well as DHAS suggests an adrenal etiology of menstrual dysfunction and hirsutism (see Table 9-3). Plasma DHAS correlates well with urinary 17-ketosteroids (17-KS) and is not subject to episodic or diurnal variation. Unlike the urinary 17-KS, DHAS demonstrates no correlation with body weight or Ponderal Index (544). Elevation of plasma DHAS makes a pure ovarian source of hyperandrogenism unlikely (581). The presence of markedly elevated levels of plasma T greater than 200 ng/dl suggests a tumor of the ovary or adrenal (634,974). An adrenal tumor is likely if there is an associated marked increased in plasma DHAS ($>800~\mu g$/dl) (385). Similarly, elevated values of plasma T ($>150-200$ ng/dl) may be seen in hyperthecosis (which probably represents a spectrum of PCOD). It must be remembered that adrenal rest tumors of the ovaries may also occur. The diagnosis of congenital adrenal hyperplasia (CAH) and hilar cell hyperplasia also must be considered. Levels of plasma T below 150 ng/dl usually are not associated with virilizing ovarian or adrenal tumors. Markedly elevated plasma levels of 17OHP are diagnostic of the 21-hydrolyxase variety of congenital adrenal hyperplasia. This may be associated with increased androstenedione and T levels, and to a lesser extent, DHAS. The inadequacies of DXM or hCG stimulation studies in evaluation of patients suspected of harboring an adrenal or ovarian tumor have been discussed in Chapter 6. It is incumbent that the physician deal directly with the possibility of a tumor of the adrenal or ovary anytime the plasma T is markedly elevated by employing appropriate radiographic, sonographic (see Table 9-5) and, if necessary, bilateral adrenal and ovarian venous catheterization techniques (as will be discussed later in the chapter). In addition, appropriate diagnostic studies to exclude tumorous or nontumorous Cushing's syndrome should be performed if clinically suspect (see later section of this chapter).

So far, the purpose of the initial blood studies was to offer a preliminary diagnostic probe of the endocrinopathy which the patient presents. Obviously, the clinical history and examination is essential in gaining an initial impression which leads to a more balanced interpretation of the laboratory data. Since further differential diag-

TABLE 9-5. Diagnostic Modalities which May Be Employed in the Differential Diagnosis of PCOD.

1 Ultrasonography of the pelvis and/or adrenals
2 Computerized tomography of the adrenals
3 Laparoscopy

nosis is purposefully left for a later section of this chapter, one may now examine ancillary tests which may be of additional value in assessing the hirsute and/or anovulatory woman. Although the following studies are not always essential they do offer additional insight into the extent of the associated endocrine dysfunction (Table 9-4).

A decreased TeBG concentration may be present in hyperandrogenemia of various etiologies. In one study, up to 36% of patients with PCOD, particularly in the absence of significant hirsutism and/or menstrual dysfunction, may demonstrate a normal plasma T (736), but the unbound (free) T is usually elevated (1002). Since perhaps 30% of patients with PCOD may not be hirsute, an elevation of unbound T may be found in many of these subjects (533) and is a better indicator of clinical androgenicity than total testosterone (662). Moll and Rosenfield (645) noted that the average free T concentration in girls reaches an adult level by mid-puberty (Tanner stage III), in association with adult serum levels of immunoreactive and bioactive LH. It is of interest that these investigators noted that the free T was the major androgen abnormality present in a series of 14 adolescent girls with PCOD (645). An overlap with normal female control values for total T (20–60 ng/dl) was found in 12 of 51 cases (23.5%) of patients with PCOD described by Raj et al. (736). Measurement of free T in this group of patients also revealed that 13 of the 51 subjects (25.5%) overlapped normal control values. Similar observations were also described by Easterling et al. (223). The association of an increased free T level in the plasma with an increased E_1/E_2 ratio is very suggestive of PCOD. An increase of plasma DHT may be found in only 36% of patients with polycystic ovaries (63). Insulin resistance may be associated with hyperandrogenism in the presence or absence of acanthosis nigricans. Impaired glucose tolerance with hyperinsulinemia following a glucose load may also be present in PCOD.

Most patients with PCOD have normal responsiveness of plasma cortisol, 17OHP, and 11-deoxycortisol (Compound S) following ACTH stimulation. Late-onset attenuated 21-hydroxylase deficiency is clinically impossible to differentiate from PCOD or those diagnosed as having "idiopathic" hirsutism. A review of several series of hirsute patients tested for the presence of late-onset attenuated 21-hydroxylase deficiency revealed its presence in 27 of 290 patients, or an incidence of 9% (148). The series described were those of Chrousos et al. (148), and others (420,541,681,732,). Once elevated androgens are noted it is recommended that an intravenous Cortrosyn® stimulation test be performed in the early follicular phase of the menstrual cycle to exlude this diagnosis (see later section in this chapter). A basal 17OHP is drawn and repeated 60 minutes after an intravenous injection of 0.25 mg Cortrosyn®. In a hypertensive hirsute patient a basal plasma level of 11-deoxycortisol (S) should be measured to exclude a late-onset 11-hydroxylase defect. A 3β-ol dehydrogenase defect may also be unmasked by ACTH testing of patients with elevated basal DHAS and/or 17α-hydroxypregnenolone levels and noting the resulting delta⁵/delta⁴ ratio pairs.

Hyperresponsiveness of plasma LH to LHRH is present in many subjects with PCOD. This is frequently correlated with the basal LH level. TRH hyperresponsiveness may be noted in subjects with PCOD, particularly those who are hyperprolactinemic. Some normoprolactinemic patients with PCOD also hyperrespond to TRH and this is considered by some to represent lactotrope hyperplasia (see Chapter 8). An absence of a normal doubling of plasma PRL following TRH testing may suggest the possibility of an occult pituitary tumor. Appropriate neuroradiological procedures, particularly computerized tomography of the sella turcica (including coronal views), are indicated to exclude an associated PRL-secreting pituitary tumor and/or a primary empty sella syndrome.

Ultrasonography of the pelvis has emerged as a helpful noninvasive technique in assessing ovarian size and shape as well as determining the presence or absence of multiple cysts (704). Most frequently this is done in conjunction with ultrasonograpy of the adrenals, to exclude the rare possibility of an adrenal neoplasm. In instances of suspected androgen-secreting adrenal tumor, computerized tomography (CT) appears to offer better resolution than sonography. CT scanning of the pelvis has also found application to gynecologic cancer with identificatiɔn of pelvic wall and para-aortic areas, sometimes with directed needle biopsy, permitting better treatment options (722).

Ultrasound examination of the pelvis has proven valuable as an ancillary aid in the diagnosis of PCOD (704,891). It is particularly useful as a precise method for the determination of ovarian size, shape and structure (Figs. 9-1 and 9-2). Furthermore, it is invaluable in assessing changes in follow-up examination of the ovaries, the presence of associated ovarian pathology or tumors, or in the differential diagnosis of a pelvic mass. In patients clinically suspected of

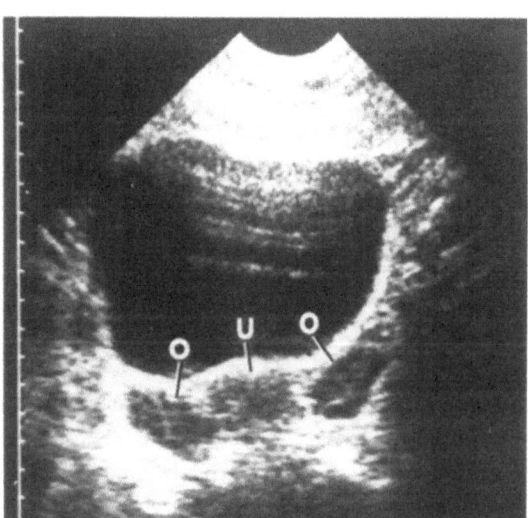

Fig. 9-1. Transverse scan of pelvis showing the uterus (u) and both ovaries (o) posterior to the bladder The ovaries are moderately enlarged and contain multiple cysts of 5–6 mm size. (Courtesy of Dr Hsu-Chong Yeh, M.D., Director of Ultrasound, Mt. Sinai School of Medicine, New York, New York)

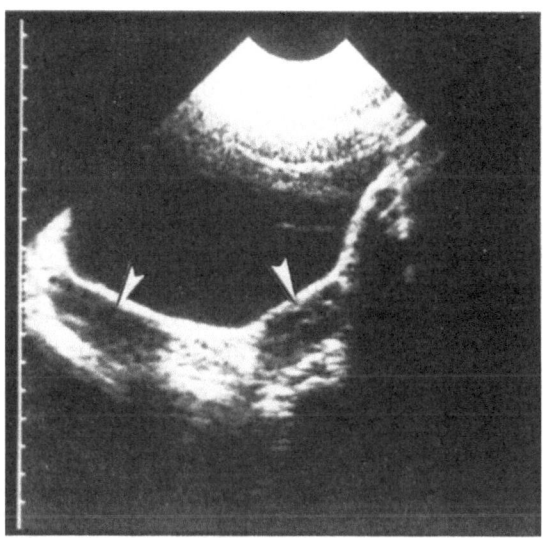

PCOD bilateral ovarian enlargement with an ovarian surface area ranging between 12 cm² – 22 cm² (mean, 17 cm²) strongly suggests PCOD (704). In instances where ovarian size is normal, the internal structure of the ovary is characterized by rounded echoless regions of variable dimensions less than 1.0 cm in size. Most polycystic ovaries show a cystic appearance with bilateral microcysts approximately 0.5 cm in diameter (Figs. 9-1 and 9-2). In a study of nine patients with bilaterally enlarged PCOD, microcysts were noted in seven patients (704). The uterine/ovarian ratio in normal subjects ranges from 1.5 – 1.8, while in PCOD with enlarged ovaries it ranges from 0.8 – 1.0 (704). The latter ratio is calculated as the maximum diameter of the uterine fundus/longitudinal diameter of the ovary.

In a study of 863 consecutive pelvic sonograms, 2.5% had evidence of polycystic ovaries (891). Real-time scanning was able to clearly detect individual cysts that ranged in size from 2 – 6 mm and arranged along the periphery of the ovary, or throughout the parenchyma. In only four instances were there no obvious clinical features present which were suggestive of PCOD. The volume of the smallest polycystic ovary was just above the upper limit of normality. All ovaries contained numerous cysts ranging from 6 to 16 in each ovary. An adequate study correlating ultrasonographic and clinical findings has not as yet been reported.

Laparoscopy and ovarian biopsy is perhaps indicated under certain circumstances (Table 9-6.)

In a series of 454 ovarian biopsies in patients with amenorrhea (primary and secondary), infertility, hirsutism, suspected neoplasm and chronic pelvic pain performed by Yuzpe and Rioux (1032), 197 biopsies were compatible with PCOD (43.3%). There was only one instance of severe bleeding requiring laparotomy. Obesity did not prevent the acquisition of adequate biopsy material for analysis. Where indicated and in those patients unresponsive to clomiphene citrate alone or in combination with hCG, adequate bilateral ovarian biopsies may be diagnostic as well as therapeutic. In the series by Yuzpe and Rioux (1032), six clomiphene-resistant patients with PCOD who underwent bilateral ovarian biopsies resumed regular menses and conceived within six months without further treatment. Other groups of investigators have also noted a therapeutic result with ovarian biopsies in patients with PCOD (680,890,894).

Fayez and Jonas (252) in a retrospective study of 74 patients conclude that laparoscopic ovar-

TABLE 9-6. Indications for Laparoscopy.

1 Avoidance of unneccessary laparotomy
2. Diagnosis of presence and extent of peritubal adhesions, or endometriosis (720)
3 As #2, several months after wedge resection, or in patients who previously failed to conceive after wedge resection
4. Diagnosis of suspicious ovarian mass with or without associated PCOD
5. Therapeutic tool for wedge resection
6 Diagnostic ovarian biopsy
7. Unexplained infertility
8 Premature ovarian failure

ian biopsy is most helpful in primary amenorrhea, and justified in secondary amenorrhea only if a histologic diagnosis of premature ovarian failure is essential. Contrary to the conclusions of Yuzpe and Rioux (1032), Fayez and Jonas (252) state that patients with ovarian hyperandrogenism need not be biopsied in that the laparoscopic appearance of the ovaries offer sufficient information and the hazards of bilateral ovarian biopsies in this group of patients outweigh their diagnostic and therapeutic benefit. Significant bleeding was noted following biopsies in 4% of the patients of Fayez and Jonas (252). They state that polycystic ovaries are difficult to grasp, more vascular and prone to bleeding. Eighteen patients with macroscopic evidence of PCOD were biopsied, following which five subjects (28%) developed regular menstrual cycles within the first six months after surgery. Ovarian biopsy was noncontributory in assessing the degrees of histologic changes in patients with macroscopic evidence of PCOD, whether the ovaries were normal-sized, enlarged or small. Similar conclusions were reported by Sutton (890), who found laparoscopic ovarian biopsies not helpful in further assessing ovarian histology in PCOD. Seventeen of 19 patients with PCOD had normal histologic findings, with significant morbidity in several patients.

It has previously been noted that there appear to be no unique histologic features of PCOD (359,852). There is a broad spectrum of patients without histologic ovarian abnormalities (457, 458) to those classically described by Stein and Leventhal (880) and extending to the changes found in hyperthecosis (13,335,446). Nine of 31 patients with clinical and biochemical PCOD had histologic examination of the ovaries, and five of the nine patients demonstrated normal ovarian histology (457). It appears clear that histologically normal appearing ovaries may be the source of ovarian hyperandrogenism with similar biochemical and clinical features as those with obvious anatomical ovarian abnormalities. The study of Kim et al. (457) has been criticized in that only nine subjects with PCOD had histologic evaluation, and that the technique of laparoscopic biopsy is limited in that only cortical rather than medullary tissue is usually examined. Similarly, a diagnosis of hyperthecosis may be missed by this technique.

An interesting study of 27 women with primary oligomenorrhea who were subjected to laparoscopy and bilateral ovarian biopsy was reported by McConway et al. (605). All had evidence of micropolycystic ovaries with increased thecal luteinization. One-third of the patients had evidence of recent ovulation as evidenced by corpora lutea and/or corpora albicantia. Three of the 18 anovulatory patients ovulated following bilateral ovarian biopsies, and no endocrinological differences were noted in the three that ovulated following biopsies as opposed to the other 15 patients that did not ovulate. Similar levels of LH, FSH, E_1, E_2, testosterone, and androstenedione were found in the ovulatory and anovulatory groups. The intriguing aspect to this study was the uniformity of histologically demonstrable PCOD in all subjects with oligomenorrhea and the associated parameters of an increased plasma LH/FSH ratio and E_1/E_2 ratio as well as an elevated androstenedione level. In a study by Wu et al. (1004), laparoscopically diagnosed PCOD had significantly higher LH/FSH ratios which were nearly double the ratios found in women with laparoscopically normal ovaries.

In a study by Maroulis (581), normal appearing ovaries were noted in instances of ovarian hyperandrogenism. It was concluded that laparoscopic evaluation of the ovaries is not as dependable as biochemical testing to determine the source of hyperandrogenism.

Understandably, the divergent data and conclusions of different investigators are difficult to merge into any meaningful consensus. It is difficult, however, to justify laparoscopy as a routine ancillary tool in the diagnosis of PCOD. Its therapeutic usefulness appears limited in PCOD.

Differential Diagnosis of PCOD

Nontumorous dependent LH-secretion of the ovaries, which is the broadest definition of PCOD, is common. Any condition causing anovulation may cause polycystic ovaries with LH-dependent hypersecretion of the ovaries constituting a large part of the hyperandrogenic state. The syndrome described by Stein and Leventhal (880) is a part of the spectrum of PCOD. On the other end of the spectrum, hyperthecosis of the ovaries may only be diagnosed histologically where it can be distinguished by the presence of isolated islands or clumps of luteinized theca-like cells deep in ovarian stroma distant from follicular and atretic cysts. Parenthetically, mild hirsutism with minor or no menstrual dysfunction (or so-called "idiopathic hirsutism"), may represent a lesser degree of LH-dependent hyperandrogenism.

A drug history should be obtained regarding prior administration of danazol, progestins (such as norethindrone and norgestrel which may be found in oral contraceptives), glucocorticoids, anabolic steroids, phenytoin, diazoxide and minoxidil.

It has been pointed out in another section that there are no distinct clinical characteristics of PCOD that are diagnostic. It has been the impression of some investigators (830) that most obese hirsute women have PCOD. From a practical consideration, the most common diseases that have to be considered in the differential diagnosis of PCOD in adolescent girls and adult women in their reproductive years who present with hirsutism and/or menstrual disturbances are listed in Table 9-7. (The differential diagnosis of amenorrhea in non-hirsute patients is considered in the last section of this chapter.)

The association of obesity and hirsutism, with hypertension and diabetes mellitus suggests hyperthecosis (838). It is essential, however, to exclude the diagnosis of hypercortisolism in the latter patients. This may be done by utilizing the following diagnostic procedures: 1) An overnight DXM–plasma cortisol study; the patient is given 1.0 mg of DXM orally the night before and a plasma cortisol is drawn the following morning; a plasma cortisol value below 6 μg/dl usually excludes Cushing's syndrome. 2) In borderline cases with no clear-cut plasma cortisol suppression following DXM, a 24 hour collection for urine free cortisol is obtained and the patient is given 0.5 mg DXM every six hours for

TABLE 9-7. Differential Diagnosis of Polycystic Ovarian Disease.

1. Adrenogenital syndrome
    (a) Congenital adrenal hyperplasia (CAH)
    (b) Adult-onset (attenuated) CAH
2. Adrenal virilizing tumor
3. Ovarian virilizing tumor
4. Cushing's syndrome
5. "Idiopathic hirsutism"
6 Ovarian hyperthecosis
7 Hilar cell hyperplasia

two days. A repeat 24 hour urine free cortisol is obtained on the second day of DXM administration. Lack of an appropriate fall of urine free cortisol to a level below 20 μg/24 hr following DXM requires thorough investigation of suspected hypercortisolism. (For full analysis of testing for Cushing's syndrome see Ref. 493.)

CONGENITAL ADRENAL HYPERPLASIA (CAH). Congenital adrenal hyperplasia is a variety of disorders of adrenal steroidogenesis which results from an inherited deficiency of one of several enzymes necessary for normal adrenal steroid synthesis. The 21-hydroxylase deficiency is transmitted as an autosomal recessive trait, with males and females equally at risk. Estimates of the incidence of this disease in Europe and the United States have been between 1 in 5000 and 1 in 15,000 (678). The gene frequency has been estimated as 1 in 100 and the carrier frequency as approximately 1 in 50. The incidence of the salt-wasting variety is 30–80% of patients with 21-hydroxylase deficiency. Less frequent enzymatic deficiences include 11-hydroxylase deficiency (76,299,681,917) and 3β-hydroxysteroid dehydrogenase deficiency (33, 771). The 21-hydroxylase form of CAH accounts for 90% or more of CAH cases. Iatrogenic 21-hydroxylase deficiency has been reported with the inadvertent administration of Danazol® during the first trimester of pregnancy. This drug may inhibit fetal adrenal enzymes causing female pseudo-hermaphroditism and salt loss with endocrinologic features of 21-hydroxylase deficiency which usually resolve within a year (131). In certain Middle Eastern groups (e.g., Moroccan Jews), 11- and 21-hydroxylase defects are equally prevalent.

The practicing gynecologist and internist does not often see the classical CAH that is seen in pediatric and adolescent practice. Instead, the type that is more frequently seen is the adult-onset attenuated CAH, usually of the 21-hydroxylase defect variety (Table 9-8).

The clinical improvement noted in 30–50% of glucocorticoid treated patients with hirsutism and oligomenorrhea had prompted an early impression that many of such patients represent an attenuated form of congenital adrenal hyperplasia (CAH). This view largely diminished following specific indicators of 21-hydroxylase deficiency such as urinary pregnanetriol and plasma 17OHP which were usually found to be

TABLE 9-8. Clinical Clues and Laboratory Studies Suggestive of Attenuated Adult-Onset 21-hydroxylase Deficiency Variety of CAH.

1. Family history of CAH
2. Short stature
3. Possible ambiguous external genitalia
4. Mild clitoromegaly
5. Borderline elevated plasma 17OHP, or 17α-hydroxypregnen-olone
6. Hyperresponsiveness of plasma 17OHP to intravenous ACTH
7. Borderline low levels of plasma gonadotropins
8. Impaired plasma LH responsiveness to LHRH
9. HLA genotyping of peripheral blood lymphocytes

within normal limits in most hirsute subjects. Despite some initial skepticism over the existence of late-onset CAH, numerous reports indicated that indeed patients may have hirsutism that develops postpuberally with similar biochemical abnormalities of classic CAH. Those with late-onset (adult) 21-hydroxylase deficiency frequently have normal or slight elevation of basal plasma 17OHP levels with striking increments of 17OHP 30–60 minutes following intravenous ACTH stimulation (85,594, 639,776) compared to mild abnormalities seen in idiopathic hirsutism or PCOD (330,353,502). Occasional basal plasma 17OHP may be elevated during the early morning hours during the peak of the adrenal circadian rhythm of ACTH (148). The clinical diagnosis of late-onset CAH is usally not made clinically. The presentation is frequently identical to that of PCOD (541) and indeed the patients with late-onset CAH may have normal or enlarged multifollicular ovaries. The delay in onset of symptoms in attenuated 21-hydroxylase deficiency is due to a milder deficiency, frequently manifesting only mildly elevated plasma T. Both classic and attenuated 21-hydroxylase deficiency may be associated with PCOD which occurs as a result of adrenal hyperandrogenism (32,76,245, 541,552). Modifying genes may minimize the clinical expression of the disease with few symptoms (515). Indeed fertility has been reported in untreated patients with 21-hydroxylase deficiency (245,515,752). The incidence of attenuated 21-hydroxylase deficiency among hirsute women ranges between 2–42% (148,541,681) with an average of 9% (148).

The classic 21-hydroxylase variety of CAH has elevated plasma levels of 17OHP, as well as

progesterone, pregnenolone and 17α-hydroxypregnenolone (Fig. 9-3) (769). The adrenal gland is a major precursor of 17α-hydroxypregnenolone in normal women, but only contributes to 50% of the plasma pregnenolone (the other 50% is derived from the ovaries). The normal adult female range for plasma pregnenolone is 30–200 ng/dl, and 30–440 ng/dl for plasma 17α-hydroxypregnenolone. McKenna et al. (614) have noted that measurement of plasma 17α-hydroxypregnenolone may be a good indicator of appropriateness of daily glucocorticoid dosage with a recommended range of 30–200 ng/dl. Acute stimulation with ACTH and the negligible response of pregnenolone and 17αOH-pregnenolone does not distinguish between adequately treated or undertreated subjects. Impaired responsiveness of LH to LHRH in CAH has been described by Klingensmith et al. (476) with a normal response following adequate adrenal suppression.

Late-onset 21-hydroxylase deficiency has frequently been genetically linked to the major histocompatibility leukocyte antigen (HLA) complex (85,523,541,639,729) analogous to the classic 21-hydroxylase deficiency (364,523). There is firm evidence suggesting that late-onset CAH is an allelic variant of CAH that results in a milder enzymatic defect. Linkage of the defect to the HLA complex has been adequately reviewed elsewhere (221,522,523,639).

The heterozygote carrier of CAH has no apparent physical or basal biochemical abnormalities. Intravenous Cortrosyn® (25 units) was administered to normal control subjects (males and females) and 13 couples (parents) of children with 21-hydroxylase deficiency (492). The mean plasma 17OHP of the controls subject was 87 ng/dl and the mean response achieved to synthetic ACTH at 60 minutes was 152 ng/dl. Basal plasma 17OHP were not significantly different in the heterozygote parents (97 ng/dl), but their mean response to ACTH was 367 ng/dl at 30 minutes. A level exceeding 1000 ng/dl was oberved in only one subject. No false positive values in the parents of children with 21-hydroxylase deficiency were noted when the cutoff point of the 17OHP response was set at 250 ng/dl, but only 15 of 26 parents were identified using this level. It is apparent that great overlap between carrier and control values following ACTH (492,513) makes it a less than perfect screening procedure for the heterozy-

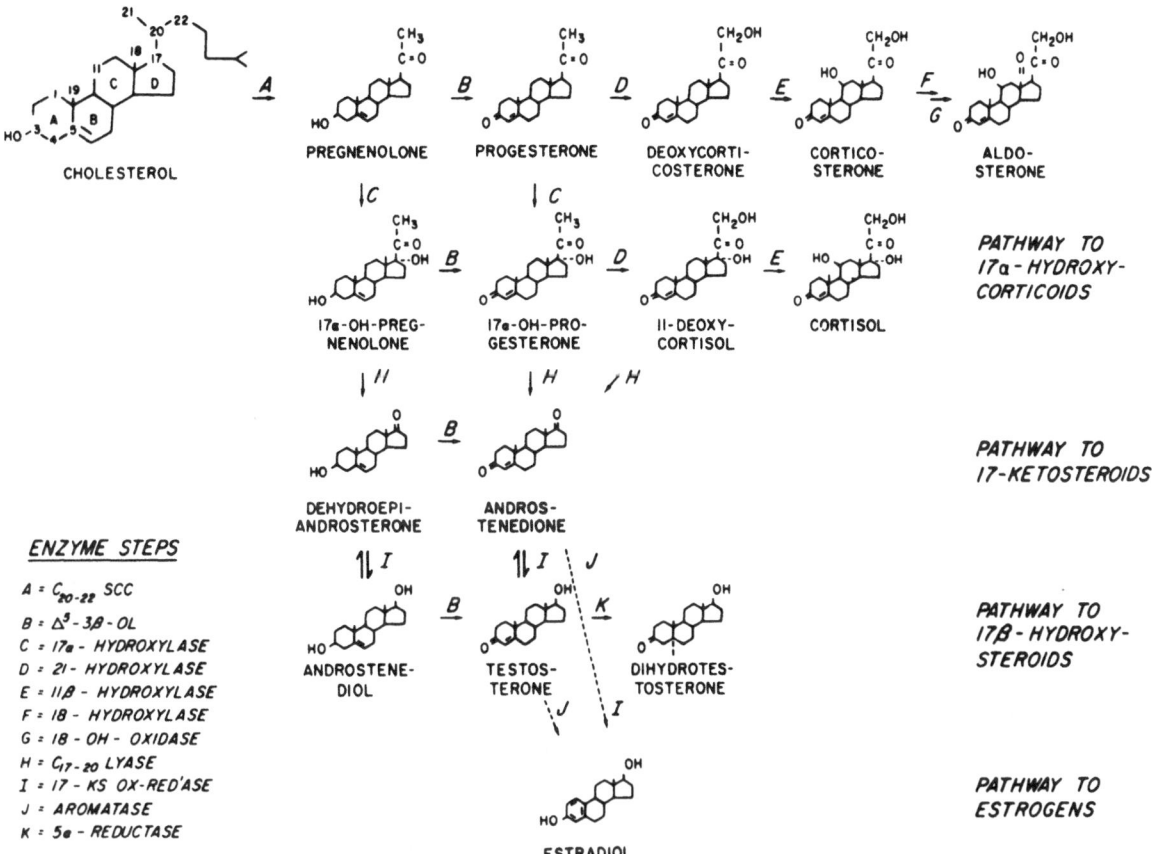

Fig. 9-3. Major pathways of steroid hormone biosynthesis. The enzyme steps are indicated by letters. (Reprinted with permission from Rosenfield RL, Miller WL. Congenital adrenal hyperplasia In: Mahesh VB, Greenblatt RB, eds. Hirsutism and Virilism. Boston: John Wright, PSG Inc., 1983 87–119.) (769).

gote carrier. Variable hyperresponsiveness to ACTH in heterozygote carriers have been noted by others (375,377,492,513,548,594). Gross-Wilde et al. (364) suggest that DXM administration the evening prior to a 60-minute Cortrosyn® test (0.25 mg intravenously) may seperate heterozygote adult females from controls about 90% of the time. It is clear that carriers have a compensated partial enzyme deficiency of 21-hydroxylase with reduced conversion rate of 17OHP to 11-deoxycortisol (S).

Another study suggests that the general population whose stimulated values of 17OHP following ACTH exceeds 700 ng/dl are probable heterozygotes of 21-hydroxylase deficiency (678).

Gutai et al. (375) employed an intravenous ACTH test and measured plasma P and 17OHP at basal and 30 minutes following ACTH injection to 30 siblings from 10 families who had at least one child with CAH. Eighteen of 30 siblings had hyperresponsiveness of P and 17OHP

to ACTH and were considered heterozygotes, while 12 were unaffected. A combined rate of increase of greater than 6.5 ng/dl/min of P and 17OHP was used to discriminate between normal controls and the CAH heterozygotes (375, 376).

In the presence of impaired 21-hydroxylation there is an accumulation of 17OHP and progesterone with decreased cortisol production. In the presence of severe enzymatic deficiency, salt-wasting results. New et al. (678) proposed that the difference in salt-wasters and simple virilizing forms of 21-hydroxylase deficiency resides in the possibility that salt-wasters have a 21-hydroxylase defect in the zona fasciculata as well as in the glomerulosa, while in simple virilizing types only the fasciculata is involved. The defect is further apparent during stimulation with ACTH when P and 17OHP rise markedly with minimal response of 11-deoxycorticosterone (DOC) and corticosterone (B).

The short arm of chromosome-6 carries the

genes for HLA, which are cell surface antigens important in transplantation. The HLA complex consists of at least four genetic loci which code for the antigens HLA-A, HLA-B, HLA-C, and HLA-D/DR (for a more detailed analysis of HLA linkage in CAH see Ref. 678). Close genetic linkage between HLA and CAH due to 21-hydroxylase deficiency has been noted since 1977. The autosomal recessive gene for the defect of 21-hydroxylase impairment in both the salt-wasting and non-salt-wasting forms of 21-hydroxylase deficiency is located close to the HLA-B locus (522,523). This serves as a marker for the CAH genotype (678). With HLA typing it is possible to predict which siblings are carriers and which are genetically unaffected. This correlates with clinical studies of family members predicted to be heterozygotes in their response of 17OHP to ACTH stimulation (548).

A cryptic form of 21-hydroxylase deficiency may occur in clinically unaffected family members of patients with classical 21-hydroxylase deficiency. Family members of an index case may have mild or usually asymptomatic 21-hydroxylase (cryptic) deficiency (678). New et al. (678) state that the genotype in family members with cryptic 21-hydroxylase deficiency is 21-OH^{CAH}/21-OH^{CRYPTIC}. Thus the family members have two recessive gene defects, i.e., a severe and mild 21-hydroxylase gene defect.

Classical CAH would comprise 21-OH^{CAH}/21-OH^{CAH}
Cryptic 21-hydroxylase. . . . .   21-OH^{CAH}/21-OH^{CRYPTIC}
Heterozygotes. . . . . 21-OH^{CAH}/21-OH^{NORMAL}
       or. . . . .   21-OH^{CRYPTIC}/21-OH^{NORMAL}

A biochemical profile in family members of classical CAH may be noted by a nanogram relating basal and ACTH stimulated values of 17-OHP, androstenedione, DHA, the ratio of DHA/androstenedione and T. The groups are distributed on a regression line as follows: classical CAH, cryptic 21-hydroxylase deficiency, heterozygotes for classical and cryptic 21-hydroxylase deficiency and those subjects genetically unaffected (by HLA) at the lower end of the regression line. The nanograms may assign the 21-hydroxylase deficiency genotype (see ref. 678). It appears that HLA typing of the family may be necessary to interpret an intermediate response of plasma 17OHP to ACTH between that of heterozygotes and mild homozygotes with 21-hydroxylase deficiency.

Late-onset 21-hydroxylase deficiency with virilization and menstrual dysfunction occurring in adolescence or in early adulthood with 21-hydroxylase deficiency has had the term "acquired" adrenal hyperplasia applied (681). This has raised the question as to whether this is the same inherited disorder as CAH with a delayed onset or a distinct entity. Initial studies by New et al. (679) indicated that it was not HLA linked. Subsequent studies by a number of groups including New and associates have suggested that late-onset 21-hydroxylase deficiency may be linked to HLA (85,505,639,678,729). Late-onset 21-hydroxylase deficiency and cryptic 21-hydroxylase deficiency are two variant forms of CAH that may be related (729). The fact that both entities appear to occur in the same family suggests that these syndromes may represent different clinical expressions of similar nonclassical 21-hydroxylase deficiency alleles (729). Further studies are needed to clarify the frequency of genetic transmission of patients with late-onset adrenal hyperplasia with 21-hydroxylase deficiency.

New et al. (678) noted the paradox of absence of clinical signs in patients with cryptic 21-hydroxylase deficiency in contrast to the virilization noted in patients with late-onset 21-hydroxylase deficiency. The latter are usually detected because of symptoms and are not family members of patients with classical CAH, whereas patients with cryptic 21-hydroxylase deficiency are usually detected as a result of CAH family studies. Prenatal diagnosis of CAH may be made by analysis of 17OHP and androstenedione of amniotic fluid. HLA genotyping of amniotic cells has also provided another method for the prenatal diagnosis of CAH in pregnancies at risk (678).

Two patients aged 17 and 22 years with attenuated CAH with elevated serum LH were noted by Rosenwaks et al. (776). They were identified by an elevated 17OHP in one subject and dramatic response of plasma P and 17OHP 30 minutes following intravenous ACTH in the other (>140 ng/dl/min). Both parents of the two subjects also hyperresponded to ACTH with an increment of 17OHP and P >6.5 ng/dl/min, indicating that the two patients had an attenuated form of congenital adrenal hyperplasia, while the parents had a heterozygous carrier state. The elevation of serum LH in the two patients may have been associated with the fact that they had an elevation of plasma estrone. Glucocorticoid treatment normalized the serum LH concentrations in the two subjects. The same group also studied nine patients with PCOD employing the ACTH stimulation test and were unable to detect any subjects with attenuated CAH.

Simultaneous measurement of plasma aldosterone, 18-hydroxycorticosterone (18-OH-B) and 18-hydroxydeoxycorticosterone (18-OH-DOC) may help identify various types of CAH (449). Twenty patients with CAH varying in age from 12–36 years were studied by Kater and Biglieri (449) and characterized by their plasma profiles of aldosterone, 18-hydroxycorticosterone and 18-hydroxydeoxycorticosterone. Their findings are summarized in Table 9-9 (449).

ACTH stimulation studies of siblings and parents of patients with CAH due to 21-hydroxylase deficiency make it clear that only the 17OHP response is useful in detecting heterozygosity. All other stimulated hormones did not discriminate between the general and heterozygous populations (548). These hormones included 17α-hydroxypregnenolone, DHA, androstenedione, testosterone, 11-deoxycortisol (Compound S), 11-deoxycorticosterone (DOC), corticosterone (Compound B) and aldosterone.

3β-HSD Deficiency. Patients with severe 3β-HSD deficency may present with Addisonian crisis in the newborn period. Inhibition of the 3β-ol step in the fetus involves the adrenal cortex as well as the gonads. A late-onset type of 3β-HSD deficiency CAH, however, has also been documented in pubertal and postpubertal females with hirsutism and/or amenorrhea who were not salt wasters (538,771). Adult-onset 3β-ol-dehydrogenase, delta$^{4-5}$ isomerase deficiency is relatively rare, and some women with a partial deficiency may undergo spontaneous sexual development, achieve and maintain a pregnancy (612). Diagnosis is made by elevation of plasma pregnenolone, 17α-hydroxypregnenolone, DHA and DHAS, with relatively low levels of delta^4 compounds such as progesterone, 17OHP and androstenedione (Fig. 9-4) (365). The 3β-ol-dehydrogenase enzyme may only be blocked with very high doses of estrogens, i.e., higher than the levels found in hirsute women (22). A compensatory elevated renin allows for adequate aldosterone formation, thereby preventing salt loss. Some children may manifest premature adrenarche, advanced linear growth and some clitoromegaly. DHAS of ovarian origin may be elevated in 3β-ol-dehydrogenase deficiency with pubertal onset (771). Basal and post-ACTH stimulated delta^5 steroids such as delta^5-pregnenolone, delta^5-17α-hydroxypregnenolone and DHA are elevated. Pang et al. (702) have proposed that patients with the salt-losing form of 3β-HSD deficiency have a defect of 3β-HSD in the zona glomerulosa as well as the zona fasciculata. The genetic locus for regulation of 3β-HSD is not linked to

TABLE 9-9. Various Mean Plasma Steroids in CAH.

Steroid	21-HYDROXYLASE DEFICIENCY (NON-SALT-WASTING). PLASMA CONC. (mean) (ng/dl)	17α-HYDROXYLASE DEFICIENCY. PLASMA CONC. (mean) (ng/dl)	11β-HYDROXYLASE DEFICIENCY. PLASMA CONC. (mean) (ng/dl)	NORMAL. PLASMA CONC. (mean) (ng/dl)
11-Deoxycorticosterone (DOC)	Increased (46)	Increased (303)	Increased (82)	(7.8)
Corticosterone (Compound B)	Normal	Increased	Decreased	(700)
18-hydroxycorticosterone (18-OH-B)	Increased (85)	Increased (327)	Reduced (5 1)	(20)
18-hydroxydeoxycorticosterone (18-OH-DOC)	Normal (8)	Increased (236)	Reduced (0.9)	(7)
Aldosterone	Increased (28)	Reduced (3.5)	Reduced (2.6)	(8)
Renin	Increased	Suppressed	Suppressed	

Modified with permission from Kater CE, Biglieri EG Distinctive plasma aldosterone, 18-hydroxycorticosterone, and 18-hydroxydeoxycorticosterone profile in the 21-, 17α-, and 11β-hydroxylase deficiency types of congenital adrenal hyperplasia Am J Med 1983, 75 43–48 (449)

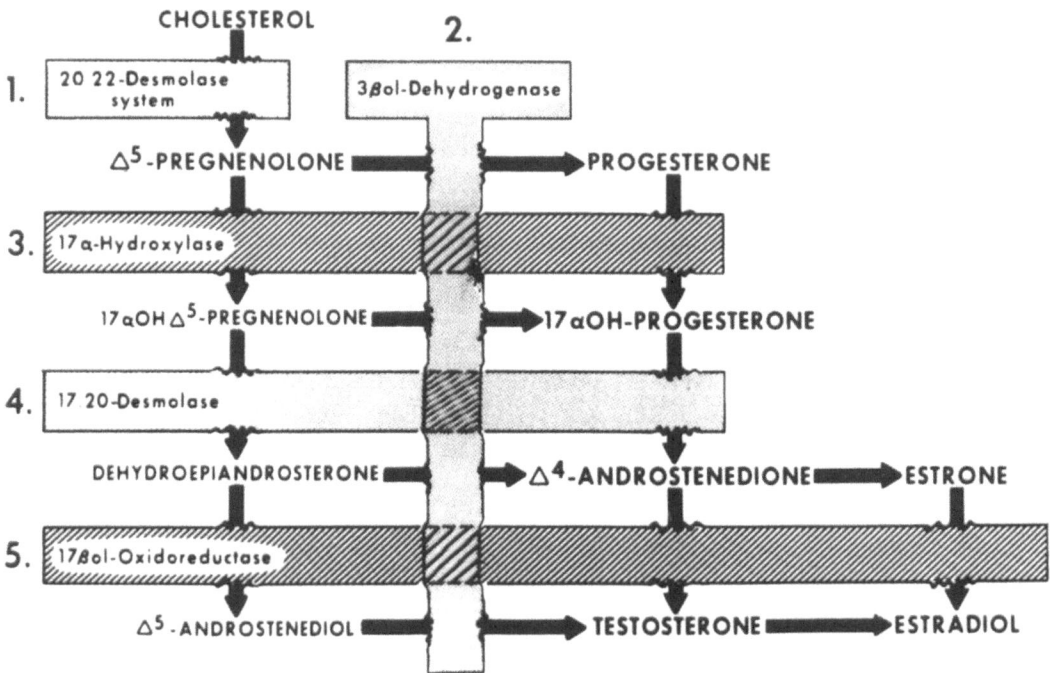

Fig. 9-4. Enzymatic defects in steroidogenesis A 3β-ol-dehydrogenase deficiency leads to an increase of delta[5] precursors and an increase of the corresponding delta[5]/delta[4] pairs (Reprinted with permission from Grumbach MM, Conte FA. Disorders of sex differentiation. In: Williams RH, ed Textbook of Endocrinology Philadelphia· WB Saunders Co , 1981 423–514.) (365)

the gene for HLA. There appears to be marked heterogeneity of CAH due to 3β-HSD deficiency (702).

Bongiovanni (92) in his review of 3β-HSD deficiency noted that its late onset in adolescent or adult females with menstrual irregularities and varying virilization mimicked a variety of ovarian and/or adrenal disorders and frequently presented with normal basal steroid levels. Of particular value in the diagnosis of this defect is the measurement of plasma 17α-hydroxypregnenolone which may be increased in the basal state as well as following ACTH stimulation (92,771). Similar increases in all delta[5]-3β-ol steroids may be demonstrated in the adrenal and ovarian steroid pathways. In view of normal levels of plasma cortisol, the defect is obviously partial and sufficiently mild so that no abnormalities are noted earlier in life, allowing for the development of normal female secondary sexual characteristics. Increased DHA and DHAS may serve as markers in a patient with hirsutism or virilization even when the patient may present with polycystic ovaries. Under these circumstances, the differential diagnosis should include the possible presence of 3β-HSD deficiency. Indeed subtle defects in 3β-HSD enzyme have attracted recent attention (433,543). Lobo

and Goebelsmann (543) employed the ratio of basal 17-OHPe/17-OHP, which in normal women was 1.2, while 20 hirsute women had a ratio of 2.8. This disparity was enhanced by ACTH stimulation so that the ratio rose to 8–14 as compared to 4.4 in normal women. In this study, five women had a ratio less than 0.5, indicative of 21-hydroxylase deficiency. High levels of 17α-hydroxypregnenolone have also been identified in some patients with PCOD by Judd et al. (433). The measurement of 17α-hydroxypregnenolone appears to be much more specific for the diagnosis of 3β-HSD deficiency than DHAS (92,771), and more frequent utilization of this steroid is indicated. Nine of 24 hirsute patients studied by Lobo and Goebelsmann (538) with elevated DHAS levels had an increased basal value of 17α-hydroxypregnenolone as well as delta[5]-androstenediol with relatively normal T and androstenedione values. The variability in clinical syndromes described in the literature may be explicable by heterogeneous defects in 3β-ol dehydrogenase.

Adult-Onset 11β-Hydroxylase Deficiency. Adult-onset 11β-hydroxylase deficiency is about as rare as 3β-ol dehydrogenase delta[4-5] isomerase deficiency with impaired conversion of 11-

deoxycorticosterone (DOC) to corticosterone (B) and 11-deoxycortisol (S) to cortisol. Glucocorticoid deficiency with poor tolerance to stress, androgen excess and mineralocorticoid excess (hypertension) may result (299). The diagnosis is made by finding a high level of plasma 11-deoxycortisol and 11-deoxycorticosterone (449). In view of mineralocorticoid excess the plasma renin is suppressed. The ovary does not require 11-hydroxylase for gonadal steroidogenesis, but is suppressed by gonadotropin suppression of adrenal androgens. With adequate glucocorticoid treatment ovarian maturation ensues with regular menstruation and reversal of possible hypertension. The 11-hydroxylase defect, a relatively rare cause of CAH which appears to be transmitted as an autosomal recessive trait, has not been linked to the HLA-B locus, and hormonal studies before and after ACTH have not been useful in detecting heterozygosity (703).

Impairment of 11-hydroxylation in nine patients with PCOD was noted by Ikkos and Dellia-Sfikaki (405) by observing a marked increase of 11-deoxycortisol (S) following ACTH stimulation. In a contradictory study of 34 hirsute women, Maroulis et al. (583) found the latter response to be present in a mild form in only 3 of 34 patients as demonstrated by an increase of the 11-deoxycortisol/cortisol ratio. Four cases of adult-onset adrenocortical 11β-hydroxylase defect were described by Cathelineau et al. (132). The ages of the cases ranged from 21–29 years, and their presentation was hirsutism with regular menses in three of four patients. Interestingly, no significant hypertension was noted. Elevated plasma ACTH values were noted, however, in three of four patients, as well as an elevation of 17OHP and androstenedione. Basal plasma 11-deoxycortisol was elevated in two patients. The above study suggests a heterogeneity of this syndrome resulting from a partial variable 11β-hydroxylation defect in the subjects tested (132).

In summary, late-onset hirsutism has been demonstrated in 21-hydroxylase deficiency (85,776), 11β-hydroxylase deficiency (299,683) and 3β-ol-dehydrogenase deficiency (771). Elevated 17OHP has been reported in patients with PCOD by Givens et al. (330), Lachelin et al. (502) and Kandeel et al. (442). A hyperresponse of 17OHP to ACTH in some patients with PCOD has been reported by Givens et al. (330) and Lachelin et al. (502), but not by Kandeel et al. (442). The employment of standard ACTH testing is recommended to exclude enzymatic defects of 21-hydroxylase and 3β-HSD in any hirsute female with or without menstrual dysfunction or signs of enlarged or sonographically suggestive polycystic ovaries.

17α-hydroxylase Deficiency. The finding of primary amenorrhea with hypertension may also be a feature of 17α-hydroxylase deficiency, an even rarer adrenal disorder than the 3β-ol-dehydrogenase or 11β-hydroxylase deficiency. In view of the elevation of the mineralocorticoid 11-deoxycorticosterone (DOC), hypertension and hypokalemia with suppressed plasma renin activity may result. Corticosterone is also increased in the plasma. This rare deficiency is also not linked to the HLA region (188). The condition is treated with glucocorticoid therapy, but estrogens are necessary to induce sexual maturation since estradiol cannot be synthesized adequately (612).

"IDIOPATHIC HIRSUTISM." The hair follicle is a derivative of the pilosebaceous apparatus and may be considered an end organ response to hormonal influences. There is no difference between the male and female in the distribution of hair follicles. The levels of circulating androgens as well as genetic or hereditary factors determine the different sexual hair patterns in normal men and women. The difference in sensitivity of Japanese women to androgens is reflected by the rarity of hirsutism and acne in these subjects. On the other hand, excessive hirsutism in hormone-dependent areas such as the face, axillae, chest and pubic areas may be a reflection of abnormal androgen metabolism. The absence of associated menstrual dysfunction or elevation of serum T or DHAS does not exclude a subtle androgen abnormality, and indeed many so-called patients with "idiopathic hirsutism" represent endocrinopathies which may be diagnosed with more refined hormonal studies (see later in section). Parenthetically, extremity hair appears to be genetic in etiology and its presence on the arms and back of prepuberal children is probably an atavistic manifestation.

Biochemically human skin is a target organ for androgens. In most androgen target tissues, including human skin, the first step in the mechanism of androgen action is the 5α-reduction of T to DHT by the enzyme 5α-reductase which is localized in microsomes and regulated by androgens. DHT is then converted to 5α-androstane-3α, 17β-diol (3α-diol) and 5α-androstane-3β, 17β-diol (3β-diol) by 3α- and 3β-ketoreductases (Fig. 9-5) (773). Little if any of the two diols are converted back to DHT in human skin. DHT and 3α-diol are potent androgens which are not secreted directly to any extent by the gonads or the adrenals. The metabolite 3α-diol is more potent than DHT in stimulating sebum production (308). DHT and 3α-diol originate mostly from 5α-reduction of T and androstenedione in hepatic and extrahepatic tissues. Androgen utilization by the skin may be gauged to some extent by plasma DHT, urinary and serum 3α-diol, and in vitro determination of skin 5α-reductase activity (595,597). There is moderate conversion to 3α-diol in the skin of human subjects of both sexes with hyper-responsiveness to androgens in patients with hirsutism and acne (1000). Recently, determination of serum 5α-androstane-3α,17β-diol glucuronide (3α-diol G) appears to correlate well with the degree of hirsutism and may best reflect androgen production in peripheral tissues (529).

The term "idiopathic hirsutism" probably applies to less than 5% of patients who present with hirsutism and/or menstrual dysfunction (782). "Idiopathic hirsutism" and PCOD are closely related and only differ in the sensitivity of the hypothalamic–pituitary unit to an abnormal steroidal milieu (922). The skin of patients with idiopathic hirsutism may convert relatively inactive androgens such as androstenedione and DHA to T, DHT and 5α-androstane-3α, 17β-diol (3α-diol). Androstenedione which is not bound to TeBG may diffuse into the skin and become converted to T and DHT (499).

Hirsute women with normal serum T levels may have hypersensitivity of the target cell to androgens, due to increased 5α-reduction of T to DHT (913). The 5α-reductase level in pubic skin fibroblasts is higher in hirsute than in normal women (663). Pubic skin fibroblasts (PSF) contain androgen receptors and are capable of responding to DHT or T treatment with increased protein synthesis or increased androgen binding. The 5α-reductase activity of PSF may be used as a marker of androgen action in vitro as well as in vivo (664).

Another possible mechanism of androgen hypersensitivity may be a primary increase in the concentration of androgen receptor. The total (cytosolic plus nuclear) androgen binding capacity of pubic skin fibroblasts from nine hirsute wome was similar to that of normal men and women regardless of the level of plasma androgens (663). It thus appears that the androgen receptor is not regulated by androgens in the skin in contrast to the 5α-reductase activity which amplifies androgen action in androgen stimulated areas such as pubic skin.

Urinary 5α-androstane-3α, 17β-diol (3α-diol)

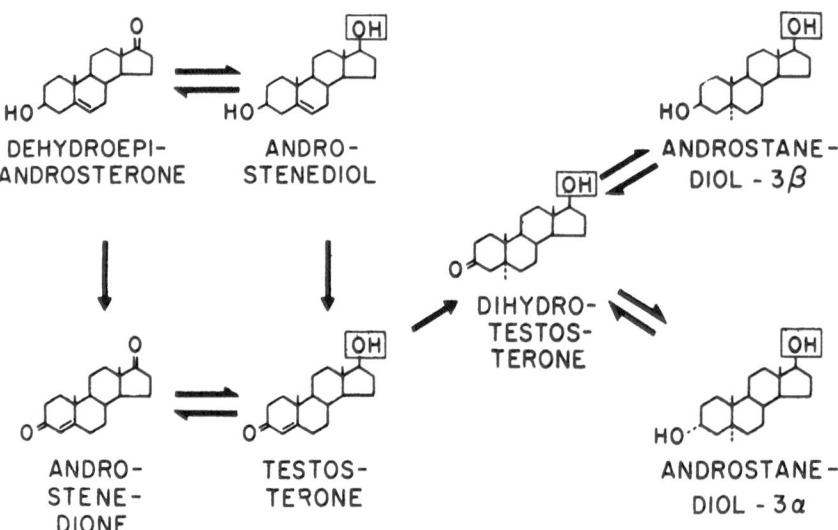

Fig. 9-5. 17β-hydroxyl pathway of androgen metabolism. DHT is converted to 3α-diol and 3β-diol by 3α- and 3β-ketoreductases. (Reprinted with permission from Rosenfield RL. Studies of the relation of plasma androgen levels to androgen action in women. J Ster Biochem. 1975, 6 695–702, Pergamon Press, Ltd) (773).

is elevated in the majority of hirsute subjects (630,1001) and may well be one of the most commonly observed abnormalities in hirsute women. The main precursor of urinary 3α-diol in premenopausal women is androstenedione, while T is the main precursor of 3α-diol in men (1001). The amount of 3α-diol in urine also reflects the testosterone 5α-reductase activity present in androgen target cells, particularly in sexual skin. Mean values for normal men were reported as 193 ± 77 $\mu g/24$ hr while normal women had levels of 44 ± 23 $\mu g/24$ hr. Forty-nine hirsute females had a significantly increased mean value of 137 ± 51 $\mu g/24$ hr (1001). Hirsute women generally have increased androstenedione production with conversion to T, as well as the contribution derived skin metabolism. The contribution of DHA and DHAS to 3α-diol is relatively low and similar in both sexes.

The most commonly elevated plasma androgen in hirsutism and one which may be elevated while many others are within normal limits is 5α-androstane, 3α, 17β-diol (3α-diol), which, as noted, reflects increased androgen formation at target level (598). The 3α-diol is derived from 3α-reductase activity and is a useful marker of androgen target tissue events, more so than DHT. The blood production rate of the potent androgen 3α-diol is similar to DHT, and most of 3α-diol is peripherally converted from secreted T (656). About 75% of 3α-diol is derived from DHT. The plasma concentration of 3α-diol in normal adult men is 15 ± 4 ng/dl. Normal adult women have 3α-diol plasma levels of 4 ng/dl, while non-hirsute patients with PCOD have mean levels of 60 ng/dl (533,656).

The target tissues generate a metabolite, 5α-androstane-3α, 17β-diol glucuronide, (3α-diol G), which arises mainly from DHT and best reflects peripheral androgen action (529,656). The markedly increased plasma levels of 3α-diol G correlated best with clinical hirsutism in a study of 12 hirsute patients with PCOD, while the levels of this metabolite were normal in non-hirsute patients with PCOD (533). The fact that similar androgen and estrogen levels may be found in hirsute and non-hirsute patients with PCOD suggests that the target tissue may determine whether hirsutism develops (533).

It has already been stressed that although the majority of patients with PCOD have elevated circulating androgen levels, up to 30% are not hirsute. Twelve hirsute (H-PCO) and non-hirsute (NH-PCO) patients with PCOD were studied by Lobo et al. (529) for the presence or absence of peripheral androgen production and activity using serum 3α-diol glucuronide (3α-diol G) as a marker. The patients were 18–26 years of age, all presented with oligomenorrhea and infertility, had an LH/FSH ratio > 3, and were slightly to moderately obese with a Ponderal Index (height in inches $\div$ cube root of the weight in pounds) < 12. Only half of the patients with PCOD had bilaterally enlarged ovaries. Results were compared to 13 normal ovulating women controls who were age- and weight-matched and studied in the early follicular phase of the menstrual cycle. Serum T, unbound T (uT) and androstenedione (A_1) were higher in both groups of PCOD patients than control subjects, but did not separate the hirsute from the nonhirsute subjects with PCOD (Fig. 9-6) (529). Mean serum DHAS and delta[5] androstenediol (A_2) were higher in the hirsute PCOD group (Fig. 9-6). Serum DHT was similar in all three groups, while 3α-diol was most elevated in the H-PCO group (Fig. 9-7) (529). The most striking difference between the H-PCO group and the other two groups was the increase in serum 3α-diol G in H-PCO to a mean of 546 ng/dl, compared to 69 and 40 ng/dl in the NH-PCO and control groups, respectively (Fig. 9-7) (529).

Lobo et al. (529) conclude that obesity and IGS may not be significant factors that separate patients with PCOD who are hirsute from those that are not hirsute. Serum 3α-diol G arises from extrasplanchnic tissues, and its elevation in hirsute women is an important reflection of androgen production (possibly DHT) in peripheral tissues. Although serum 3α-diol G is an excellent marker of peripheral androgen formation at the level of the pilosebaceous unit, it probably is not the cause of hirsutism. The mean serum levels of 3α-diol G in normal adult males is 197 ng/dl (656), which is lower than that found in the hirsute PCOD group. The calculated blood PR of 3α-diol in young men appears to be between 200–300 $\mu g/day$ (656) while the MCR is 1798 l/day. The data of Lobo et al. (529) confirm the premise that the presence of hirsutism is not only a function of circulating androgen levels, but is also determined by the extent of androgen production in peripheral tissues.

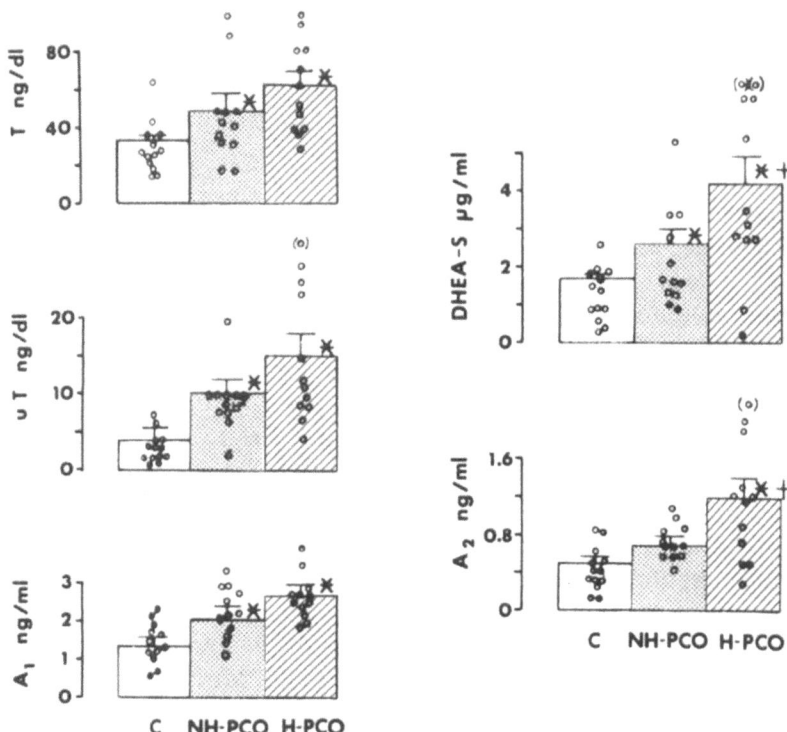

Fig. 9-6. Serum testosterone, free testosterone, androstenedione, DHAS, and delta5-androstenediol in controls (C), NH-PCO, and H-PCO patients * = significantly different levels compared to controls + = significantly different levels between NH-PCO and H-PCO groups. Individual subjects are depicted together with the SEM. (Reprinted with permission from Lobo RA, Goebelsmann U, Horton R. Evidence for the importance of peripheral tissue events in the development of hirsutism in polycystic ovary syndrome. J Clin Endocrinol Metab. 1983, 57.393–397.) (529).

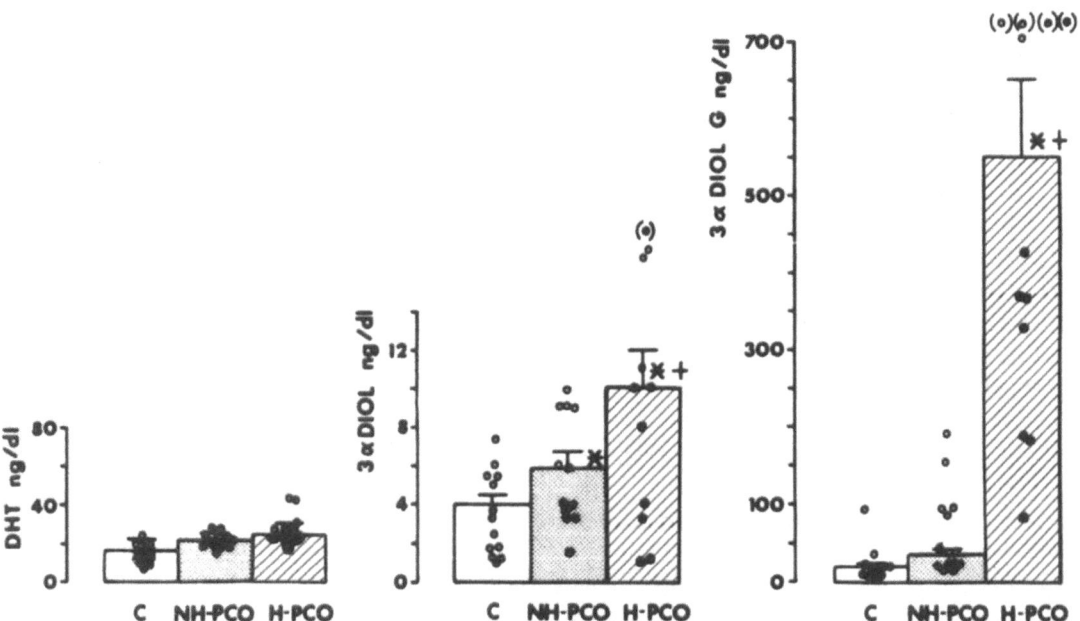

Fig. 9-7. Serum DHT, 3α-diol, and 3α-diol G in controls (C), NH-PCO, and H-PCO patients. * = significantly different levels compared to controls + = significantly different levels between NH-PCO and H-PCO groups Individual subjects are depicted together with the SEM (Reprinted with permission from Lobo RA, Goebelsmann U, Horton R. Evidence for the importance of peripheral tissue events in the development of hirsutism in polycystic ovary syndrome. J Clin Endocrinol Metab. 1983; 57.393–397.) (529)

The absence of an androgen receptor results in insensitivity of androgens, as in the complete form of the testicular feminization syndrome. The capacity of the target cell to utilize androgens depends on the ability to form DHT from T or from inactive precursors. Also needed is the cytosolic receptor which binds DHT and transfers it to the nucleus to promote specific androgen action.

VIRILIZING OVARIAN AND ADRENAL TUMORS. The elevation of plasma T is of some help in the differential diagnosis between PCOD and a virilizing ovarian or adrenal tumor. Markedly elevated plasma T values above 200 ng/dl may be found in tumorous virilizing syndromes. However, there are patients with hyperthecosis who also may have markedly elevated plasma T levels. Under these circumstances ultrasonography of the adrenals and ovaries should be performed, and where indicated CT scan of the adrenals. It can be appreciated that baseline ultrasonography is frequently of importance particularly where there is a suspicion of an ovarian tumor which may occasionally be associated with PCOD. Clinically any rapidly progressive change in severity of hirsutism, usually in association with secondary amenorrhea and clitoromegaly, is highly suggestive of a virilizing ovarian or adrenal tumor. A tumor is suspect when virilization occurs with amenorrhea, generalized scalp hair loss, acne, male escutcheon, increased musculature, deepening of the voice and clitoral hypertrophy. An adrenal mass may sometimes be palpable. It can often be readily seen on ultrasonography or CT scan of the adrenals.

In a review of clinical features of 34 adult females with virilizing adrenal adenomas, Gabrilove et al. (297) underscored the fact that elevated plasma T is almost invariably present in such tumors in levels similar to those found in ovarian sources of virilization. Most patients with virilizing adrenal tumors presented with amenorrhea, clitoromegaly (27 of the 34 patients), marked hirsutism and deepening of the voice. Acne and breast atrophy were less frequent. Seven of 34 patients with virilizing adrenal adenomas had hypertension. Fourteen of 16 patients in whom plasma T was measured had a striking elevation, and of interest was the fact that seven patients with virilizing adrenal tumors had neutral 17-ketosteroids below

15 mg/24 hr. The tumors varied in size from as little as 1×1 cm to $13-16$ cm in diameter. Close to 100% of the tumors were localized by ultrasonography and computerized tomography (297). In the occasional instance of a very small tumor, the diagnosis may be established by selective venous angiography for radiographic delineation as well as for measurement of the adrenal venous effluent on both sides (297,298). Gabrilove et al. (297) further stressed that an adrenal tumor must be carefully excluded before laparotomy is performed for a presumptive ovarian source of hyperandrogenemia. The use of suppression and stimulation tests by some investigators prompted ovarian ablative precedures instead of adrenalectomy. It is now quite obvious that most subjects with adrenal virilizing tumors (6 of 7) respond to hCG stimulation testing (297). No consistent pattern was noted following ACTH stimulation. The use of DXM-suppression testing yielded equivocal or slight suppression in five subjects, no effect in five others and some increase of plasma T in one subject. Estrogen-suppressive testing demonstrated a reduction of plasma T in two of five patients. Plasma DHAS or androstenedione is increased in approximately 50% of patients with virilizing adrenal adenomas (354). Hypertension in virilizing adrenal adenomas may be associated with elevated 11-deoxycorticosterone (DOC) elevation (297). The clinical features of patients with adrenocortical carcinomas are similar to those of adenomas other than the fact that the onset is usually abrupt with a more dramatic picture of virilization, balding, breast atrophy, increased musculature, deepening of the voice and clitoromegaly.

The radiologic finding of an adrenal mass in a patient with a variable degree of hirsutism or virilization warrants diagnostic measures to exclude hypercortisolism. This can not be overemphasized, since failure to make this diagnosis may result in acute adrenal insufficiency following tumor extirpation. Some of the diagnostic steps are outlined earlier in this chapter. In instances where selective venous catheterization is performed, sampling of the effluent for cortisol levels should be routinely performed. Parenthetically, the more widespread use of computerized tomography of the adrenals has demonstrated the not infrequent presence of nonfunctioning adrenal adenomas, most of which are benign. The nonfunctioning character of these lesions, however, must be confirmed by thorough hormonal studies. Finally, the fact that the majority of adrenal carcinomas do not demonstrate evidence of adrenal hyperfunction makes surgical excision of the lesion the only reliable way to exclude a malignant neoplasm.

An adrenal tumor should be strongly suspected in instances of rapid virilization with or without associated Cushing's sydrome. Although markedly elevated serum DHAS levels $>700 \mu g/dl$ are frequently found in patients with virilizing adrenal tumors, there are reports of testosterone-secreting adrenal tumors with normal urinary 17-ketosteroid and/or serum DHAS levels (297,334,438,802,865,974).

Twelve patients with nontumorous ovarian hyperandrogenism (9 with PCOD and 3 with hyperthecosis) as well as three patients with virilizing ovarian tumors were studied by Wiebe and Morris (978). This group employed a plasma T/androstenedione (A_1) ratio in assessing the changes in the ratio in the three disease states. The ratio was calculated as follows:

$$\frac{\text{Plasma T} \div \text{upper normal concentration T}}{\text{Plasma } A_1 \div \text{upper normal concentration of } A_1}$$

The three patients with virilizing ovarian tumors as well as 16 other cases culled from the literature revealed T/A_1 ratios greater than 1.5 (range 1.8–22) in 15 of 19 patients. An adnexal mass was palpable in only eight patients. However, in four ovarian tumors the T/A_1 ratio approached 1.0 (978), as in eight of nine patients with PCOD. In three cases with hyperthecosis the T/A_1 ratio was greater than 1.5 (range 2.6–6.7). Plasma DHAS was not elevated in three instances of virilizing ovarian tumors where it was measured (978). In hyperthecosis, androstenedione production exceeds T production but it is usually less than the increased androstenedione production seen in PCOD. In virilizing ovarian tumors the delta^5 pathway is favored leading to delta^5-androstenediol and then to T with relatively less delta^4 conversion to androstenedione → T.

Two adrenal-like tumors of the ovaries had a T/A_1 ratio less than one, suggesting that the major androgens that were secreted by the tumors were DHAS and androstenedione (978). An elevated DHAS level greater that 700–800 $\mu g/dl$ can be seen in the presence of an adrenal tumor or adrenal rest tumor of the ovary. The T/A_1 ratio may possibly be a useful ancillary study in the diagnosis of an ovarian masculinizing tumor (978). The absence of an elevated T/A ratio, however, does not necessarily exclude the presence of a virilizing ovarian tumor.

In a review of 43 cases of virilizing ovarian tumors by Meldrum and Abraham (634) only seven patients (16%) had peripheral T concentrations less than 200 ng/dl. No correlation was noted between tumor size and peripheral T levels. Unlike the frequency of markedly elevated plasma T levels in patients with virilizing ovarian tumors, only 1 of 159 patients with nontumorous hyperandrogenism had a T level as high as 150–200 ng/dl (634). Selective adrenal and ovarian vein catheterization may be of value in localizing the site of the tumor, particularly in those instances where the tumor may not be palpable or obvious on ultrasonographic examination. The ovarian venous concentration of T usually exceeds 2000 ng/dl, particularly in the presence of tumors less than 5.0 cm in diameter (634).

Stromal luteinization associated with virilization may occur in the presence of benign or malignant non-masculinizing ovarian tumors (primary or metastatic) (408,810). It must also be remembered that patients with PCOD are at risk for the development of functional or nonfunctional ovarian tumors, most frequently dermoid cysts (287). Detailed descriptions of the clinical characteristics and histopathology of virilizing ovarian tumors may be found in excellent reviews (270,809,995).

Human chorionic gonadotropin stimulation does not afford a reliable test to distinguish between an ovarian and adrenal source of androgens. Non-invasive localizing techniques such as CT scanning of the adrenals can localize small adrenal tumors. In the presence of uncertainty regarding the diagnosis of an adrenal tumor, selective adrenal venous studies must be performed (297).

VIRILIZATION DURING PREGNANCY. Apart from the fact that some patients with PCOD are ovulatory and are capable of conceiving there is little data available on the outcome of pregnancies in patients with PCOD. As yet there are no reports of masculinization of a female infant in patients with non-tumorous PCOD. The chorionic gonadotropin stimulus of pregnancy may induce ovarian stromal hyperandrogenemia in normal subjects as well as those with PCOD. Clinical observation of ovarian size with ultrasonography as well as analyses of serum androgens should be performed to avoid unnecessary surgical intervention. Virilizing syndromes during pregnancy are usually not due to PCOD, but result from luteomas of pregnancy, and occasional benign and malignant virilizing tumors of the ovary. Less than 5% of pregnancy luteomas have been associated with virilization. Luteomas of pregnancy usually regress following delivery, and therefore surgery is not often indicated.

In a review of 25 documented cases of virilization occurring during pregnancy, three had associated hyperthecosis (693). Magendantz et al. (563) described three other patients with virilization during pregnancy associated with PCOD. The common features of all three cases was rapid onset of virilization during the latter part of pregnancy with increased clitoral size, deepening of the voice, increased hair growth and unilateral ovarian enlargement. All three patients had normal term deliveries. Although all patients had bilateral ovarian enlargement, the fact that more marked unilateral enlargement was noted made exclusion of a virilizing ovarian tumor necessary by subsequent oophorectomy in one, and bilateral wedge resection in the other two patients (563).

HYPERTHECOSIS. Hyperthecosis was first described as a syndrome by Culiner and Shippel (181). The clinical picture is that of severe hirsutism, mild clitoromegaly, obesity, temporal balding, oligomenorrhea, and refractoriness to clomiphene citrate therapy (251,446,670). Obesity, diabetes mellitus and hypertension occur with greater frequency in hyperthecosis, but the disease may occasionally be associated with regular menses (1,839) and fertility (98, 122,123). The clinical and laboratory features of hyperthecosis are usually similar to those of PCOD (335,435) but the former are not only severely hirsute and balding but also virilized (clitoromegaly).

Ovaries of patients with hyperthecosis frequently do not tend to be cystic. Ovaries in hyperthecosis may be normal sized or enlarged (13,53,335,446,670). Since ovarian size and gross morphology may be normal (1,13), therapy cannot be gauged by the appearance of the ovaries at laparotomy or laparoscopy. There is associated histologic evidence of large granular or vacuolated lipid-containing cells which are distributed in clusters in the hyperplastic ovarian stroma at a considerable distance from the follicles. The stroma is firm with yellow areas containing nests of large clear luteinized cells with round vesicular nuclei and prominent single nucleoli (446). Occasionally cystic follicles similar to that of PCOD may be present (335, 704,809,838) which are frequently surrounded by a thickened luteinized theca interna (251). Luteinized atretic follicles may also be present. A hilus cell tumor or hyperplasia must be excluded after careful sectioning of the ovaries particularly in women over 40 years of age (53, 881). In some instances hilar cell hyperplasia (881) may co-exist with hyperthecosis (809) or the "gonadotropin-resistant ovary syndrome" (633). Unless bilateral ovarian and adrenal catheterization studies are performed in virilizing syndromes, small hilar cell tumors may be missed and bilateral ovarian wedge resection will be unsuccessful in the treatment of these women. Hilar cell tumors are usually less than 1.0 cm, unilateral and benign, may contain Reinke crystalloids, and must be considered in virilized perimenopausal or older women (574, 856,881). Of interest is the association of endometrial hyperplasia in 50% of patients with hilar cell tumors (48).

Hyperthecosis and PCOD are inseparable other than the virilization and the histologic finding of scattered nests of polyhedral luteinized cells in the ovarian stroma which is characteristic of hyperthecosis. Hormonally they have similar patterns of LH, FSH and T (335), and they may occasionally and transiently respond to bilateral ovarian wedge resection. Inappropriate gonadotropin secretion with increased LH may also be found in hyperthecosis (335, 446,971,985). Following wedge resection of the ovaries, four of five patients with hyperthecosis demonstrated normal LH levels and no change in FSH levels (446). Improved menstrual function was also described in a patient with hyperthecosis following ovarian wedge resection by Givens et al. (335) with resulting normal LH and FSH levels. Some, however, have concluded that PCOD and hyperthecosis are indeed two separate disease entities which may differ from one another histologically as well as by the frequent failure of clomiphene citrate or wedge resection to be effective in inducing ovulation (251). However, in the absence of a specific clinical or biochemical difference between the two, hyperthecosis should be properly retained in the spectrum of PCOD. As with PCOD, a familial tendency has been described in hyperthecosis (127,335,435), and no correlation between histologic findings and clinical evidence of hyperandrogenicity is present in either disease process (435,971).

Scully (124) and Judd et al. (435) found no increase of serum LH in their patients with hyperthecosis. Despite the normal levels of LH reported by Judd et al. (435), an increased LH/FSH ratio was present in two sisters with hyperthecosis. Following wedge resection no significant changes in the LH levels were noted, while the FSH concentration appeared to increase in one of the two patients. Androgens soon returned to preoperative levels with no improvement of clinical symptoms (435).

Studies of peripheral and ovarian venous concentrations of various steroids were described in two virilized patients with hyperthecosis by Abraham and Buster (1). The patients were 36 and 42 years of age, with normal menses, and one was parous with severe hirsutism and clitoromegaly. Both ovaries appeared grossly normal at laparotomy, as has previously been described by Bardin et al. (53). The 36-year-old obese patient had a well differentiated adenocarcinoma of the endometrium. DHAS levels were normal (1,66), while elevated serum values of 90–130 ng/dl, and 40–50 ng/dl, were noted for T and DHT, respectively. The 17OHP and P levels were also elevated, while 17α-hydroxypregnenolone and pregnenolone levels were normal. The ovarian–peripheral venous gradient was elevated for 17OHP, T and DHT. Following bilateral oophorectomy the levels of T, DHT, P and 17OHP were markedly reduced (1).

Variable ranges of serum T may occur in hyperthecosis (1,13,53,251,335,435,446,670). Abraham and Buster (1) postulated that a preferential androgen pathway from the delta[5] pathway occurs in hyperthecosis via 17α-hydroxypregnenolone to DHA, and then to delta[5]-androstenediol and to T, therefore bypassing androstenedione. The latter steroid may at times be relatively normal in hyperthecosis (1,66). No explanation was offered for the

suppressed DHAS observed in these two patients.

Six nulliparous obese virilized women with hyperthecosis were studied by Aiman et al. (13). Their age range was 13–28 years and one presented with primary amenorrhea, with oligomenorrhea in the others. Wedge biopsies were performed on four patients and another had bilateral oophorectomy. Grossly all ovaries were enlarged with thick gray surfaces beneath which a few follicle cysts were present measuring up to 5 mm in diameter. Similar histopathological changes were noted in all five patients, consisting of superficial collagenization of the ovarian cortex with only several developed follicles and follicular cysts present. Although the granulosa cell layer was not prominent, the theca cells were prominent and luteinized. Nests of luteinized theca cells were present in the cellular cortical stroma which stained readily with oil red O stain for lipid. The mean production rate of T for the six women with hyperthecosis was 2.1 mg/day, or eight times more than that found in normal ovulatory women and two times the average PR of T found in PCOD (54, 485). An increased PR of T in hyperthecosis has also been found by Bardin et al. (53), Judd et al. (435) and others (66,810). Aiman et al. (13) correlated the severity of the hirsutism and virilization in his patients with hyperthecosis to the T production rate. The mean MCR of the six women was 1238 l/day (approximately twice the normal female MCR) with an average serum T concentration of 180 ng/dl (range, 44–284 ng/dl). An increased MCR of T was also found by Judd et al. (435) and Belisle et al. (66). All six patients had increased androstenedione production rates, with a mean value of 8.5 mg/day, compared to 2.6 mg/day in normal women. The MCR of androstenedione was only slightly increased to a mean of 2338 l/day, and the mean serum concentration of androstenedione was 369 ng/dl (13). In five of the six women only 6–17% of the plasma T was derived from androstenedione. In patients with hyperthecosis, less than one-third of the total plasma PR of T comes from prehormones (androstenedione > DHA) while two-thirds is derived from direct glandular secretion, either ovarian or adrenal. The marked, albeit, transient fall in plasma T and androstenedione after wedge resection in patients with hyperthecosis implies that the ovaries of these women are the principal source of excess T and androstenedione. A large gradient in the latter two steroids was noted in one patient between ovarian and peripheral venous plasma. This has also been found by Bardin et al. (53), Abraham and Buster (1), and Belisle et al. (66). Similar findings were found by Nagamani et al. (670), who also noted an increased ovarian venous gradient for DHT, P and 17OHP. It is quite clear from ovarian-peripheral venous gradients that the major source of androgens in women with hyperthecosis arises from the ovaries (1,13,53,66,670). A significant adrenocortical contribution to the androgens in hyperthecosis is unlikely (13).

Estrone was the principal estrogen produced in these women and was formed from extraglandular sites from plasma androstenedione. Variable elevated or normal levels of estrone have been described in hyperthecosis with an increased E_1/E_2 ratio (335,670). This abnormal pattern of estrogen production may account for the fact that endometrial carcinoma has been reported frequently in a relatively small number of women with hyperthecosis whose endometrial histology has been described. In reviewing the literature of the endometrial histology of 17 women with hyperthecosis, Aiman et al. (13) found five with endometrial hyperplasia and three with endometrial carcinoma.

Endocrine studies were performed in five nulliparous, obese, infertile women with hyperthecosis aged 24–36 years by Nagamani et al. (670). All but one patient was hirsute since onset of menarche, and none responded to clomiphene citrate up to 200 mg/day for five days. Only one of the five patients had an elevated LH/FSH ratio (16/6.7 mIU/ml). Serum levels of T and DHT were markedly elevated, with mean values of 186 and 54 ng/dl, respectively. One patient had a serum T value of 270 ng/dl with a serum DHT level of 99 ng/dl. Serum androstenedione levels were slightly elevated in two subjects, while the serum P and 17OHP levels were increased (mean, 98 ng/dl and 309 ng/dl, respectively). Ovarian venous T, DHT and androstenedione were elevated in all five subjects tested (670), whereas normal ovaries do not secrete DHT to any extent. The significant peripheral-ovarian venous gradient for DHT suggests the presence of 5α-reductase activity in hyperthecosis (670). There was a nor-mal response of serum LH and FSH to LHRH in 3 patients tested (670). All ovaries were enlarged 2–3 times size. Four of the five patients had no follicular cysts present similar to the findings of others (1,13,53,66,335,670). The concentration of androstenedione/T in ovarian venous plasma is 25/1 in normal women, while all five patients reported by Nagamani et al. (670) had a ratio of 2/1–5/1. The significant peripheral ovarian venous gradient of P and 17OHP was also noted in their patients, suggesting again an increased utilization of the delta⁵ pathway leading to T (1).

The virilization and markedly elevated T levels in some patients with hyperthecosis makes it imperative that a diagnosis of a virilizing tumor be excluded. Normal levels of T, however, have been reported (123,251,335). Testing of hyperthecosis patients with hCG has demonstrated variable responses of T and is of little differential value (Table 9-10).

Significant reduction of hirsutism may occur in patients with hyperthecosis who undergo bilateral oophorectomy, unlike those who have bilateral ovarian wedge resection performed (985).

Some males in families with hyperthecosis may be mildly hypogonadal. This has also been suggested in PCOD family members by Cooper et al. (160). Some adult males in families with hyperthecosis have been reported to have an elevation of LH/FSH and decreased germ cells

TABLE 9-10. A Summary of Variable Plasma Testosterone Responses to Different Testing Modalities which Are of Limited Usefulness in the Differential Diagnosis of Hyperthecosis, and Virilizing Adrenal and Ovarian Tumors.

HYPER-THECOSIS	VIRILIZING ADRENAL ADENOMA	VIRILIZING OVARIAN TUMOR
Response to hCG (66,98,251, 446,971)	Response to hCG (87,195,281, 297,334,506, 850,865,974)	Response to hCG (333,700,929)
No response to hCG (1,53,122)	E₂ suppression (334,506,974)	E₂-progesterone suppression (333,988)
E₂ suppression (53)		Response to ACTH (300,865,929)
Lack of E₂ suppression (122)		Response to DXM suppression (455,865,929)

of the testes. Chromosomal abnormalities were not observed by Givens et al. (335), and X-linked inheritance was excluded by the finding of male-to-male transmission of the disorder. An autosomal-recessive inheritance pattern was also excluded by the finding of patients with oligomenorrhea and/or hirsutism in several generations of families. An autosomal dominant pattern may be present, but an X-linked mode also cannot be entirely excluded. (See Chapter 5.)

Differential Diagnosis of Non-Hyperandrogenic Amenorrhea

Prolonged absence of menstrual cycles in non-hirsute women necessitates a diagnostic strategy which should include laboratory evaluation (Table 9-11).

As previously noted, some women with PCOD may have minimal or no significant hirsutism and the presentation of secondary amenorrhea may not be uncommon. Absence of withdrawal bleeding following the administation of 10 mg medroxyprogesterone acetate for five days usually correlates with poor estrogen elaboration (< 40 pg/ml of plasma E_2) or the presence of uterine pathology (e.g., endometrial atrophy and Asherman's syndrome). Hypothroidism (primary or secondary) should be excluded by appropriate thyroid-function testing (T_4, TSH, T_3). Galactorrhea in association with amenorrhea and hyperprolactinemia may occur in PCOD but should alert the clinician to the possible presence of a prolactin-secreting pituitary adenoma or suprasellar lesions (craniopharyngiomas, meningiomas, suprasellar extension of pituitary tumors, chordomas, internal hydrocephalus, or a primary empty sella syndrome). A drug history of prior oral contraceptive use, or the use of other drugs such as phenothiazines, tranquilizers, cimetidine, reserpine, or methyldopa should be sought. Similarly,

women should be questioned regarding prior radiation or chemotherapy for a variety of hematologic or malignant disorders. Significant weight changes, psychological stresses and disorders, a history of a postpartum hemorrhage or complication, visual disturbances, polydypsia, changes in facial appearance, reduction of axillary or pubic hair, episodes of hypotension and lightheadedness, intractable headaches, hypopigmentation, asthenia and reduced sexual interest and initiative, all may be manifestations of hypothalamic–pituitary involvement which may be the basis for the secondary amenorrhea (147,637,744,1039). In the absence of severe weight loss, hypothyroidism, psychogenic stress or drugs which may suppress gonadotropin and/or increase serum PRL, repeated low LH and FSH (hypogonadotropic) determinations necessitate cone-down views of the sella turcica and/or CT scanning of the sellar and suprasellar areas to exclude space-occupying lesions and microadenomas of the pituitary. Further testing should include evaluation of visual fields, a 24-hour urine free cortisol and where indicated, tests of antidiuretic hormone adequacy, ACTH and growth hormone reserve (e.g., insulin tolerance test). TRH and LHRH testing is of value in further defining pituitary reserve of PRL, TSH, LH and FSH, but is not always diagnostic or helpful in differentiating between patients with hypothalamic involvement from those with pituitary dysfunction. Bergh et al. (75) found LHRH testing to be of little diagnostic value in the investigation of amenorrhea. Indeed, from a functional point of view the hypothalamus and pituitary act in concert and as a unit, and testing with TRH and LHRH affords more information relating to pituitary function when an adequate pituitary response is observed. This is particulary true for LHRH testing, and is similar in some respects to clinical observations seen in patients subjected to ACTH or TSH testing. Clearly, an inadequate response to a single bolus of tropic stimulation is insufficient for definitive diagnosis. Since there are occasional PCOD patients with primary amenorrhea, the differential diagnosis between hypothalamic–pituitary dysfunction and PCOD may at times be difficult. As noted previously, this is further complicated by the occasional association of pituitary tumors and PCOD. This is obviously more than of academic interest, in that some of the previously mentioned disease states may be associated with

TABLE 9-11. Initial Laboratory Evaluation of Non-hirsute Women with Secondary Amenorrhea.

1. Plasma LH and FSH
2. E_2
3. T_4, TSH
4. Prolactin

TABLE 9-12. Laboratory Evaluation of Patients with Hypergonadotropic Amenorrhea.

1 Plasma E_2
2. X-ray evidence of cardiovascular renal malformations (in patients <63")
3 Sex chromosome karyotype
4 Ovarian biopsy (laparotomy, laparoscopy)
5. Evidence of associated autoimmune diseases: Addison's disease Hashimoto's thyroiditis
6. Electromyographic evidence of muscular dystrophy (where indicated)

progressive or rapid visual impairment and/or reduced adrenal reserve which if not detected may be the cause of serious and life-threatening consequences.

The finding of elevated (hypergonadotropic) levels of serum LH and FSH is indicative of ovarian failure and warrants the following studies, which are outlined in Table 9-12.

Patients with hypergonadotropic amenorrhea, either primary or secondary, may be diagnosed by the finding of elevated levels of serum LH as well as FSH. Hyperresponsiveness of the LH to LHRH is usually noted and an increased prolactin reponse to TRH has also been described in sporadic cases with primary ovarian failure (391). Specific diagnosis may be identified by the availability of improved cytogenetic techniques and gonadal visualization and biopsies. It has been increasingly evident that in the category of hypergonadotropic amenorrhea there exists an approximate 30% incidence of phenotypically and cytogenetically normal females who have pure gonadal dysgenesis with streak gonads (857). Intermittent menstruation to the time of presentation may be present in up to 40% of patients with chromosomally competent ovarian failure (608). Although chromosomally competent forms of gonadal failure with XY karyotypes are infrequent, the risk of development of subsequent tumor in a dysgenetic gonad with a Y cell line prompts prophylactic

removal of both rudimentary streak gonads. The latter consideration does not apply to gonads of patients with ovarian failure of sex chromosome karyotypes such as 45, X or sex chromosome mosaicism as in 45, X/46, XX or other defects (608). Short stature and a varied frequency of somatic anomalies may be a clue to the existence of chromosomally incompetent ovarian failure.

Ovarian biopsy is important in differentiating between gonadal dysgenesis and the "Savage syndrome." The latter has also been called "gonadotropin-resistant ovary" syndrome, and biopsy in these patients reveals large numbers of primordial follicles unlike their relative absence in gonadal streaks. The "Savage syndrome" appears to be associated with an ovarian cell membrane receptor defect to gonadotropins which is partial in most instances (608). It appears that some of these patients will menstruate spontaneously and a few may conceive (698). The entity of autoimmune ovarian failure should be considered in a patient with documented autoimmune disease such as Addison's disease, Hashimoto's thyroiditis, idiopathic hypoparathyroidism, pernicious anemia and insulin-dependent diabetes mellitus (55). Tang and Faiman (901) conclude that antigonadotropin receptor factors play a role in only a few cases of premature ovarian failure, possibly only in those cases associated with other autoimmune diseases. It is clear that at the present time it is not possible to differentiate premature menopause (secondary amenorrhea with elevated gonadotropin levels prior to the age of 35 years) from the gonadotropin-resistant ovary syndrome by noninvasive means. Further studies will also be necessary to correlate serologic findings with the presence of follicles in ovarian biopsy material so that differences between the gonadotropin-resistant ovary syndrome and premature menopause due to depletion and/or atretic follicles may be distinguished without resorting to surgery.

Treatment of Polycystic Ovarian Disease 10

The treatment of polycystic ovarian disease is directed towards the following features which are present alone or in variable combinations in most patients with this syndrome:

1. Anovulation
2. Hirsutism
3. Dysfunctional bleeding

Patients with PCOD frequently present with irregular menses, or secondary amenorrhea in association with varying degrees of hirsutism. In the absence of significant hirsutism, treatment is directed to interruption of the chronically unopposed effect of estrogens on the endometrium. The persistence of the abnormal hormonal milieu predisposes the patient to the risk of endometrial cancer and possibly breast cancer. Thus even if the patient does not wish to become pregnant at the initial presentation, she is a candidate for treatment to insure withdrawal bleeding at intervals not greater than two months. If the patient wants to conceive, medical therapy is directed to the induction of ovulation. The presence or absence of hyperprolactinemia is also an important factor in deciding the modality of treatment in such patients. Prolonged intervals of amenorrhea with or without galactorrhea, particularly in those patients who may have been on previous oral contraceptive therapy, makes further investigation necessary to exclude co-existing pituitary tumors or hyperplasia. The latter characteristically are associated with moderately high levels of serum prolactin, and frequently do not respond to progestin withdrawal therapy or ovulation induction with clomiphene citrate.

Hirsutism is often the most distressing symptom in patients with PCOD, manifesting itself in negative behavior patterns both socially and psychosexually. The patient often has a distorted sense of body image; anxiety concerning their sexuality, as well as their fertility potential. A realistic and sympathetic approach to this endocrine and cosmetic problem necessitates accurate assessment of the degree of hirsutism present, ethnic origin, and previous response of the hair growth to such temporary procedures as waxing, depilatories or shaving. Similarly, the previous effects of electrolysis should be noted as well as the duration and frequency of such treatments. The endocrine evaluation should be helpful in deciding upon the appropriate treatment of the hirsute patient with PCOD, and combined with electrolysis, may offer significant reduction of the hirsutism.

Successful weight reduction of obese patients with PCOD may have a beneficial effect on menstrual dysfunction as well as on the hirsutism (461). It warrants emphasis that weight reduction is an essential part of the initial management of the patient. Treatment directed to pregnancy induction or hirsutism is facilitated after weight normalization.

Prolonged and frequent episodes of menstrual flow secondary to anovulation may characterize some patients with PCOD. Failure of the hypothalamic–pituitary unit to respond to the positive feedback effect of estrogen may be partially responsible for dysfunctional uterine bleeding. It is not infrequent to see patients with dysfunctional uterine bleeding alternate with episodes of oligo-amenorrhea. In the absence of the usual hormonal changes present in ovula-

TABLE 10-1. Therapeutic Modalities for the Treatment of Anovulation and/or Hirsutism Associated with PCOD.

ANOVULATION OR INFERTILITY	HIRSUTISM
1. Clomiphene citrate	1. Spironolactone
2. Glucocorticoid	2. Estrogen–progestin combination
3. Bromocriptine	3. Glucocorticoid
4. Gonadotropins	4. Medroxyprogesterone acetate
5. Tamoxifen citrate	5. Cyproterone acetate
6. ? Spironolactone	6. LHRH-agonists
7. LHRH	7. Cimetidine
8. Wedge resection of ovaries	8. ? Bromocriptine

tory cycles which prompt regular cyclic shedding of the endometrium, anovulatory patients, particularly those with high sustained levels of estrogens, develop spontaneous uterine bleeding due to excessive endometrial growth. Random endometrial bleeding may occur without the vasoconstrictive rhythmicity to help hemostasis. Medical therapy is necessary to affect a more orderly series of events leading to normal induction of withdrawal bleeding. Persistence of abnormal bleeding despite medical therapy is an indication for diagnostic procedures to exclude the possible presence of endometrial cancer, or other local or systemic diseases.

An outline of various therapeutic approaches to the treatment of the patient with PCOD is presented in Table 10-1. Treatment is directed either to anovulation (or infertility) or to the hirsutism.

The numerical order of the author's preference is indicated in the table. Occasionally combined treatment is employed (e.g., bromocriptine and spironolactone, bromocriptine and clomiphene or clomiphene and hCG).

Clomiphene Citrate

Clomiphene citrate is an orally active synthetic nonsteroidal weak estrogen with chemical similarities to diethylstilbestrol and chlorotrianisene (Tace®). Its similarity of structure to an estrogen allows clomiphene to act as a competitive inhibitor of estradiol-binding receptors and bind to estrogen receptors in the hypothalamus and anterior pituitary. The concentration of cy-

toplasmic estrogen receptors is reduced by inhibition of estrogen receptor replenishment in the hypothalamus and pituitary, as well as by competitive inhibition of endogenous estrogen at receptor sites of the ovary, uterus and cervix. By inhibition of the negative feedback mechanism of endogenous estrogens an elaboration of LHRH occurs with augmentation of LH and FSH release by the anterior pituitary. The subsequent follicular augmentation of serum estradiol induces a hypothalamic positive feedback with an ovulatory surge of gonadotropins. The ovulation is a reflection of follicular maturation induced by the rise in serum gonadotropins, particularly FSH (1013). Withdrawal bleeding following progesterone therapy (5–10 mg medroxyprogesterone acetate orally for 4–5 days) is an excellent indication that the patient will probably respond to clomiphene therapy. Other tests considered to be predictors of clomiphene responsiveness appear to be too impractical for ordinary practice. Such tests consist of positive feedback adequacy (829), and of differential LH and FSH responsiveness to LHRH before and after treatment with estrogen (443). The pituitary gonadotropin response to LHRH itself is not always helpful (315). It appears easier to test the ovulatory response to clomiphene itself rather than attempt more complicated procedures which may or may not indicate possible response to clomiphene. A strategy for treatment with clomiphene citrate is depicted in Fig. 10-1 (642). Clomiphene citrate is given orally in a dosage of 50–200 mg/day for 5 days starting from the fifth to the ninth day of a spontaneous or progesterone-induced menstrual cycle. The peak serum LH and FSH peaks usually occur seven days after cessation of the clomiphene treatment (day 16 of the cycle). Similar qualitative and quantitative measurements of LH and FSH occur in both PCOD patients and normal controls (1015). Although a biphasic basal body temperature curve may be present in association with elevation of plasma progesterone or biopsy presence of a secretory endometrium, luteinization of the follicle without ovum release has been documented (869). This may perhaps account for some of the disparity between apparent ovulatory rates and pregnancy rates in patients treated with clomiphene citrate.

The utilization of clomiphene citrate in the oligomenorrheic patient who does not seek fertility is inappropriate since it is transient and lasts only one cycle, and the increased LH stimulation by the drug may further increase the hirsutism (869).

Complications of clomiphene citrate treatment include vasomotor flushes (10%), visual symptoms such as scintillation and light halos, hair loss (<1%), abdominal bloating and discomfort. The latter may indicate a possible hyperstimulation syndrome of the ovaries. Its occurrence should mandate avoidance of intercourse and undue physical exercise and the drug is withheld while the ovaries regress in size. Although the visual symptoms are reversible, their presence should prompt immediate discontinuance of treatment.

Follicular maturation sufficient for ovulation induction may be gauged by serial serum FSH levels, particularly on the fifth day of clomiphene administration. Clinical evaluation for ovulation induction may be performed by serial examination of the treated patient from the 10th to the 21st day following clomiphene citrate administration. A change in the appearance of the cervix and ferning of the cervical mucus is usually indicative of adequate follicular maturation and estrogen production. Clomi-

phene may have an anti-estrogenic effect on cervical mucus with thick and scanty mucus and loss of ferning, resulting in poor sperm penetration. This may occur in 10–15% of clomiphene treated patients as determined by a post-coital test (379). Treatment of inadequate cervical mucus has been attempted by the administration of 0.3–0.6 mg conjugated estrogens from day 9 to day 15 of a clomiphene treated cycle (407,960). Theoretically, small doses of estrogens for several days following clomiphene administration may stimulate a more adequate mucus production without inhibiting ovulation (585) but this has been questioned by others (697). Garcia et al. (306) recommend the use of 5000 IU of human chorionic gonadotropin (hCG) at the time of optimal mucus or presumed ovulation with an additional 5000 IU after five days of basal body temperature elevation to insure adequacy of the luteal phase following clomiphene treatment. The high incidence of abortions in clomiphene-induced pregnancies may be related to luteal defects which may occur with clomiphene treatment. Fifty percent of patients with post-clomiphene endometrial biopsies demonstrate a defective endometrial pat-

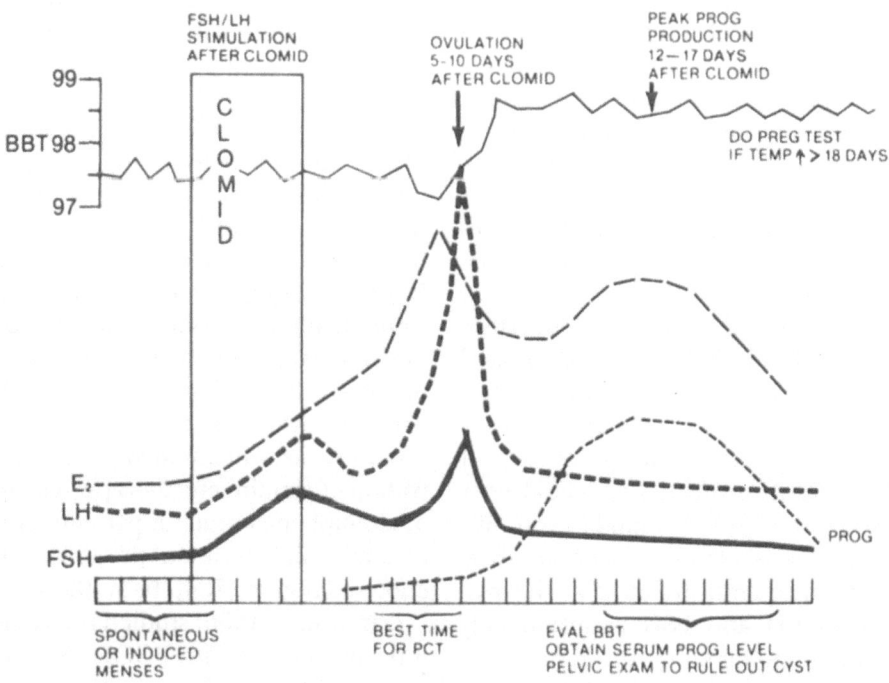

Fig. 10-1. Serum LH, FSH, E$_2$ and progesterone levels before, during and following treatment with clomiphene citrate (With permission, from Mishell DR Jr, March CM. Induction of ovulation. In. Mishell DR Jr, Davajan V, eds Reproductive Endocrinology, Infertility and Contraception. Philadelphia. F.A. Davis Co., 1979 317–337.) (642).

tern. Improvement of follicular function and therefore the corpus luteum function has been attempted by adjunctive therapy with hCG which may reproduce the LH surge (306,898). Ultrasonic assessment of follicular size, so that at least one follicle of 18 mm or more has developed, is valuable in allowing precise timing of the hCG injection in clomiphene–induced cycles with significant increase in ovulation and pregnancy rate (697).

Yen (1013) states, however, that the use of hCG together with clomiphene citrate has no rationale in PCOD, and may interfere with the adequacy of response to clomiphene. (An analysis of the results of sequential clomiphene and hCG, as well as clomiphene and human menopausal gonadotropin is described in a later section of this chapter). Other alternatives include increasing the dosage of clomiphene citrate and/or its duration of treatment to 10 days (306). The use of progesterone vaginal suppositories, 50 mg daily, has also been of some benefit in patients with a possible luteal phase defect associated with clomiphene therapy.

Monitoring for luteal phase adequacy during ovulation induction with clomiphene citrate is usually done by a determination of serum progesterone 5–10 days prior to the first day of the next menses (898). A mid-luteal endometrial biopsy may interfere with early nidations with reduced pregnancy rate in hMG-induced ovulatory cycles in which this procedure is carried out and is therefore not usually preferred as a diagnostic tool for evaluating the adequacy of the luteal phase. After six induced ovulatory cycles with clomiphene citrate and a normal hysterogram, laparoscopy is advised if conception has not occurred (898).

Yen et al. (1028) studied seven amenorrheic patients with proven PCOD who were treated with clomiphene citrate 50–100 mg for five days. An ovulatory response was noted in six of the seven patients treated. A mean increase of 166% and 139% of serum LH and FSH over basal levels, respectively, was found four to five days after initiation of clomiphene citrate therapy. This was subsequently followed by the ovulatory surge of LH and FSH approximately seven days following cessation of therapy. An associated maximal rise in serum progesterone was frequently noted three to five days after the LH surge, an interval of time occurring earlier and declining more rapidly than the levels seen in normal ovulatory cycles. Normal ovulatory

women with normal luteal function achieve a steady rise in P concentration after the LH surge with a peak six days after the LH surge which is maintained for four to five days. A maximal rise of serum P below 5 ng/dl and duration of a luteal phase less than 12 days is inadequate and indicative of defective corpus luteum function (1028). In the study of Yen et al. (1028), more than half of the PCOD patients studied had an inadequate luteal phase following clomiphene citrate treatment. It appears that treatment of PCOD with clomiphene citrate is associated with a significant incidence of luteal insufficiency (a luteal phase of 11–12 days or less) (943) and a disparity in a high "ovulation" and low pregnancy rate (144). It should be stressed that lack of conception following an apparent ovulatory response to clomiphene may also suggest the presence of infertility factors other than anovulation (784). This may include pelvic disease (tubal adhesions, endometriosis), cervical pathology or a significant male factor (379). Gysler et al. (379) state that nearly 90% of patients who ovulate following clomiphene treatment are able to conceive if a correction is made for associated infertility factors in such patients (most of whom did not have PCOD). They also question the validity of Marik and Hulka's "luteinized unruptured follicle syndrome" (578) which proposes follicle luteinization and progesterone secretion without ovulation as a frequent occurrence in infertile females.

It appears that the majority of patients with PCOD will ovulate following clomiphene citrate therapy (144). An initial course of therapy consisting of 50 mg of clomiphene citrate a day for five days is recommended for one to two cycles. If ovulation does not occur with a 50 mg dose of clomiphene, the dosage is increased by 50 mg increments the following cycles to a maximum of 200–250 mg/day for five days. Clinical evaluation of ovarian size is necessary to detect unusual ovarian enlargement prior to readministration of clomiphene therapy. The success rate of clomiphene citrate in patients with PCOD is generally high in view of the adequacy of endogenous estrogens (784,1015,1028).

Garcia et al. (306) studied the response of 35 infertile patients with PCOD to clomiphene citrate. Although 26 of 35 patients (74%) achieved ovulation, only 10 pregnancies occurred and four of these miscarried. An abortion rate of 25.3% was reported in a total of 63 pregnancies achieved with clomiphene citrate treatment in a diverse group of patients with anovulatory infertility (306). Despite the fact that 131 of the 159 patients (82%) with anovulatory infertility ovulated following clomiphene citrate therapy, only 63 became pregnant (48%). The success rate of clomiphene citrate appears to be related to the etiologic factor involved in the infertility. Patients with premature menopause, luteal phase defects, hyperprolactinemia, unexplained infertility and normal menstrual function are not likely to respond to clomiphene citrate administration.

In 1967, a summary of clomiphene treatment of patients with "Stein-Leventhal syndrome" reported that 359 of 436 patients ovulated after one course of treatment with an aggregate response of 95% to further treatment with clomiphene (428). Raj et al. (737) treated 55 infertile patients with PCOD with clomiphene citrate alone or with adjunctive therapy and noted that 91% ovulated and 51% conceived. Forty-three of the 55 patients had significantly enlarged ovaries. Clomiphene citrate alone was successful in inducing ovulation in 30 of the 43 patients (70%), and conception occurred in 17 of the 30 patients (57%). Clomiphene citrate induced ovulation in only one of six patients with "Type II" PCOD (adrenal etiology), while prednisone succeeded in achieving ovulation in 8 of 12 such patients. Conception only occurred in only two of the eight patients with a predominant adrenal component to the PCOD. The authors advocate the use of estrogen–progestin combination therapy to those patients who do not desire to become pregnant (737).

In properly selected patients with anovulation, 70–80% ovulate (340,869) and approximately 40% become pregnant following clomiphene treatment (869). The multiple pregnancy rate is 8%, almost entirely twins. This twinning rate contrasts to the general incidence of 1%. Most of the pregnancies (75%) occur during the first three treatment cycles. There is no increased incidence of fetal malformations in patients who conceive following clomiphene citrate (402,496,778). A higher incidence of multiple gestation occurs in PCOD as compared with other anovulatory patients with varying diagnoses (340,402). Goldfarb and Crawford (340) noted that 21.6% of 37 pregnancies induced with clomiphene in patients with PCOD resulted in multiple gestations, and appeared not to be dose-related. On the other hand, the same study revealed that only 12 among 131

other patients with anovulation and poor corpus luteum function resulted in multiple gestations. Ovarian enlargement also tends to be more frequent in patients with PCOD receiving clomiphene treatment (an incidence of 5%). This usually resolves spontaneously within one to four weeks.

In a report of 4098 patients treated with clomiphene citrate (558), 827 patients with PCOD were studied. Ovulation following therapy with clomiphene citrate occurred in 76.2%, while only 33% achieved pregnancy within six months (558). The disparity between ovulation and pregnancy was quite similar to that observed in clomiphene-treated women with other etiologies of anovulation (340,869).

Clinical experience with clomiphene citrate has indicated that obese women may require larger doses of clomiphene for ovulation induction (835). Lobo et al. (535) performed a prospective two-year study of 158 anovulatory women, most of whom appeared to have PCOD on the basis of an elevated LH/FSH ratio. Ninety-five percent of clomiphene-treated patients in this series ovulated. A positive correlation occurred between body weight and obesity and the dose required to achieve ovulation. Only 20% of patients weighing over 200 pounds were able to ovulate following a five-day course of 50 mg clomiphene citrate daily, and only another 20% ovulated when the dose was increased to 100 mg daily. Once ovulation occurred, obesity did not have any influence on the ability to conceive. Body weight and obesity did not differ in those that conceived from those that did not conceive with either 50 mg daily or a 250 mg daily dosage of clomiphene. PRL levels were in the normal range and did not show any correlation with the clomiphene dose required for ovulation induction. There also was no correlation between the serum LH, increased LH/FSH ratio and the dosage of clomiphene citrate necessary for induction of ovulation. Women who failed to ovulate with clomiphene or those who required 100–250 mg of clomiphene daily for ovulation had higher mean levels of serum DHAS than normal ovulating control subjects. Obesity may be associated with an abnormality of the hypothalamus and/or pituitary which may reflect partial resistance to clomiphene citrate (535).

Dupon et al. (220) studied the sequential changes of plasma androgens during spontaneous and clomiphene-induced ovulatory cycles in four normal and five anovulatory women. Three of the latter five women were diagnosed as having PCOD. Clomiphene citrate was administered in a dosage of 100–200 mg daily for five consecutive days. Four of five clomiphene-induced cycles demonstrated an increase in plasma androstenedione above pretreatment levels within three days after cessation of clomiphene treatment. This occurred prior to the thermal nadir of the basal body temperature graph. A lesser increase of plasma testosterone was apparent and was associated with an increase of the free testosterone index. The latter data indicated to the investigators a probable increased T production associated with clomiphene treatment in their relatively small series of oligomenorrheic patients. A return to pretreatment levels, however, was usually observed at the onset of the menses. In contrast to the clomiphene-treated women no significant elevation in T or androstenedione was apparent during normal spontaneous menstrual cycles, other than a modest midcycle rise of plasma androstenedione. Dupon et al. (221) explain the abnormally elevated androgen concentrations in some of their oligomenorrheic patients as reflecting ovarian hypersecretion in response to clomiphene-induced gonadotropin stimulation. It is possible that ovarian hyperandrogenism, which may be induced by clomiphene in PCOD, may interfere with normal follicular maturation, thereby reducing the frequency of ovulation and pregnancy.

Further data supporting the concept of ovarian hyperandrogenism playing a significant role in the reproductive failure associated with clomiphene treatment has been presented by Lawrence et al. (510). These investigators confirmed an absence of a rise in plasma T or androstenedione following clomiphene treatment of normal ovulatory women with luteal insufficiency. A slight increase of plasma T and androstenedione was noted following clomiphene treatment in 14 nonhirsute women with normal sized ovaries and amenorrhea–oligomenorrhea, while a significant increase in these androgens occurred in 13 clomiphene treated patients with PCOD at the presumptive pre-ovulatory and presumptive luteal phase. Although the ovulation rate was similar in both groups (75%) the pregnancy rate in those that ovulated was 75% in the nonhirsute amenorrhea–oligomenorrhea group and only 21% in patients with

PCOD. An analysis of plasma androgen values by Lawrence et al. (510) indicate that those that conceived had lower baseline level of androgens than those that failed to conceive. An exaggerated androgenic response to clomiphene appears to occur mainly in those patients who present with elevated androgen levels prior to treatment. It is clear that the incidence of low pregnancies in apparent successfully achieved ovulation may be related to the hyperandrogenism present in PCOD (510,1003). Preliminary suppression of the elevated androgens with a combination of estrogen–progestin or glucocorticoid therapy may therefore be of value prior to treatment with clomiphene citrate or other ovulation-inducing agents.

The combined administration of dexamethasone (DXM) and clomiphene citrate to anovulatory patients with adrenal or combined adrenal and ovarian dysfunction has been advocated by Fayez (253). He found that patients with a functional adrenal component to anovulation responded favorably when DXM was used as an adjuvant to clomiphene therapy. A combination regimen of clomiphene citrate and DXM 0.5 mg nightly for six weeks was administered to 12 normoprolactinemic women with PCOD in whom 250 mg clomiphene daily for five days and 10,000 IU hCG failed to induce ovulation (537). After the initial two weeks of DXM treatment withdrawal bleeding was induced with a progestin. This was followed by 250 mg clomiphene daily for five days, which was followed by 10,000 IU hCG five to seven days later. With this combination treatment regimen, 6 of 12 patients ovulated, with one pregnancy. The authors advocate the combination of clomiphene–DXM in clomiphene-resistant patients, particularly those with elevated DHAS levels. Decreased levels of T and unbound T following two weeks of DXM therapy was found in four ovulatory women prior to clomiphene treatment, with a significant reduction of elevated DHAS in these subjects. The authors further suggest that significant elevation of DHAS rather than T be used as a guide in selecting women for combined treatment with clomiphene and DXM prior to embarking on a course of gonadotropin therapy. The dosage of 0.5 mg DXM had no effect on serum LH, FSH, E_2, unbound E_2 or PRL (537). Administration of clomiphene during DXM treatment caused an increase of T and unbound T in the ovulatory patients after an initial suppression following two weeks of DXM treatment. Pharmacological doses of DXM (8.0 mg/day for five days) suppress the pituitary response of LH to clomiphene (862).

Koike et al. (482) studied 23 infertile patients with normoprolactinemic amenorrhea who were clomiphene failures and who responded to progesterone withdrawal. Sixteen of 21 patients had a relatively high serum LH with a normal FSH level. On day 2 of a spontaneous or induced menstruation, 2.5 mg bromocriptine was given daily for two days, and this was increased to 2.5 mg twice daily for 12 days. Clomiphene citrate 150 mg/day was given from day 5 to day 9 of the cycle. Fourteen patients (61%) ovulated following treatment, and 3 of the 14 women conceived (21%). There was no difference in responders and nonresponders in the pretreatment levels of LH, FSH or PRL. These investigators suggest that bromocriptine restores the responsiveness of the hypothalamic–pituitary–ovarian axis to clomiphene (482). The low pregnancy rate in this series may have been present due to associated oligospermia in four husbands.

In addition to its primary use as an ovulation-inducing agent, clomiphene may also be employed as a diagnostic tool and as adjunctive therapy of infertility (306). Its use as a therapeutic test of hypothalamic–pituitary–gonadal competence was reported by Wentz et al. (972), who studied a 6–8 hour pulsatile response of FSH and LH to an intravenous bolus of 100 μg LHRH before and after clomiphene citrate administration to 17 patients with secondary amenorrhea and oligomenorrhea. Five oligo-amenorrheic patients with polycystic ovarian disease were also studied. Following clomiphene administration the LH and FSH pulse frequency in five patients with PCOD was unchanged. PCOD patients who were clomiphene responders demonstrated a decreased LH peak and a decreased increment of LH and FSH to LHRH testing after clomiphene treatment. Wentz et al. (972) considered that the LHRH response following clomiphene administration detected abnormalities of negative and positive feedback stimulation. Hyperresponsiveness of LH to LHRH before and after clomiphene treatment in patients with PCOD who fail to ovulate may reflect a defect of the positive estrogen feedback mechanism. Similarly, an ab-

sence of a response to LHRH before and after clomiphene administration indicates a probable pituitary defect.

Estrogen–Progestin Combination

Although empiric use of glucocorticoids is not indicated in the treatment of hirsutism in the absence of a specific adrenal factor, suppression of ovarian steroidogenesis leading to hyperandrogenism may be indicated (223,854).

Goldzieher (341) states that the treatment of choice of hirsute patients with PCOD who do not wish to conceive at the time of their presentation is the use of an oral contraceptive agent of sufficent potency to suppress LH and subsequently ovarian androgen production. This implies the initial use of at least 80 μg of ethinyl estradiol for several cycles. He lists the therapeutic advantages of combination estrogen–progestin therapy as follows: (1) normalization of the elevated LH secretion; (2) subsequent lessening of ovarian hyperstimulation leading to a reduction of ovarian androgen production; (3) reduction of plasma androgens, which results in a decrease of androgenic symptoms such as acne, seborrhea, hirsutism and weight gain—a decrease in free T and the MCR of T also results (129) with an increased level of plasma TeBG; (4) estrogens apparently inhibit the conversion of T to DHT in the skin (320); (5) estrogens may have an inhibitory effect on adrenocortical activity possibly resulting in reduced adrenal androgen secretion; and (6) contraceptive steroids insure cyclic shedding of the endometrium which may be useful to prevent endometrial hyperplasia. However, Goldzieher (341) clearly noted that in the absence of clinical studies of the natural course of PCOD in the treated or untreated state, no firm conclusions are possible regarding the appropriateness of any form of therapy for PCOD. From what will be presented in this section it does appear that contraceptive steroids offer some advantages in the treatment of normoprolactinemic patients with PCOD. Caution should be exercised in administering estrogens to any woman with hypertension, marked obesity, a history of heavy cigarette or alcohol consumption, diabetes mellitus, or associated hyperprolactinemia. The well known side-effects of these compounds are reviewed elsewhere (343,870).

Administration of relatively modest doses of progestins alone does not alter pituitary–adrenal function (326). This has been demonstrated by the cyclical administration of 1.0 mg norgestrel daily for 21 days to normal women (326), as well as by 0.5 mg norethindrone daily (507). Norgestrel does not alter plasma LH, FSH, cortisol, or cortisol-binding globulin (326). The TeBG binding capacity may be significantly reduced by treatment with norgestrel and this is associated with a reduction of plasma levels of T, E_2 and E_1. Progestins compete with T for 5α-reductase in androgen target tissues resulting in decreased DHT formation (987). The decreasing order of biologic activity of progestins is as follows: norgestrel, ethynodiol diacetate, norethindrone acetate, norethindrone, megestrol acetate, norethynodrel and dimethisterone (987).

Mestranol appears to be stored more avidly in body depots than ethinyl estradiol, but the two estrogens are equipotent in their action on the endometrium and their pituitary inhibition (343). Some have claimed that ethinyl estradiol is twice as potent as mestranol in animals and humans (146). Amounts of estrogen and of progestin, insufficient to inhibit ovulation individually, when combined synergize in their pituitary inhibitory effect, thereby forming effective contraceptive compounds. Hormonal treatment of hirsutism with a combination estrogen–progestin has no effect on previous established hair, but may inhibit new hair growth after 6–12 months.

Controversy exists regarding the problem of post-pill amenorrhea following the use of contraceptive therapy in PCOD. Unfortunately, there is an absence of a well defined description of the natural history of PCOD, i.e., the untreated patient as opposed to those treated with an oral contraceptive or other modalities (342). A controlled clinical trial is needed in order to define the possible role of sex steroid therapy and its effects on subsequent fertility or other factors such as prolactin secretion.

A combination of mestranol 0.1 mg and norethindrone 2.0 mg was administered for 17–21 days to seven patients with PCOD by Givens et al. (332). The combination therapy effectively reduced plasma androstenedione and T by 58% and 65%, respectively. An increase of TeBG with an associated decrease in free testosterone

was also noted by these investigators (20). All elevated values were brought to normal levels during treatment. Suppression of the two androgens correlated with suppression of LH and occurred by the third week of treatment (332). The proportionate increase of the LH/FSH ratio, however, persisted during treatment, while a mean LH suppression of 71% was achieved with a mean FSH suppression of 31% (332). A greater increase of TeBG has been found in women receiving the combination of mestranol 0.1 mg and norethindrone 2.0 mg than with ethinyl estradiol 0.05 mg and norgestrel 0.5 mg (328). Normalization of plasma T and androstenedione occurred in approximately 80% of 39 consecutive women with diverse etiologies of hirsutism and oligomenorrhea during treatment with either combination estrogen–progestin regimens. These investigators suggest that hirsute women with elevated T and androstenedione levels following a three-week course of therapy should have the androgen levels restudied after two to three cycles of therapy (328).

Patients with PCOD and hirsutism or severe acne were treated with 100 mg estradiol pellet therapy subcutaneously in the lower abdominal wall at six-month intervals, with administration of 10 mg oral medroxyprogesterone acetate for the first seven days of the month to ensure regular cyclic withdrawal menstruation (301). All five patients with PCOD demonstrated regression of the bilaterally enlarged ovaries to normal size with improvement in hirsutism and acne following estrogen treatment.

The use of low-estrogen dosage oral contraceptive to suppress free T concentrations in nine subjects with PCOD was tested by Talbert and Sloan (899). Treatment consisted of 35 μg ethinyl estradiol combined with 0.5 mg norethindrone. While unbound T was reduced in eight of nine subjects studied, the total T was generally unchanged (possibly reflecting the uniform increase in TeBG secondary to the estrogen). No details on the effects of therapy on hirsutism was given in their study. Easterling et al. (223) noted a 58% mean reduction of unbound T in 15 subjects with PCOD following three months or more of an oral contraceptive combination of 80 μg mestranol and 1.0 mg norethindrone. No specific details on the effect on hirsutism was given in this report but the authors claimed that improved acne, hirsutism and decreased ovarian size occurred as a result of the combination estrogen – progestin treatment. It appears that more specific data is necessary to assess any efficacy of such treatment for the hirsutism in PCOD.

Poor results on suppressing excessive hair growth were noted with the administration of 0.5 mg betamethasone daily at bedtime for four months to seven hirsute patients (129). Empiric administration of combination estrogen – progestin therapy with a daily dose of 0.5 mg betamethasone for six months is frequently effective in reducing elevated T levels. Ten patients so treated had a reduction of the T production rate from 0.53 mg/day to 0.15 mg/day, with moderate improvement in hirsutism in 6 of 10 subjects (129).

Some investigators have noted that women taking estrogen oral contraceptives have reduced plasma DHAS levels (105,258,561,979). Fern et al. (258) demonstrated that plasma DHAS as well as androstenedione concentrations are decreased in oral contraceptive users. Similarly, androgen precursors such as plasma pregnenolone and 17α-hydroxypregnenolone are also reduced in such patients. Mean plasma DHAS in the control subjects decreased from 229 μg/dl to 134 μg/dl while plasma androstenedione decreased from a mean level of 299 ng/dl to 151 ng/dl following administration of Ortho-Novum 1/50® for a period of at least six months duration (258). There is experimental support suggesting that contraceptive steroids may exert an effect on adrenocorticosteroid synthesis at the level of pregnenolone formation via an effect on cytochrome P450 oxidase. Confirmatory studies of the suppressive effect of oral contraceptive treatment on DHAS was described by Madden et al. (561), who found a mean serum DHAS concentration that was 57% lower than normal ovulatory controls in the women who were taking oral contraceptive therapy (mestranol 80 μg and norethindrone 1.0 mg). No significant variations of DHAS during the menstrual cycle were noted in the ovulatory women. In view of the relatively long half-life of DHAS of 6 – 8 hours, no marked distinct pattern for episodic secretion of DHAS was identified (561). The reduction in DHAS with combination estrogen – progestin therapy does not occur as a result of an increased MCR.

A direct adrenal effect or a decreased ACTH release has been postulated (258,561,979). Improvement in cystic acne with reduction of serum DHAS was noted by Marynick et al. (590), who used daily 50 μg ethinyl estradiol combined with 1.0 mg ethynodiol diacetate.

It is of importance to appreciate a possible role of progestins in the suppression of adrenal androgens in that some reports have demonstrated no effects of estrogens on serum DHAS levels in castrate women receiving 200 μg ethinyl estradiol daily for three weeks (753), women receiving ethinyl estradiol 50 μg daily for 4 – 6 weeks (22), and postmenopausal women on stilbestrol or conjugated estrogens (4). No effect of acute or chronic administration of ethinyl estradiol on 3β-ol-HSD activity was noted in four ovariectomized women by Anderson and Yen (22). This was reflected by an absent effect on basal levels of the ratio of plasma concentrations of the delta^5/delta^4 steroid pairs. In vitro studies by Yates and Deshpande (1009) of E_1 and E_2 as noncompetitors of 3β-ol-HSD activity of human adrenal tissue have been previously noted (Chapter 6).

Decreased adrenal androgen secretion with age is reflected by a decrease in the plasma delta^5-steroid levels in postmenopausal women. Controversy exists, however, in that decreased estrogen levels have been postulated to account for the reduction of DHA and DHAS by Abraham and Maroulis (4) while this has not been confirmed by others (22,950).

Different observations were recorded in an age-matched control study of women on various contraceptives from six months to five years and normal controls (105). The mean level of DHAS in the treated group was 130 μg/dl, while that of the control group was 100 μg/dl. The percentage binding of DHAS to plasma proteins was not different in control subjects from those taking oral contraceptives. Although there was no clear relation between the estrogen content of the oral contraceptives and the reduction in plasma DHAS, a higher estrogen concentration (75 μg or greater) was associated with a greater reduction of DHAS than the 50 μg dosage form. Interpretation of results may have been clouded by the variety of oral contraceptives used and also by the various types and concentrations of progestins employed.

Further studies of the effectiveness of oral

contraceptive treatment in a well controlled series of patients with PCOD are needed.

Glucocorticoid

In 1953, Jones et al. (426) reported on the treatment of follicular phase defects with cortisone. Subsequently other reports have indicated the beneficial effects of cortisone treatment in suppressing plasma androgens of infertile patients with hirsutism and patients with polycystic ovarian disease (362,393,717,852,1035). Perloff et al. (717), in 1965, noted that the beneficial effect of prednisone on female infertility (41% pregnancy rate in "Stein-Leventhal" syndrome) may be due to its suppressive effect on plasma androgen concentrations. Steinberger et al. (884) studied 48 hirsute hyperandrogenic infertile women who were treated with 7.5 mg prednisone daily for a minimum of two months. Only 20% of women were not suppressed to T levels below 40 ng/dl and were considered to have an ovarian source of androgens. Normality of menstrual cycles occurred frequently during therapy, and a 44% pregnancy rate was achieved. A significant correlation was noted between the degree of T suppression, the shortening of the follicular phase and the lenghtening of the luteal phase (760).

Zarate et al. (1035) reported a pregnancy rate of 36% with prednisone therapy, and their series included some with failures following wedge resection of the ovaries. Rodriguez-Rigau et al. (760) noted that the use of 5 – 10 mg prednisone daily induced ovulation in 5 of 14 amenorrheic hirsute women and 10 of 11 anovulatory patients. A maximal effect was noted within two months. A subsequent report by the same group confirmed the adequacy of glucocorticoid treatment, which equaled the therapeutic effects of wedge resection in patients with PCOD (851,852).

Eight of 22 patient with PCOD with enlarged ovaries responded to prednisone therapy (36%), while the presumed ovulation rate was 45%. One woman who did not previously respond to wedge resection and another that failed to respond to clomiphene citrate conceived on treatment with prednisone (1035). Smith et al. (852) reported an ovulation and pregnancy rate in PCOD similar to that of patients who under-

went wedge resection, by employing 10 mg prednisone daily for 3 – 6 months.

As noted in Chapter 6, the effects of glucocorticoids may not necessarily be only on suppression of adrenal androgen production, but on ovarian androgen production as well (463). (Its efficacy in suppression of circulating androgens is also reviewed in Chapter 6.) There is incontrovertible evidence that this form of treatment suppresses plasma T in most hirsute patients and patients with PCOD (2,52,393, 713,852,884). A direct effect of prednisone on the hypothalamic – pituitary – ovarian axis can not, however, be excluded (760). Large doses of DXM (2.0 mg every six hours for five days) impair the pituitary LH and FSH response to LHRH (862).

Steinberger et al. (883) compared the incidence of spontaneous abortions in clomiphene-treated subjects to prednisone-treated subjects with ovulatory dysfunction. The control subjects receiving no therapy had a 14% abortion rate while the prednisone- and clomiphene-treated subjects has an abortion rate of 18% and 26%, respectively. The abortion rate in the prednisone-treated patients was not statistically different from control subjects. The incidence of twins in the clomiphene treated group was 5.9%, while the prednisone treated group had an incidence of 1.2%. The authors stress the beneficial effects of low dose glucocorticoid therapy in female infertility associated with hyperandrogenism and ovulatory dysfunction. It cannot be stated with clear-cut certainty that those patients who responded to glucocorticoids had a predominant adrenal source of androgens since the possibility exists that glucocorticoid therapy may also exert a direct effect on ovarian androgen production (418,463). Thus the interpretation of results employing DXM suppression as a guide to treatment is unclear in view of the apparent suppression of androgens of ovarian origin with DXM (463). Random fluctuations of plasma T of significant magnitude in hirsute women also make short-term DXM suppression studies suspect (409). It is also clear that the measurement of plasma testosterone before and after hCG stimulation while on DXM suppression is of no value in assessing appropriate therapy for PCOD (976).

A given dose of glucocorticoid is more effective in its ACTH-suppressive effect if it is administered at night. Occasionally a single dose of

0.5 mg DXM at night is adequate for suppression of hyperandrogenemia. Doses of DXM greater than 0.5 mg at bedtime may cause adrenal suppression and lead to side effects such as facial mooning. Patients should be warned of the need for steroid coverage during stress or surgery. Although corticosteroids may suppress the increased androgen production rate they have little or no effect on the growing hair itself. Thus the effect on menstruation appears to be more favorable than improvement in the hirsutism (409,976).

The possible role of hyperandrogenism in clomiphene resistant cases of infertility warrants a trial of glucorticoids in such patients prior to gonadotropin therapy. Toaff et al. (915) found androgenic hyperactivity in 35 of 60 patients with clomiphene resistant anovulation. Twenty-seven of these 35 patients had laparoscopic findings suggestive of PCOD (77%). An excellent response was noted following 0.5–1.0 mg DXM daily for 2–3 months. In the event that ovulation did not ensue, clomiphene citrate was added. Of 34 treated patients, 22 conceived (64.7%), while seven ovulated without becoming pregnant. Treatment consisted of DXM alone in 11 patients, combined DXM and clomiphene citrate in 19, DXM-hCG in two, and hCG alone in two (915).

Hatch et al. (385) also recommend the use of glucocorticoids to anovulatory infertile patients who are resistant to clomiphene. The dosage of 0.25 mg DXM given at night is increased to 0.75 mg until the androgens "normalize" (385).

Recognition of untreated adult-onset congenital adrenal hyperplasia is important since if pregnancies do occur there is an increased risk of spontaneous abortion (261), which may be prevented by glucocorticoid treatment. Sarris et al. (792) presented data on 30 patients with mild adrenal hyperplasia aged 17–33 years, most of whom were hirsute and oligomenorrheic. Ten of the 30 untreated patients had a total of 22 pregnancies, only two of which resulted in the delivery of liveborn infants, the other 20 having ended in abortions (91%). Obesity was present in five of the 30 patients and regular menses in five patients. Enlarged ovaries were noted in four patients. Two patients had primary amenorrhea, and the others had onset of menarche ranging from 10–16 years with a mean of 12.6 years. Five of the 30 patients had primary infer-

tility and another eight had secondary infertility averaging 3.7 years. The criteria of adrenal hyperplasia was based solely on elevated 17-ketosteroids above 15 mg/24 hr (range 15.2–35.4 mg/24 hr). Prednisone therapy was employed in a dosage of 2.5–10.0 mg/day. Eighteen of 20 patients with oligomenorrhea demonstrated ovulatory cycles within one month of treatment, while five with primary and secondary amenorrhea developed ovulatory cycles within one to two months of treatment. All 13 patients that presented with infertility became pregnant, the majority within three months of therapy. Of the 53 pregnancies, five ended in abortions (9.4%), while 47 had normal deliveries (88.7%). Supplemental cortisone was administered during labor. Forty-three percent noted improvement of hirsutism with long-term treatment. No teratogenic effect of glucocorticoids was noted, and this is similar to the data of Speroff (871).

Three months of treatment with DXM to 34 patients with idiopathic hirsutism and regular ovulatory cycles was associated with a significant suppression of plasma T, DHT, DHA, DHAS and androstenedione (652). Improvement in hirsutism was noted in 58% of patients. Those who responded to DXM had similar basal androgen levels and similar responses to ACTH and DXM. It is not improbable that "idiopathic hirsutism" (i.e., hirsutism without evidence of menstrual dysfunction or enlargement of ovaries) and PCOD reflect different aspects of the same disease entity of systemic androgen production. The circulating androgens are increased in PCOD, and to some extent the anatomical changes in the ovaries may reflect the effects of hyperandrogenemia. The evidence to support this concept may be derived from experimental data which indicate that thickening and capsular fibrosis of the ovaries may be induced by administration of androgens (807) and in that polycystic ovarian changes may result from adrenal hyperandrogenemia (32,76,541, 552).

Lachelin et al. (501) studied the effects of 1.0 mg DXM nightly for one month on basal levels and diurnal fluctuations of serum androgens and cortisol in four patients with PCOD and four normal women. These investigators demonstrated that only a minimal suppressive effect of 15% and 7% from basal testosterone and androstenedione levels, respectively, were noted in subjects with PCOD. Significant suppression of cortisol, DHA and delta⁵-androstenediol was also noted, as well as an obliteration of the diurnal fluctuations of these predominantly adrenal steroids. Their conclusion, based unfortunately on only four subjects with PCOD, is that DXM-suppressive therapy in PCOD appears to be less effective than treatment with oral contraceptives (332). Their conclusion does appear to be valid if a significant adrenal factor is excluded. It must be stressed again that neither routine ACTH testing nor DXM suppression studies accurately assess the significance of the adrenal factor in patients with PCOD.

Medroxyprogesterone Acetate (MPA)

Gordon et al. (351) demonstrated the effectiveness of medroxyprogesterone administration in reducing plasma T in normal men and women by acting as a potent suppressant of LH release. The administration of MPA results in an approximate 40–50% reduction of serum LH in normal women and patients with PCOD (350). Gordon et al. (351) reported that MPA treatment induces hepatic testosterone A-ring reductase activity resulting in an increased MCR of testosterone. Administration of a daily dose of 40 mg MPA orally for 4–6 weeks to six women with PCOD resulted in a 43% reduction in plasma T, a 23% increase in its MCR and a 33% decrease in the production rate of testosterone (350). Its use in PCOD has also been reported by Wortsman et al. (997), who studied 21 patients with PCOD whose diagnosis was confirmed by laparoscopy. All had oligomenorrhea or amenorrhea and 19 were hirsute. Depo-medroxyprogesterone acetate (depo-MPA) was administered intramuscularly in a dosage of 400 mg every two weeks for nine months. By the sixth to seventh month of treatment ovarian size was clinically decreased and confirmed by laparoscopic evaluation. A marked improvement in hirsutism was apparent between 6–9 months following institution of therapy. Six of the 21 patients had no improvement in the hirsutism during treatment with depo-MPA. A decline in serum LH and T levels of 70% and 40%, respectively, was noted after three months of treatment, while FSH and E_2 levels declined by 50% after six months of treatment (997). The reduction of serum LH preceded that of FSH

and was more pronounced during therapy with depo-MPA. A persistence of the gonadotropin-suppressive effect of depo-MPA was noted in that suppression of ovarian size remained for two years following cessation of treatment. Most of the patients remained amenorrheic during treatment or had occasional menstrual spotting.

A study of 24 hirsute women by Correa de Oliveira (170) treated with 100 mg depo-MPA intramuscularly every 15 days for 2–6 months also revealed improvement in hirsutism in 23 patients associated with a reduction in plasma T values. Three of 17 patients tested had abnormally elevated plasma T levels following completion of treatment. In only one subject was there no change in the elevated T value following six months of treatment with MPA. During therapy the patients remained amenorrheic. Return of menses occurred five months following cessation of treatment in two subjects who wanted to become pregnant.

Twenty-three patients with hirsutism and moderately elevated plasma T levels were treated for three months with 10 mg of medroxyprogesterone acetate orally three times a day for three months or more (234). Sixteen patients had oligomenorrhea, and four were amenorrheic. The mean pretreatment plasma T level of 133 ng/dl was reduced to 57 ng/dl after a trial of MPA therapy for 2–3 months (a reduction to 40% of the basal value). Twenty-one of the 23 patients had a decrease of plasma T to the normal range (<70 ng/dl). In 12 patients the DHT was reduced from a mean pretreatment level of 29 to 19 ng/dl. The apparent free testosterone concentration was also reduced from a mean pretreatment value of 1.00 to 0.69 ng/dl (normal adult female range was reported as 0.20–0.75 ng/dl). Three months following discontinuation of MPA treatment, plasma T values returned to pretreatment levels in 54% of patients. Ten of 20 patients in the above series of Ettinger and Golditch (234) developed regular menses during treatment with MPA, while amenorrhea developed in 2 of 16 subjects with pretreatment oligomenorrhea. In addition, three subjects with previous oligomenorrhea developed prolonged irregular spotting during treatment.

Some of the disadvantages of MPA therapy are its induction of amenorrhea, weight gain and headaches, and a long delay in the elimination of the tissue deposits of MPA (341). MPA has also been shown to decrease the percentages of binding of T and DHT to TeBG (268).

The use of medroxyprogesterone acetate may be an alternative in those patients where use of oral estrogen-containing contraceptive drugs are contraindicated or where side effects develop with other drugs such as spironolactone.

Cyproterone Acetate (CPA)

Cyproterone acetate (CPA) is a potent anti-androgen and progestin with reported effectiveness in the treatment of hirsutism and acne (382,409). One of the effects of CPA is a competitive inhibition of DHT binding to its cytosol receptor. CPA was first recognized as a progestin but was subsequently noted to have peripheral antiandrogenic and antigonadotropic properties. In view of animal experiments which have demonstrated the effectiveness of CPA in preventing the masculinization of male fetuses at a critical time in pregnancy it is of utmost importance to ensure the avoidance of the medication to pregnant women (382). The drug is administered orally 50–150 mg/day from day 5 to 14 of the menstrual cycle, together with 50 μg estinyl estradiol daily from day 5 to 25. CPA accumulates in fatty tissues and remains active for eight days after administration. Menstrual bleeding usually occurs 3–6 days after discontinuation of the estrogen. The addition of estrogen to cyproterone acetate prevents ovulation and the development of hypoestrogenism.

Compilation of data from five German centers revealed that CPA was most effective in the treatment of acne and seborrhea, while a distinct beneficial effect on hirsutism was noted in only 50% of patients after six months of treatment, and 69% after treatment which exceeded nine months (382). The main side effects include tiredness and an increase in body weight in approximately 20% of patients. A reduction in libido may occur in 10% of treated subjects. Additional side effects may include breast discomfort, nausea, headache, depression, irregular uterine bleeding and sleep disturbance (382). The loss of libido may be attributed to the antiandrogenic property of the drug, while the tiredness and increased body weight may be related to the progestational activity of CPA. The

regimen outlined by Hammerstein et al. (382) precludes the use of the combination CPA and estinyl estradiol treatment to those women who have medical contraindictions to estrogen therapy (hypertension, diabetes mellitus, hyperlipemia and obesity).

Dewhurst et al. (204) administered 100 mg CPA daily (days 5–14 of the cycle) and 50 μg ethinyl estradiol (days 5–25 of the cycle) to seven patients with PCOD for a period of six months. All demonstrated improvement in hirsutism. Cessation of treatment resulted in resumption of hair growth after three months. These investigators advocate an intermittent 3–6 months of treatment followed by a three-month period without CPA treatment.

Kuttenn et al. (498) administered 50 mg CPA daily from days 5 to 25 of the menstrual cycle along with 3.0 mg 17β-estradiol administered percutaneously from day 16–25. This regimen was given to 20 hirsute women, nine of whom had PCOD, while the other eleven patients had normal ovulatory cycles with normal levels of LH and T. Patients were treated for 3–20-month periods. Seborrhea and acne decreased dramatically after one month, while hirsutism frequently improved after the third month of treatment. Following nine months of treatment all patients had improvement of hirsutism. Plasma T and androstenedione were reduced to mean levels less than 30 ng/dl and 70 ng/dl, respectively, in both groups of hirsute females after three months of treatment. The pretreatment values of T and androstenedione were 64 ng/dl and 251 ng/dl, respectively. During the ninth month of treatment plasma T and androstenedione values were 21% and 17% of the mean basal values, respectively. A significant reduction of plasma LH and E_2 was noted, while FSH, urinary free cortisol, and urinary 5α-androstane-3α,17β-diol (3α-diol) were unchanged. Although these investigators found no clinical evidence of adrenal insufficiency, others have noted ACTH suppression which may last for months following withdrawal of the drug (316,424). Appropriate glucocorticoid coverage should be given to these patients prior to surgery for an interval of time no less than one year following treatment with CPA.

A recent study by Gaspard (308) reveals that a contraceptive combination of 2 mg CPA and 50 μg ethinyl estradiol (Diane®), which is taken from day 5–25 of the menstrual cycle, is a very effective form of therapy for severe resistant acne and seborrhea. It is obviously less effective in the treatment of hirsutism than larger doses of CPA.

The effectiveness of CPA in both PCOD and in idiopathic hirsutism suggests two levels of action: (1) suppression of ovarian androgen secretion and (2) a peripheral antiandrogenic effect (498). After three months an antigonadotropic effect is shown by the decrease in plasma T, androstenedione, E_2 and LH. Even when plasma T and androstenedione levels are normalized, clinical improvement continues, suggesting a peripheral effect of CPA on skin cytosolic receptors. The combination of CPA and E_2 percutaneously has a contraceptive effect due to its antigonadotropic action with an increased coagulation effect on the cervical mucus and induction of atrophy of the endometrium.

The drug is not yet available for use in the United States, but appears as an effective agent in the treatment of hirsutism. Its combination regimen with estrogen makes it necessary to follow the usual precautions for the latter, even if administered percutaneously.

LHRH Agonists

Theoretically LHRH agonists hold great promise in the treatment of PCOD since increased elaboration and pulsatility of endogenous LHRH may be a key factor in the pathogenesis of the disease. Ory (699) suggests that pulsatile LHRH therapy may be effective in stimulating ovulation in clomiphene resistant patients with PCOD. A modified insulin delivery pump system may be used for this and such compact devices are available (811). Previous experience with a long-acting LHRH agonist to ovulatory women with endometriosis revealed a reduction of serum E_1 and E_2 as well as a reduction of androstenedione and T (632). The effect of an LHRH agonist (GnRH-a) was studied by Chang et al. (137) in five patients with PCOD, six ovulatory women during the first few days of their menstrual cycle and eight young women who had bilateral hysterectomy and oophorectomy for benign gynecological disease. Each subject received 100 μg GnRH-a subcutaneously for 28 consecutive days. The patients with PCOD as well as normal subjects had an elevation of serum LH following one month of treatment

which was not statistically different from each other. Similarly the serum FSH levels were reduced by GnRH-a in ovulatory controls to levels seen in women with PCOD who demonstrated no change in FSH following treatment. A reduction in the pulse amplitude of LH was noted in both groups following treatment with the GnRH-a. After an abrupt rise of E_2 and E_1 following two weeks of treatment in ovulatory women which was not observed in PCOD patients, there followed a marked fall of both estrogens in both groups to levels seen in oophorectomized women. While only a modest reduction of androstenedione and T occurred in normal ovulatory women at the end of the GnRH-a treatment, patients with PCOD showed a reduction of both androgens to levels seen in normal subjects and oophorectomized women. However, unlike androstenedione and T, the levels of DHA and DHAS were unaffected at the completion of treatment and a similar ACTH response (10 μg/hr for four hours intravenously) of DHA and DHAS was noted before and after the administration of the GnRH-a in both PCOD and ovulatory subjects.

A divergent response of GnRH-a resulting in a persistently elevated LH and suppressed FSH level occurred in all subjects of this study (137). This suggests that GnRH itself may modulate gonadotropin secretion resulting in a differential release of LH and FSH. Unlike the initial rise of serum E_1 and E_2 in normal women, patients with PCOD demonstrated a progressive reduction of estrogens after the initiation of treatment. The reduction of serum androstenedione and T in patients with PCOD resulted from suppression of the ovarian contribution to these androgens, while no adrenal effect on DHA and DHAS was noted. The suppression of both ovarian estrogens and androgens suggested effective suppression of ovarian steroid secretion. This could occur via desensitization of the gonadal response to persistent nonpulsatile LH levels and/or direct inhibition of ovarian steroid synthesis (399). The suppression of the androgens androstenedione and T to levels noted in oophorectomized subjects suggests that the five patients studied by Chang et al. (137) had elevated androgens of ovarian origin. A separate and coexisting disorder of the adrenals accounted for the elevation of serum DHA and DHAS noted in the five subjects which was unaffected by administration of GnRH-a. Thus suppression of ovarian steroidogenesis with this treatment does not appear to influence adrenal androgen secretion in PCOD. ACTH excess is also not responsible since basal levels of ACTH are similar in patients with PCOD and normal subjects (139). It is likely that diagnostic separation of ovarian from adrenal secretion may be accomplished by the use of this GnRH agonist. The search for other more selective LHRH agonists in the treatment of PCOD may well be rewarding.

Cimetidine

Vigersky et al. (957) employed cimetidine, a histamine H_2 receptor antagonist, as an antiandrogen in the treatment of hirsute women, four of whom had PCOD. The dosage administered was 300 mg, five times daily, for three months. A significant reduction in the rate of hair growth was observed while no effect on serum androgens was noted. Serum LH, DHT, T, free T and urinary 17-ketosteroids were unaltered during treatment. Four of the five patients that responded to cimetidine had a greater than 50% reduction in the rate of hair growth (facial, thigh or chest hair). Decreased oiliness of face and skin was also noted. Cimetidine may block androgen action by inhibiting binding of DHT to androgen receptors (283).

Spironolactone

Spironolactone, an aldosterone antagonist, may be of benefit in the treatment of hirsutism via competitive inhibition with the intracellular androgen receptor in human hair follicles. Spironolactone also inhibits the first step of the binding of T and/or DHT to prostate, adrenal, skin and other target tissue cytosol and nuclear androgen receptors (172). Since an elevated intraovarian androgen concentration inhibits follicular maturation (551), it is possible that the antiandrogenic effect of spironolactone within the ovary may facilitate resumption of cyclic ovarian function. Some investigators have postulated inhibition of 21-hydroxylase, or of 17,20-desmolase activities by spironolactone (549,889). A loss of activities of cytochrome P-450 enzymes that catalyze the hydroxylation of steroids in the adrenals and gonads has also been demonstrated

(635,636,889). It appears that spironolactone acts as a potent antiandrogen by (1) suppression of biosynthetic pathways leading to testosterone, (2) increased peripheral conversion of T to estradiol, and (3) competitive inhibition of the binding of DHT to intracellular receptors. Boisselle and Tremblay (91) administered a dosage of 25 mg twice daily to six hirsute females and 10 normal controls. A 50% reduction of urinary 17-ketosteroids was noted after six months of therapy and was associated with a decrease in the T production rate. A significant fall in the blood production rate of T was noted as early as seven days after initiation of spironolactone therapy in normal subjects. An increased MCR of testosterone with an approximate 50% reduction in T production rate and plasma concentration of T was noted in normal as well as hirsute women following six months of therapy. This was associated with a reduced rate of hair growth and a decrease in the diameter of the hair shaft occurring within 4–5 months of initiation of spironolactone treatment. Normal adult female volunteers did not show a significant reduction of plasma T after five days of the spironolactone regimen although an increase of P and 17-OHP was noted.

The therapeutic effect of spironolactone was studied in 30 hirsute nonobese patients (many with PCOD) by Shapiro and Evron (823), who administered 100 mg twice a day from day 4–22 of each cycle for a period of 6–13 months. Improvement in hirsutism was frequently evident 3–5 months after institution of therapy. After 13 months of treatment, hirsutism improved in 23 of 30 patients. Disturbed menstrual abnormalities were regulated in four patients, and improvement of hirsutism occurred in women with elevated or normal serum T concentration. Those with elevated serum T levels had a mean T reduction of 80% following 6–9 months of treatment. Although serum LH was unchanged, serum FSH was significantly reduced and estradiol increased during therapy. Eight of 30 women complained of metrorrhagia during therapy, which necessitated reduction of the dosage to 100 mg/day. Hair density grading revealed improvement after six months of therapy, and this was associated with a reduction in acne. In another study Evron et al. (243) attempted to determine whether suppression of androgens by spironolactone might restore ovulation and normal menstrual cycles in anovulatory hyperandrogenic women. Spironolactone was administered from the 5th to the 21st day of the menstrual cycle to 13 hirsute and oligomenorrheic women in a dosage of 100–150 mg/day for six cycles. Five of the 13 women had PCOD on the basis of laparoscopy. Spironolactone treatment caused a significant reduction of serum LH, T and urinary 17-ketosteroid values. The mean pretreatment level of T of 70 ± 8.0 ng/dl was suppressed to 25 ± 3 ng/dl. LH values normalized during treatment from a pretreatment level of 27.2 ± 0.3 mU/ml to a post-treatment level of 12.4 ± 1.0 mU/ml, while FSH levels were unchanged. A slight reduction of PRL was noted in the subjects although basal values were in the normal range. Values of serum P increased as a result of induced ovulation. Nine of 13 women (70%) showed improvement of hirsutism, and 11 of 13 had regular cycles restored (85%) with induction of ovulation and absence of serious side effects (243). The reduction of LH levels by Evron et al. (243) may have been induced by suppression of androgens and/or their peripheral conversion to estrone. In normal volunteers, spironolactone elevated or did not change the LH/FSH ratio (549), while Rose et al. (767) found elevated plasma LH levels in hypertensive males receiving spironolactone. The latter group also found elevated blood E_2 and reduced T levels with an increased MCR of T. An intermittent type of spironolactone therapy may lessen the tendency to electrolyte imbalance or menstrual disturbances.

Cumming et al. (182) administered 100–200 mg spironolactone daily to 12 amenorrheic women with PCOD for seven days. Subsequently 3- and 12-month treatments of the drug were administered to 20 patients, 10 of whom were amenorrheic with PCOD and 10 of whom had regular menses with "idiopathic hirsutism." A brief elevation of LH regressed to normal one week after cessation of the treatment with spironolactone, while no change occurred in serum PRL, FSH, DHA, E_1 or E_2. There was, however, a transient rise in 17-OHP and progressive decline of serum T and androstenedione which reached their nadir one week following cessation of therapy. Long-term administration of the drug for 3–12 months resulted in an improvement of hirsutism in 19 of the 20 patients with PCOD as well as those with "idiopathic hirsutism" and regular menses. A 40% maximum

decrease of hair-shaft diameter occurred at 6 months, with no further change with continued treatment to 10 months. Improvement or decrease in oiliness of skin and acne was reported in 11 patients. The reduction in quantity and quality of facial hair growth in patients with PCOD was associated with a lowering of circulating total and free T by approximately 50% and 30%, respectively, after three months of treatment (182). The latter levels, however, remained significantly higher than those found in patients with "idiopathic hirsutism" treated with spironolactone. A significant reduction of serum androstenedione from a mean of 300 ng/dl to approximately 200 ng/dl was noted after three months of therapy of patients with PCOD, while the levels of androstenedione remained unaltered (approximately 150 μg/dl) in patients with "idiopathic hirsutism." The mean TeBG concentration was unchanged in both groups of patients under treatment with spironolactone for 12 months, as were levels of DHAS, DHA, cortisol, LH, P, and 17OHP. Cyclic menses occurred during treatment in 6 of 10 amenorrheic women with PCOD while ovulatory women had unaffected menses. The early effects in causing an elevation of 17OHP together with a reduction in androgen levels of T and androstenedione after 7–14 days may suggest, as previously stated, that spironolactone inhibits the cytochrome P-450 dependent 17,20-desmolase enzyme system. Adrenal androgens appear to be unaffected by treatment in view of normal levels of DHA, DHAS and cortisol (182). In addition to the reduction of androgens, the effect of spironolactone was also operative in women with "idopathic hirsutism" with relatively normal androgen levels, thereby suggesting an additional direct inhibitory effect of spironolactone on the hair follicle.

Milewicz et al. (640) reported on the use of spironolactone in 34 severely hirsute women with PCOD who had menstrual abnormalities. Hormonal studies were compared to values obtained prior to administration of 100 mg/day of spironolactone. Following three months of treatment all patients demonstrated a significant decrease of hirsutism, particulary facial hirsutism. Only 1 of 25 patients developed ovulatory cycles, while the others had regular cyclic anovulatory menses every 22–25 days. No liver or electrolyte abnormalities were noted. No significant change in body weight was observed, and a reduction in libido was present in only one patient. The levels of LH and FSH were unchanged over the three-month treatment period, while a modest reduction of serum PRL was noted during treatment from a mean value of 11.4 ng/ml to 8.6 ng/ml. Three of four additional hyperprolactinemic patients with PCOD studied by this group (range of serum PRL 25–30 ng/ml) experienced a moderate reduction of the serum PRL level to a range of 9–20 ng/ml. The effect of spironolactone on serum androgens was significant (Table 10-2) (640).

The basal T, androstenedione and DHAS levels of the 34 patients with PCOD were statistically different from control subjects and the values were significantly suppressed following three months of treatment. The suppression of androgens confirmed the clinical data of Rose et al. (767). The latter study, however, demonstrated increased conversion of T to E_2, while the data of Milewicz et al. (640) failed to demonstrate increased levels of urinary estrogens. Furthermore, the study of Ober and Hennessy (694) also noted a reduction of E_2 levels during spironolactone treatment in the two-patients treated with the drug.

A combination treatment of bromocriptine and spironolactone to two women with PCOD has been described by Blum et al. (88). The combined treatment consisted of 15–20 mg/day of bromocriptine and 100 mg/day of spironolactone. One patient was a 21-year-old hirsute female with menstrual dysfunction with a plasma PRL of 29 ng/ml, a plasma T of 100 ng/dl, and an LH/FSH ratio of 18.0/8.0 mU/ml. Although slight improvement was noted in the hirsutism following treatment with 15 mg bromocriptine for five months, the addition of 100 mg/day of spironolactone resulted in ovulatory cycles and significant reduction of hirsutism at the second month of treatment. One year after institution of combined therapy the patient was maintained on 5 mg/day bromocriptine and 50 mg/day spironolactone. Repeated trials to reduce the drug regimen resulted in the appearance of increased facial hirsutism. Another patient, a 32-year-old female with ovarian hyperthecosis and plasma T values ranging from 100–150 ng/dl, had wedge resection of the ovaries with unremitting hypertension and persistence of the elevated plasma T. Institution of bromocriptine 20 mg/day caused a response of her blood pressure without improvement of the hirsutism. The addition of 100 mg/day spironolactone resulted in a marked reduction of hirsutism but menses remained anovulatory. The actions of the two drugs appear to be complimentary. Bromocriptine may decrease hirsutism and lower the T level in the plasma of PCOD subjects, possibly by reducing increased plasma prolactin and LH (429). Spironolactone further reduces the action of androgens at receptors, reducing their synthesis, increasing their MCR and increasing the conversion of T to estradiol (767). The reduction of the T/E_2 ratio in adult males treated with spironolactone accounts for the gynecomastia and impotence which may occur with this drug (767).

Additional reports have described the beneficial effects of spironolactone in patients with PCOD (89,694). The reduction of serum LH in the patient with ovarian hyperthecosis described by Blum et al. (89) may have been due to the addition of bromocriptine to the management of the patient, which probably suppressed LH since it acts as a dopamine agonist. Judd et al. (429) have demonstrated that dopamine (DA) suppresses plasma LH in agonadal (ovariectomized) women with elevated LH and FSH levels more than normal women on day 2 of

TABLE 10-2. Serum Androgens (mean ± S.D.) in Patients with PCOD Before and After Spironolactone Therapy.

	N (PTS.)	T (NG/DL)	ANDROSTENEDIONE (NG/DL)	DHAS (μG/DL)
Pretreatment	34	112.0 ± 32.0	315.3 ± 78.8	293.0 ± 50 0
Post-treatment	34	72.6 ± 22 8	208.1 ± 59.1	197.5 ± 41.1
Controls	50	55.0 ± 25.7	97.5 ± 42.5	233.0 ± 40.0

With permission from Milewicz A, Silber D, Kirschner MA Therapeutic effects of spironolactone in polycystic ovary syndrome Obstet Gynecol 1983; 61 429–432) (640)

their cycles. On the other hand, the mean suppression of serum PRL with DA is greater in normal women than in agonadal subjects. It appears that spironolactone offers a relatively safe and effective therapy for patients with PCOD. It is of particular usefulness in hirsute patients and frequently causes resumption of menses, although ovulation is not often observed.

Bromocriptine

Bromocriptine (2-bromo-alpha-ergocryptine) is an ergot derivative with dopamine receptor agonist effects that lowers serum prolactin levels. Its actions can be explained by prolonged stimulation of DA receptors on pituitary lactotropes. The dose of bromocriptine that reduces serum PRL is 10 times lower than that which improves the symptoms of Parkinson's disease. A broad spectrum of pituitary lactotrope sensitivity to bromocriptine, and by analogy to endogenous dopamine, has been suggested by Thorner et al. (910). Bromocriptine is available as the methane sulfonate (mesylate) in 2.5 mg tablets and 5.0 mg capsules. Mild side effects occur early and include nausea, vomiting, orthostatic hypotension and nasal stuffiness. Vascular effects such as Raynaud's phenomenon and erythromelalgia of the lower extremities may occur occasionally, as well as neuropsychiatric symptoms in 1% to 2% of patients (709). Other rare side effects may occur such as exacerbation of angina, blurring of vision, dyspnea and rarely gastrointestinal hemorrhage (113).

Infertility is one of the more important consequences of hyperprolactinemia and may be present even if plasma PRL levels are only slighty elevated. Bromocriptine is effective against infertility due to hyperprolactinemia. About 20% of patients with PCOD may have elevated plasma PRL levels (709) and bromocriptine frequently restores fertility in these instances (78). Patients are usually advised to employ contraception until a resumption of menstrual flow follows institution of treatment. A subsequent delay in menses may indicate pregnancy and if pregnancy is confirmed the drug may be discontinued. In a large series of women treated with bromocriptine during the early weeks of pregnancy, no increased incidence of spontaneous abortions or of congenital malformations was noted (932). Bromocriptine

rarely restores fertility in infertile women with PCOD whose plasma PRL levels are not elevated (709).

Some normoprolactinemic patients have been reported to respond to bromocriptine (816,921). Van der Steeg and Coelingh Bennink (941) studied 19 women with normoprolactinemic post-pill anovulation with no roentgenographic evidence of a pituitary tumor and noted a response in 14 of 19 patients treated with bromocriptine. Onset of menses occurred at a mean of 32 days after institution of 1.25 mg bromocriptine twice a day with meals. The mean reduction in serum PRL by bromocriptine was greater in non-responders than responders (6.5–8.0 and 2.5–4.0 ng/ml, respectively) (941). In another report, Seppälä et al. (814) noted that treatment with bromocriptine resulted in ovulation in 4 of 11 anovulatory patients with basal plasma prolactin values below 15 ng/ml. These patients had associated weight loss and/or post-pill anovulation. Twenty-three patients with amenorrhea (including 9 post-pill, 8 weight-related, and 5 postpartum) were treated with bromocriptine by Seppälä et al. (816). Eleven patients had elevated basal PRL levels, including the eight patients with galactorrhea. The mean basal level of PRL in the normoprolactinemic group was 12.5 ng/ml, with an E_2 level of 59.6 pg/ml. The E_2 levels increased in both hyperprolactinemic and normoprolactinemic subjects. The normoprolactinemic group had an increase from a mean basal E_2 value of 59.6 pg/ml to 186.5 pg/ml, while the mean E_2 value in the hyperprolactinemic subjects rose from 27.0 pg/ml to a level of 97.8 pg/ml after 3–5 weeks of bromocriptine treatment. Treatment did not significantly alter the levels of serum LH and FSH in both groups. Menstruation was restored in 5 of 12 normoprolactinemic subjects whose amenorrhea was associated with self-induced weight loss. Van der Steeg and Coehlingh Bennink (941) interpret the above findings as probably due to stimulation of LHRH by bromocriptine. It appears that bromocriptine may be effective in diverse hypothalamic etiologies of amenorrhea or anovulation such as post-pill amenorrhea, weight-related amenorrhea or amenorrhea following emotional stress. It is possible that the drug may also exert a direct hypophyseal effect with induction of a preovulatory LH surge (941). A valid criticism of the studies of Seppälä et al.

(814) and van der Steeg and Coehlingh Bennink (941) is that they were uncontrolled studies (421).

In view of the episodic nature of PRL secretion single morning specimens of PRL may not accurately reflect the cumulative 24-hour secretion. To avoid stress hyperprolactinemia and the random pulsatile secretion of PRL, three to four speciments should be drawn over a fixed period of time (e.g., one hour) and pooled (421). One of the mechanisms where there may be a return of ovulatory menses in normoprolactinemic amenorrheic women treated with bromocriptine may be the presence of enhanced PRL secretory capacity in these patients. Corenblum and Taylor (167) attempted to define the normoprolactinemic patients with amenorrhea who responded to bromocriptine from those who did not. All the 14 amenorrheic women had demonstrable galactorrhea on physical examination and none had weight loss, recent pregnancy or a history of drug ingestion. Basal serum PRL and FSH were normal on at least three occasions. Four of the 14 patients had elevated levels of serum LH, and normal levels were observed in 10 subjects. Sellar tomograms were normal in all subjects tested. Medroxyprogesterone acetate 10 mg/day orally for five days achieved withdrawal bleeding in all subjects. After a TRH stimulation test (200 μg intravenously), and a chlorpromazine (CPZ) stimulation test (25 mg intramuscularly), all 14 patients were treated with 2.5 mg bromocriptine twice daily. Nine of the 14 women treated with bromocriptine demonstrated evidence of ovulatory cycles and five conceived. Five of the 14 women did not have a return of menses. There was no difference in clinical characteristics between the women who achieved menstruation with treatment and those who did not, and serum PRL levels ranged between 3–14 ng/ml during bromocriptine therapy in both groups. TRH responsiveness was exaggerated with a mean peak PRL value of 88 ng/ml in the women responsive to treatment, unlike the mean PRL peak of 32 and 26 ng/ml in the nonresponders and control subjects, respectively. Hyperresponsiveness to CPZ was noted in six responders to bromocriptine, while the nonresponders had a peak PRL level similar to control subjects. It must be stressed that the study by Corenblum and Taylor (167) only included patients with amenorrhea and unexplained galactorrhea. Hyperre-

sponsiveness of pituitary lactotropes occurred following TRH and CPZ stimulation in the bromocriptine responders, suggesting enhanced PRL secretory capacity in those patients. The normal basal levels of serum PRL in the latter patients and normal or elevated gonadotropin levels suggest normal hypothalamic DA content. Furthermore, absence of a primary hypothalamic dopaminergic dysfunction is suggested by hyperresponsiveness of both TRH and CPZ. It is possible that the group of normoprolactinemic subjects with amenorrhea and galactorrhea studied by Corenblum and Taylor (167) may have a disorder at the level of the lactotrope or possibly increased hypothalamic serotoninergic activity.

In a study of serial PRL measurements throughout the menstrual cycle, small but significant transitory preovulatory hyperprolactinemia was noted in 45 of 48 patients with idiopathic infertility (69). The latter patients had evidence of ovulation and adequacy of luteal phase, but the mid-cycle hyperprolactinemia exceeded that recorded in 28 previously fertile control subjects. While 18 of the 45 infertile patients demonstrated the hyperprolactinemia only at mid-cycle, 27 of the 45 patients also demonstrated more significant hyperprolactinemia during the late luteal phase as well. Treatment with bromocriptine was followed by conception in 18 of these 45 patients. The investigators concluded that minimal hyperprolactinemia of short duration can affect reproduction by its possible effect on fertilization, implantation, embryogenesis or on the corpus luteum of pregnancy. Confirmation of these interesting findings should be attempted.

A report by Lenton et al. (518) of 40 normoprolactinemic ovulatory women with unexplained infertility of 2–10 years duration and normal luteal function noted a 63% cumulative pregnancy rate after 10 months of bromocriptine therapy. No matched controls were studied in the latter study. A double-blind study of 47 patients with unexplained primary infertility and normal serum prolactin levels and matched controls treated with 2.5 mg bromocriptine twice a day for six months demonstrated no difference in cumulative pregnancy rate between the two groups (999). Similarly, Saunders et al. (794) described the results of bromocriptine treatment of 15 normoprolactinemic women with a defective luteal phase. The results were disappointing, and the possibility exists that 15 mg/day of bromocriptine may have been an excessive dosage since 7.5 mg/day of bromocriptine may reduce serum progesterone (803). A previous study by Crosignani et al. (179) failed to demonstrate any difference between bromocriptine and a placebo in patients with normoprolactinemic amenorrhea. It appears that the use of bromocriptine for unexplained normoprolactinemic infertility is questionable, and therapy should be reserved for those patients with documented hyperprolactinemia.

Falaschi et al. (248) studied 47 patients with PCOD and 13 normal controls with a short-term bromocriptine suppression test consisting of 2.5–7.5 mg/day for 13 days. Basal prolactin levels ranging between 20–50 ng/ml were present in 27% of PCOD patients, with a mean level of 29.4 ± 3.1 ng/ml. Basal plasma T levels in this group was 107.8 ± 7.0 ng/dl. There was a significant reduction of plasma prolactin to 3.6 ± 0.2 ng/ml and 1.9 ± 0.1 ng/ml after 7 and 13 days of bromocriptine, respectively, while T levels were suppressed to 57.0 ± 3.3 ng/dl and 50.8 ± 4.7 ng/dl after 7 and 13 days of bromocriptine treatment, respectively (248). These investigators suggest that the dopamine agonist may inhibit the high pulsatile LH levels via a hypothalamic effect, thereby reducing ovarian androgen stimulation.

Successful treatment of infertility in hyperprolactinemic PCOD patients with bromocriptine has been described by others (913). Six of eight normoprolactinemic subjects with galactorrhea and/or amenorrhea responded to bromocriptine treatment with return of normal menstrual function and three of four who were infertile conceived with bromocriptine treatment (912).

Studies of del Pozo and Falaschi (197) have stressed the successful treatment of hyperprolactinemic PCOD subjects with administration of bromocriptine. Eight of 10 anovulatory or amenorrheic subjects with a mean basal plasma PRL level of 29.7 ng/ml became ovulatory with basal body temperature and plasma progesterone confirmation following daily doses of 3.75–7.5 mg for several months. This was associated with a mean 40% reduction of plasma T as well as a reduction of plasma LH levels and attenuated LH pulsatility (197), although chronic dopaminergic stimulation with bromocriptine failed to alter cyclic LH secretion in normal

ovulatory women (588) or in a diverse group of hyperprolactinemic women studied (241). Administration of bromocriptine has no effect in suppressing LH release in the latter group of subjects, possibly because there is already maximal endogenous LHRH inhibition by the enhanced DA turnover in hyperprolactinemic subjects. It appears that bromocriptine in hyperprolactinemic subjects with PCOD is effective and is the preferred treatment. Further confirmatory studies of its effect on plasma T and LH in PCOD are needed.

Administration of 2.5 mg bromocriptine for 2 weeks to hyperprolactinemic and normoprolactinemic subjects with amenorrhea (non-PCOD) did not demonstrate a reduction of serum T and DHT levels despite normalization of the mean PRL levels from 234 ng/ml to normal levels (817). Normal levels of T and DHT were noted in the hyperprolactinemic subjects before treatment with bromocriptine. The study of Seppälä et al. (817) negates any effect of bromocriptine on T and DHT and the possible role of these androgens in enhancing the secretion of PRL in their subjects. There is, however, enhanced LH sensitivity to a four-hour dopamine infusion in patients with PCOD (1011). It appears that bromocriptine may exert a dopaminergic mechanism which results in decreased LHRH activity in patients with PCOD.

It is clear that bromocriptine administration is the treatment of choice for hyperprolactinemic patients with PCOD. Insufficient data does not justify its use in normoprolactinemic subjects with polycystic ovaries.

Gonadotropins

Infertile patients with PCOD who do not ovulate after repeated trials of clomiphene or a combination of clomiphene and hCG may be considered as candidates for gonadotropin therapy with human menopausal gonadotropin (hMG) alone or usually in combination with human chorionic gonadotropin (hCG) therapy. The expense and more importantly the risks of complication make careful patient selection essential prior to treatment with gonadotropins. Combination hMG–hCG therapy stimulates ovarian follicular growth and maturation resulting in ovulation. Close monitoring of serum estrogens as well as ovarian size is necessary to avoid serious complications resulting from such therapy.

It appears that women with PCOD are at risk to develop the hyperstimulation syndrome following treatment with gonadotropins (177, 312). By utilizing rapid serum estrogen determinations the untoward effects of gonadotropin treatment may be minimized. Wang and Gemzell (961) treated 41 infertile patients with PCOD who failed to ovulate or conceive with clomiphene therapy. Clomiphene failure was defined as a lack of an ovulatory response or conception to a dose of clomiphene of at least 150 mg for five days with 10,000 IU hCG intramuscularly on the day of maximum cervical mucus production. Gonadotropin therapy was administered intramuscularly following a spontaneous menstrual period or a progestin-induced flow. Treatment was usually started with 2 ampules of hMG (a combination of 75 IU of FSH and 75 IU LH per ampule) daily. This was given until the plasma E_2 level reached 600–800 pg/ml, at which point ovulation was induced with 5,000 or 10,000 IU hCG 24–48 hours after the last hMG injection. The patient was instructed to have intercourse for three consecutive days starting the day before the hCG injection. Usual indices of ovulation were followed which included an elevation of basal body temperature (BBT), and a serum progesterone level above 10 ng/dl. In the absence of ovarian enlargement a repeat injection of 5000 IU hCG was given one week later. The results of treatment are summarized in Table 10-3 (961).

Twenty-seven of the 41 infertile patients with PCOD (65.9%) conceived with gonadotropin treatment (Table 10-3). Eleven of the 41 patients had a previous history of ovarian wedge resection and 10 were hyperprolactinemic. Three patients were hospitalized because of severe ovarian hyperstimulation and recovered following conservative treatment. One of the three patients aborted at seven weeks of gestation. Mild ovarian hyperstimulation occurred in six additional patients (7.8%). Three of the latter six patients failed to conceive following hMG–hCG treatment (961). The mean effective dose of hMG used in the treatment of 40 patients with PCOD was 1650 IU with a range of 500–4500 IU (928). The hyperstimulation syndrome was more apparent in those patients with PCOD who ovulated but did not become pregnant on previous clomiphene therapy. PCOD patients who did not ovulate with clomiphene were less likely to develop this complication with hMG–hCG (961). A review of the diagnosis and management of the hyperstimulation syndrome may be found elsewhere (804, 869). Wang and Gemzell (961) reviewed the clinical results of hMG–hCG in women with PCOD and noted that of 724 patients described in the literature the ovulation rate ranged between 76–95%, while the pregnancy rate varied between 21–65% (311,696,738,908,928, 961). Two-hundred and five of the 724 patients (28%) conceived following treatment with gonadotropins, and the multiple pregnancy rate ranged between 13.6–36.3% (311,908,961). No increased incidence of congenital malformations has been described (869). An abortion rate of 24–39% has been reported in hMG–hCG-treated patients with PCOD (311,908,961).

In view of the fact that many patients with PCOD have elevated serum levels of LH, a number of patients ovulated following hMG alone without additional hCG. This is of practical im-

TABLE 10-3. Results and Complications of hMG–hCG Treatment in Women with PCOD.

	PCOD WITH PRIMARY AMENORRHEA	PCOD AFTER WEDGE RESECTION	PCOD WITH HYPER-PROLACTINEMIA	OTHERS	TOTAL
No. of women	4	11	10	20	41
No. of treatment cycles	12	23	19	35	77
No. of pregnant women	1(25%)	5(45.5%)	5(50%)	16(80%)	27(65 9%)
No. of pregnancies	1(8 4%)	5(21.7%)	6(31.6%)	18(51 4%)	29(35.8%)
No. of complicated treatments	1(8.3%)	2(8.7%)	2(10.5%)	4(11.4%)	9(11.7%)
Mild hyperstimulation	1	2	2	1	6(7.8%)
Severe hyperstimulation	0	0	0	3	3(3.9%)

From Wang CF, Gemzell C The use of human gonadotropins for the induction of ovulation in women with polycystic ovarian disease. Fertil Steril 1980, 33 479–486 With permission of the publisher, The American Fertility Society (961)

portance since intercourse is thus advised throughout administration of hMG.

A pregnancy rate of 33% in patients with PCOD was described by Gemzell (311) following gonadotropin therapy, with an abortion rate of almost 40%. Some of the patients with PCOD who were unsuccessfully treated with gonadotropin therapy became pregnant within six months by ovulating spontanenously (311).

The use of clomiphene citrate 50–100 mg/day for five days prior to hMG–hCG treatment has been advocated by some investigators in an attempt to reduce the amount of gonadotropin required for ovulation induction (453,469, 869,960).

A report by Kemmann et al. (454) of 24 women with clomiphene resistant polycystic ovary syndrome noted a 100% ovulation rate with a conception rate of 58% after an average of 2.4 gonadotropin treatment cycles. Twin pregnancies occurred in 36%, while spontaneous abortions were noted in 21%. Part of the reason such a high pregnancy rate was achieved may have been due to the careful exclusion of associated factors which may have made conception more difficult. HMG treatment was discontinued once the serum E_2 level reached 800–1200 pg/ml, following which 10,000 IU hCG was given 48 hours later. A repeat hCG injection of 2,500–10,000 IU 48 hours after a previous hCG injection was required in 2 of 14 cycles which resulted in conception. Moderate ovarian enlargement of 4–8 cm was noted in 11 of 24 patients during the luteal phase. One subject had 10 cm ovarian enlargement without the presence of ascites. It appears that close surveillance of the patient's response to hMG–hCG with clinical and laboratory facilites for such treatment limits the use of such a modality to specialized centers equipped for this service.

The addition of 0.5 mg DXM during hMG–hCG treatment to PCOD patients who failed to conceive with clomiphene citrate and hMG–hCG alone has been suggested by Evron et al. (242). The conception rate reported by these investigators was 74%. Ovarian hyperstimulation syndrome occurred in only 1 of 27 infertile patients with PCOD (242).

Unlike clomiphene-induced hyperandrogenemia, patients with PCOD are less likely to have a significant increase of serum T and androstenedione following hMG–hCG treatment (1003).

Raj et al. (738) described the use of human pituitary FSH obtained from the National Pitui-tary Agency of Baltimore, Md., to 10 infertile clomiphene failures with PCOD. Eighteen treatment cycles were employed utilizing daily injections of 40–80 IU FSH starting on day 6 or 7 of a progestin-induced menstrual period. An hCG injection of 8,000 or 10,000 IU was used to trigger ovulation unless the total urinary estrogen exceeded 150 μg/24 hr. In these 18 cycles, 14 ovulations occurred with five cases of mild ovarian enlargement. A more gradual urinary estrogen response was noted in the FSH-treated patients with PCOD than hMG-treated cycles who frequently demonstrated an abrupt rise of urinary estrogens on treatment.

The use of chronic low-dose FSH therapy without the addition of hCG has been reported in two patients with PCOD by Kamrava et al. (441). Both patients were clomiphene resistant with hCG adjunctive therapy, and both conceived with therapy. The dosage of FSH consisted of 40–80 IU daily intramuscularly for 3–6 weeks depending on the ovulatory response as noted in BBT and cervical mucus. Following the presence of ovulation the FSH was discontinued. Exogenous FSH treatment resulted in an initial decrease in serum androstenedione, E_1 and LH, with an increase in E_2. Subsequent to the initial decline in LH levels the LH showed substantial peaks that were associated with ovulatory changes in the BBT chart. This was associated with a slight increase of serum T during ovulation and the luteal phase of the cycle. A gradual rise of serum FSH was noted during therapy. As previously noted in Chapter 6, endogenous FSH is reduced in PCOD resulting in inappropriate follicle maturation which is further inhibited by intraovarian androgens. Since sufficient endogenous LH is present in patients with PCOD, it appears that the addition of exogenous FSH alone may be sufficient to reverse the relative FSH deficiency found in this syndrome. The use of FSH alone appears to offer less hyperstimulation and multiple pregnancies than other modalities such as hMG–hCG or clomiphene citrate.

Tamoxifen Citrate

Tamoxifen citrate (TMX) is a nonsteroidal antiestrogen which is used in the palliative treatment of advanced breast cancer in postmenopausal women. Studies utilizing TMX in the induction of ovulation have been reported

(477,560,783,813,897,984). Some anovulatory patients who failed to respond to clomiphene have been noted to respond to TMX. Two reports specifically describe several patients with PCOD who ovulated following administration of 20–40 mg of tamoxifen for 4–5 days (477, 560). These patients were among a larger group of anovulatory patients treated with the drug. In a report by Klopper and Hall (477), three patients with PCOD ovulated following TMX and one of the three patients became pregnant. Ovulation occurred 6–20 days (median 10 days) following the start of TMX treatment for 4 days. A study by Macourt (560) of four patients with polycystic ovarian disease revealed ovulation in all four, with pregnancy in three of four patients treated. The dosage of tamoxifen used ranged between 10–40 mg twice daily from days 3–7 of the cycle. No multiple pregnancies occurred and three of five anovulatory patients of diverse etiologies who were clomiphene failures ovulated following tamoxifen. The hyperstimulation syndrome is very infrequent with TMX therapy.

Studies of normal premenopausal volunteers indicate that tamoxifen induces an increase in serum estradiol greater than that of a control cycle (363,836). The rise in serum LH, FSH and progesterone is similar in TMX-treated and control cycles. A mid-cycle decrease of serum prolactin has been described by Groom and Griffiths (363). They suggest that TMX may act directly on the ovary to stimulate estradiol release, and perhaps the reduced prolactin concentration permits augmented ovarian stimulation with normal concentration of gonadotropins. There is recent experimental and clinical data suggesting that bromocriptine therapy may be enhanced with tamoxifen (200).

In a recent report of 22 anovulatory women (none of whom had documented PCOD) treated with tamoxifen 40 mg/day for five days from day 5 to 9 of the menstrual cycle, Tajima and Fukushima (897) noted ovulation in 33 of 46 treated cycles in 16 women. Four of the latter patients became pregnant. Daily hormonal profiles were performed in this study and compared to normal controls. Serum FSH and LH rose slightly during or subsequent to TXM administration, followed by an increase in serum E_2 which triggered an LH surge. Serum PRL did not show any change after TXM treatment. No difference was found in FSH concentrations during the follicular phase of TXM-induced ovulatory cycles and normal cycles. Studies of the luteal phase in TMX-induced ovulatory cycles also did not show any differences in duration (mean = 14 days) or in P concentration when compared to normal ovulatory women. The authors concluded that although the initial effect of TMX appeared to be on the hypothalamic–pituitary unit (897), a subsequent action on the ovary is possible with simultaneous recruitment of multiple ovarian follicles (836, 897).

Preliminary data in several of our clomiphene-resistant subjects with PCOD treated with 40–80 mg tamoxifen daily from days 3–7 following a spontaneous or progestin-induced menses, reveal minimal efficacy in inducing ovulation in such patients (285). A significant reduction in mid-cycle serum PRL was noted, confirming previous data in normal subjects (363). Further trials are necessary before TMX can be recommended in clomiphene-resistant patients since several toxic effects such as transient thrombocytopenia and leukopenia may occur (<5%). Hot flashes and nausea may also occur in 13–16% of treated patients.

Wedge Resection of Ovaries

In view of the almost exclusively medical management of infertility in polycystic ovarian disease the role of bilateral ovarian wedge resection has been appropriately minimized. Early studies indicated reduced ovarian androgen production following wedge resection (101). The fact that postoperative adhesions have been demonstrated as a complication of wedge resection makes this modality of treatment rarely indicated.

Cohen (153) analyzed 740 patients with PCOD who underwent wedge resection of the ovaries, mostly for infertility, although 20% were performed for hirsutism. Seventy-five percent of all patients who were operated established regular menses following surgery with a corrected live birth rate of 56%. Primary failures were noted in 17%, while secondary failures occurring after six months postoperatively were present in another 17% of patients. Laparoscopic wedge resection with drainage of follicular subcapsular cysts yielded the highest corrected live birth rate (75%), while a wedge resection with wide hilar excision yielded a 56%

corrected live birth rate. An incidence of 44% corrected live birth rate was noted in the classical wedge resection, and 56% achieved regular menses. The least percentage of primary and secondary failures (total of 17% after six months) occurred in the group of patients who had wedge resection with adequate excision of the stroma and hilum. Gonadal mass reduction of androgen-producing tissue is more likely to result in ovaries which are more responsive to endogenous gonadotropin. The 6% abortion rate in the review of the 740 patients with PCOD who had ovarian surgery compares favorably to the much higher abortion rate described following medical ovulation induction. There were no cases of ectopic pregnancies in the surgical cases, and the twinning rate was 8% (153). A later study by Adashi et al. (12) reported an 8% incidence of ectopic pregnancy following wedge resection, and a 47.8% conception rate.

The surgical morbidity with bilateral ovarian wedge resection is 2% (hemorrhage, infection and ovarian failure). It appears, however, that ovarian wedge resection is significantly complicated by the development of intrapelvic adhesions (12,109,470,916,968). Peritubal and periovarian adhesions may account for the lower pregnancy rate than ovulation rate following surgery. The surgical precautions to reduce adhesion are detailed in the paper of Cohen (153) which also includes the operative techniques stressed by Stein. Some surgeons have proposed laparoscopy 6–8 weeks following ovarian surgery to ensure the absence of significant adhesions (893).

Concern regarding post-wedge resection adhesions leading to infertility was already voiced in the late 60's (470). All 59 of a series of 173 patients (34%) who had a prior wedge resection of the ovaries one year or more before an endoscopy or laparotomy performed mostly for infertility were found to have postoperative adhesions (109). Among these 59 patients were 12 who became pregnant the first year after surgery and who later became infertile. A follow-up of patients by Buttram and Vaquero (109) indicated that when pregnancy occurred it did so in the first year or not at all. Even though pregnancy resulted, it was followed by infertility. The 34% postoperative adhesion rate is a rather conservative one since a number of patients were lost to follow-up. Only 42.6% of those de-

siring pregnancy conceived within the first year following surgery without any subsequent conceptions. Of the 173 patients, ovarian wedge resection had no effect on menstruation in 6.3%, while in 31.8% the effect on menstruation was only temporary. The authors advocate good hemostasis, avoidance of unnecessary trauma and reducing the number of raw surfaces that are left exposed to minimize formation of adhesions (109).

It is of interest that even the minor trauma of laparoscopic biopsy in six women unresponsive to clomiphene citrate and hCG initiated menses and resulted in pregnancy without further treatment (1032).

A summary of findings of the results of wedge resection of the ovaries in 1079 cases culled from the literature by Goldzieher and Axelrod prior to 1962 (347) revealed the development of regular cycles in 6–95% of cases (mean = 80%), and a pregnancy rate of 13–89% (mean = 63%). The improvement in hirsutism was generally poor, with positive results in less than 20% of patients. It has become clear that failure of medical therapy does not always imply failure of surgery, and vice versa (341).

Studies of serum LH and FSH following wedge resection of the ovaries in eight clomiphene-resistant patients with PCOD reveal no significant changes up to the time of the midcycle LH peak which occurs 13–25 days after surgery in the patients that apparently ovulated (434). Significant decreases of T and androstenedione occur postoperatively, while androstenedione levels resume preoperative levels within a month. The reduction of serum T postoperatively appears to be more sustained. This pattern of androgens is present in patients that ovulate following wedge resection as well as in those that do not. Judd et al. (434) explained the above findings as indicating that the results of local intraovarian changes in androgens are responsible for the induction of ovulation rather than central effects in view of lack of significant changes in circulating gonadotropins. Others have also noted a reduction of serum T following ovarian wedge resection (437,527,861) with a decrease in the blood production rate of T measured 7–10 days after wedge resection (10,861).

Two intraovarian factors may be responsible for postoperative ovulation resulting from bilateral wedge resection (434): (1) increased local intraovarian blood flow allows increased delivery of gonadotropins to the follicles, and (2) an acute localized reduction of androgenic tissue decreases the local inhibitory effect of androgens on follicular maturation.

Serum LH, FSH and T are usually not different in normoprolactinemic and hyperprolactinemic subjects with PCOD (553). The percentage of regular menses following wedge resection of ovaries is higher in the normoprolactinemic group (45 of 74 patients) than with the hyperprolactinemic subjects with PCOD (3 of 12 patients). Hyperresponsiveness to LHRH is present in both groups. Three of the 12 hyperprolactinemic subjects with PCOD in the above series had an abnormality of the sella turcica (553). This may indicate pituitary hyperplasia and/or adenoma formation (75,249).

In a unique report, long-term follow-up (mean = 5.7 years) of 29 patients with PCOD treated with wedge resection of the ovaries revealed the establishment of normal menstrual cycles in 26 patients (390). In 13 patients who desired to become pregnant, 10 conceived, with one abortion. Weight-reduction was noted in eight of nine patients who were obese preoperatively, although hirsutism was not affected (390).

In conclusion, the use of wedge resection of the ovaries should be considered only as a relatively late option to achieve conception and should be performed by one experienced with careful surgical techniques to minimize trauma and adhesions. This may be accomplished by means of improved surgical techniques employing microsurgery (224). The use of a follow-up laparoscopy several months later appears indicated.

Hypothesis and Summary 11

Type I polycystic ovarian disease (PCOD-I) is classically described by the association of bilateral polyfollicular ovaries (PFO), infertility, menstrual dysfunction and hirsutism (880). A disease spectrum has emerged which is commonly associated with a varying incidence of obesity, hyperandrogenemia, increased peripheral conversion of androgens into estrogens, and an elevated luteinizing hormone (LH) to follicle-stimulating hormone (FSH) ratio (1011). Although the etiology of PCOD-I is unclear, the spectrum of disorders, ranging from some patients with "idiopathic hirsutism" to hyperthecosis, involves an abnormal hypothalamic–hypophyseal–ovarian axis; this differs from type II polycystic ovarian disease (PCOD-II) which initially involves an adrenal steroidogenic defect (37). It is suggested that both PCOD-I and PCOD-II consist of two stages: a causative "generator" stage and an "effector" stage manifested by a positive-feedback cycle between the ovary and the hypothalamic–pituitary unit (629). It is proposed that one of the etiologies (or "generator") of PCOD-I is an aberrant puberal hypothalamic gonadostat to ovarian feedback (629).

The Generator Stage of PCOD

The frequency of perimenarchal hirsutism and obesity in PCOD suggests puberal dysfunction (hypothalamic–pituitary–ovarian and/or adrenal). Normal puberty is characterized by an intrinsic CNS-controlled diminished hypothalamic–hypophyseal sensitivity (increased go-nadostat set-point) to negative feedback of gonadal steroids on LHRH release resulting primarily in increased FSH secretion; this is subsequently followed by gradual development of a competent positive feedback of gonadal steroids on gonadotropin surges and the appearance of episodic LH secretion (367). Experimentally, the initiation of puberty in the female rhesus monkey depends upon the maturation of the CNS which modulates the pattern of LHRH presentation to the pituitary gland (982). In the human, puberal diminution of intrinsic CNS inhibition of LHRH secretion gradually leads to the appearance of episodic LHRH release (366). In contrast to tonic LHRH release patterns where LHRH receptors are down-regulated, the puberal onset episodic of LHRH release sensitizes the pituitary gonadotropes to LHRH. This occurs by permitting regeneration of LHRH surface membrane receptors between the LHRH pulses, thereby enhancing pituitary gonadotropin secretion (366). Since patients with PCOD-I characteristically display increased amplitude and frequency of LH pulses throughout adolescence and adulthood, it appears that regulatory events for gonadotropin release are altered. The reasons for this event may involve aberrant hypophyseal set-points to ovarian feedback. A pathological decreased rate of normal augmentation of gonadostat set-point to negative ovarian feedback results in a diminished FSH release in early puberty, while a coincidental further decrease in set-point for positive feedback facilitates secretion of cyclic LH during late puberty. An abnormal net effect of high LH and low FSH secretion (IGS) may ensue at the time of puberty. Hypophyseal set-point aberrations leading to puberal IGS may result from abnormal development of the pituitary gland, hypothalamus or higher brain centers, and perhaps may be genetically predetermined. In essence, PCOD-I may be caused by an abnormal CNS mechanism responsible for regulating gonadostat set-point during puberty.

In contrast PCOD-II is caused by adrenal steroid biosynthetic enzymatic defects resulting in elevated androgens, reduced steroid-hormone-binding globulin (SHBG) binding capacity, and increased unbound (free) testosterone, delta[5] androstenediol and estradiol (538).

The Effector Stage of PCOD

It has been hypothesized that the generator stage in PCOD-I produces a puberal state of IGS. A series of events follow which lead to a perpetuation of IGS. Decreased serum FSH and high levels of LH-stimulated intraovarian androgens suppress granulosa cell aromatase activity resulting in a decline of follicular maturation and estradiol production (551). The high levels of serum LH may also cause down-regulation of granulosa cell receptors. The combina-

tion of low FSH and high LH secretion rates (IGS) synergize to induce polyfollicular ovaries in various stages of growth and atresia. The state of LH-dependent ovarian hyperandrogenism (thecal and stromal) enhances granulosa cell production of inhibin, a nonsteroidal suppressant of FSH release (Fig. 11-1) (143,273,577). The elevated levels of ovarian androgens, primarily androstenedione (> testosterone), are aromatized peripherally into estrone (E_1) > estradiol (E_2), respectively (341). As a result, SHBG (TeBG) becomes saturated and SHBG binding capacity becomes reduced resulting in high acyclic production of unbound E_1 and E_2 (539). Observations suggest that chronically elevated E_2 levels augment pituitary sensitivity to LHRH resulting in an increased amplitude and frequency of LH pulsatile release (532,742). In contrast, high acyclic E_1 levels diminish FSH secretion without affecting LH secretion (138). The consequence of increased acyclic estrogen production is also apparent by its effect on hypothalamic dopamine. Studies in the rat indicate that dopaminergic neurons may inhibit LH release either directly or indirectly via paracrine neuromodulation of LHRH neurons in the lateral palisade zone of the median eminence (ME_1) (733). The elevated estrogen levels which

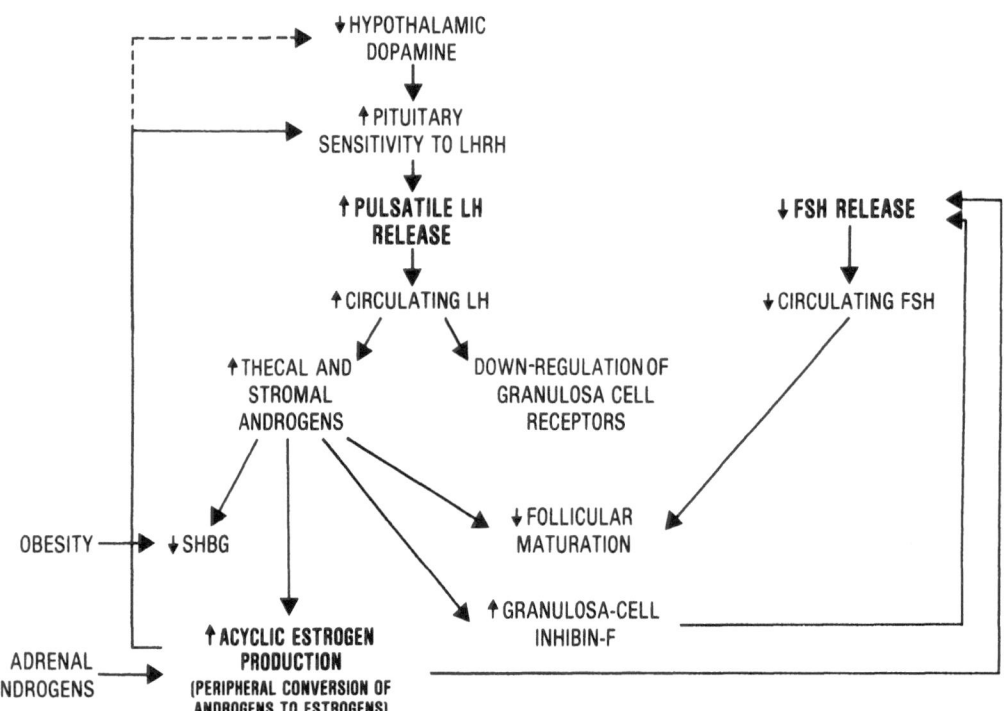

Fig. 11-1. Series of events which are associated with inappropriate gonadotropin secretion in PCOD.

occur as a result of increased extraglandular conversion of androgens exert on inhibitory effect on hypothalamic dopaminergic tone. The latter further enhances pituitary gonadotrope sensitivity to LHRH in PCOD resulting in exaggerated pulsatile LH release (658,733). As a consequence, the net result of all these factors is an augmented LH/FSH secretion rate ratio, or IGS. To summarize, the cyclic effector stage of PCOD consists of (1) an initial (generative) IGS, (2) PFO, (3) hyperandrogenemia, (4) peripheral aromatization into $E_1 > E_2$ and (5) consequential IGS.

Clinical Manifestations

Hyperandrogenemia and resulting hirsutism is the hallmark of the effector stage of PCOD. Polyfollicular ovaries represent an IGS effect and the source of hyperandrogenemia. Peripheral conversion of androgens into estrogens appears to occur mainly in adipose tissue. Obesity is not found uniformly in PCOD but its presence contributes to elevated acyclic production of E_1 and E_2. Data suggest that the unopposed effect of E_2 stimulates adipocyte replication (765). The decrease in cyclic E_2 and progesterone coupled with an increase in acyclic E_1 predisposes to chronic anovulation and infertility, dysfunctional bleeding and an increased incidence of endometrial carcinoma (1011). Low circulating FSH levels which decrease follicular maturation and aromatase activity by promoting an androgenic intrafollicular microenviroment result in decreased ovarian estradiol production and anovulation (230). Thus it is not surprising that chronic low-dose FSH therapy is an effective treatment for ovulation induction (441).

It has been proposed that PCOD-I is the result of an aberrant puberal gonadostat to ovarian feedback, and a reliable history obtained from parents frequently reveals the presence of premenarchal obesity and hirsutism (1011). Premenarchal histological findings suggest that the prepuberal ovary is not quiescent. Necropsy studies of 121 infants and children revealed graafian follicles and thecal luteinization in 84 and 68 instances, respectively (490). The estimated incidence of 3.5–7.0% of PCOD in the general population (715,859) may reflect those females with an abnormality of neural and/or hypothalamic development. It is not unlikely

that the true incidence of PCOD may be higher than 7%, and that indeed most patients may be asymptomatic or have only minimal symptoms. The presence of mild hirsutism, thinning scalp hair, chronic cystic acne and dysfunctional bleeding should alert the astute clinician to look for evidence of an increased LH/FSH ratio.

PCOD-II occurs in a variety of adrenal steroidogenic enzymatic disorders which produce increased androgens (538). Increased peripheral conversion of androgens to estrogens may also lead to IGS and associated ovarian hyperandrogenism. Most commonly, elevation of DHAS may be present with hyperresponsiveness of serum progesterone (P) and 17-α-hydroxyprogesterone (17OHP) to ACTH stimulation (37). Many also differ clinically from PCOD-I patients in their tendency to lesser obesity, oligomenorrhea rather than amenorrhea, and increased severity of hirsutism (37).

Hyperprolactinemia with or without galactorrhea may be found in 20–40% of patients with PCOD (341). Chronic hyperestrogenemia may result in lactotrope hyperplasia and possible acceleration of the growth of a pre-existing occult pituitary adenoma (290). The galactorrhea–amenorrhea syndrome in the patient with PCOD is associated with an absence of IGS. Hyperprolactinemia enhances negative feedback and/or decreases positive feedback of E_2 on LHRH, thereby resulting in the reduction of serum LH and E_2 (947). PCOD patients with hyperprolactinemia and amenorrhea should be carefully studied with computerized tomography of the sella turcica to exclude pituitary adenomas (284,290,497) which usually respond to medical treatment with dopamine agonists.

Summary

It is hypothesized that the spectrum of polycystic ovarian disease may perhaps result from an aberrant hypothalamic gonadostat at puberty (398). Abnormal neural development in the brain may decrease the hypophyseal set-point for negative and positive ovarian hormone feedback. This generates an inappropriately elevated hypophyseal luteinizing hormone (LH) secretion. The inappropriately elevated LH/FSH ratio is termed inappropriate gonadotropin secretion (IGS). The events which create the initial state of IGS are referred to as the "generator" stage. IGS is maintained by ovarian-derived hyperandrogenemia, increased peripheral aromatization of androgens (Fig. 11-1), and reduced testosterone-binding globulin (TeBG) (or steroid-hormone-binding globulin, SHBG) resulting in elevated free testosterone (T), serum estrone (E_1) and unbound estradiol (E_2) levels. E_1 preferentially suppresses release of hypophyseal FSH, while E_2 exerts positive feedback on LH pulsatile release by increasing pituitary sensitivity to luteinizing hormone-releasing hormone (LHRH). Reduced circulating FSH levels decrease granulosa cell aromatase activity sufficiently to cause suboptimal conversion of LH-induced thecal androgens into estrogens. As a result, chronic intrafollicular hyperandrogenemia with associated arrested follicle maturation results in enhancing the production of inhibin-F by the granulosa cells. This further suppresses pituitary FSH release (Fig. 11-1). The elevated circulating LH/FSH ratio stimulates early development and proliferation of multiple immature follicles causing the appearance of polyfollicular ovaries in various stages of growth and atresia. In the "effector" stage of PCOD, a vicious cycle is fashioned whereby IGS causes polyfollicular ovaries and increased ovarian androgen production (androstenedione > T) which, in turn, promotes IGS. One of several possible etiologies of the disease spectrum of PCOD may involve an aberrant puberal gonadostat-to-ovarian feedback that establishes a persistent faulty hypothalamic–hypophyseal–ovarian axis.

References

1. Abraham GE, Buster JE. Peripheral and ovarian steroids in ovarian hyperthecosis. Obstet Gynecol. 1976; 47:581–586.
2. Abraham GE, Maroulis GB, Buster JE, et al. Effect of dexamethasone on serum cortisol and androgen levels in hirsute patients. Obstet Gynecol. 1976; 47:395–402.
3. Abraham GE, Chakmakjian ZH, Buster JE, et al. Ovarian and adrenal contributions to peripheral androgens in hirsute women. Obstet Gynecol. 1975; 46:169–173.
4. Abraham GE, Maroulis GB. Effect of exogenous estrogen on serum pregnenolone, cortisol and androgens in postmenopausal women. Obstet Gynecol. 1975; 45:271–274.
5. Abraham GE. Ovarian and adrenal contribution to peripheral androgens during the menstrual cycle. J Clin Endocrinol Metab. 1974; 39:340–346.
6. Abraham GE, Chakmakjian ZH. Serum steroid levels during the menstrual cycle in a bilaterally adrenalectomized woman. J Clin Endocrinol Metab. 1973; 37:581–587.
7. Abu-Haydar N, Laidlaw JC, Nusimovich B, et al. Hyperadrenocorticism and the Stein-Leventhal syndrome (abstr). J Clin Endocrinol Metab. 1954; 14:766.
8. Ackerman GE, Smith ME, Mendelson CR, et al. Aromatization of androstenedione by human adipose tissue stromal cells in monolayer culture. J Clin Endocrinol Metab. 1981; 53:412–417.
9. Adams TE, Norman RL, Spies HG. Gonadotropin-releasing hormone receptor binding and pituitary responsiveness in estradiol-primed monkeys. Science. 1981; 213:1388–1390.
10. Adams TE, Spies HG. Binding characteristics of gonadotropin-releasing hormone receptors throughout the estrous cycle of the hamster. Endocrinology. 1981; 108:2245–2253.
11. Adams TE, Spies HG. GnRH-induced regulation of GnRH receptor concentration in the phenobarbital-blocked hamster. Biol Reprod. 1981; 25:298–302.
12. Adashi EY, Rock JA, Guzick D, et al. Fertility following bilateral ovarian wedge resection: a critical analysis of 90 consecutive cases of the polycystic ovary syndrome. Fertil Steril. 1981; 36:320–325.
13. Aiman J, Edman CD, Worley RJ, et al. Androgen and estrogen formation in women with ovarian hyperthecosis. Obstet Gynecol. 1978; 51:1–9.
14. Aiman J, Nalick RH, Jacobs A, et al. The origin of androgen and estrogen in a virilized postmenopausal woman with bilateral cystic teratomas. Obstet Gynecol. 1977; 49:695–704.
15. Alger M, Vazquez-Matute L, Mason M, et al. Polycystic ovarian disease associated with hyperprolactinemia and defective metoclopramide response. Fertil Steril. 1980; 34:70–71.
16. Allen WM, Woolf RB. Medullary resection of the ovaries in the Stein-Leventhal syndrome. Am J Obstet Gynecol. 1959; 77:826–834.
17. Ances IG, Haskins AL, Ganis FM. Metabolism of ovarian steroids in a patient with chronic familial anovulation. Am J Obstet Gynecol. 1970; 108:1130–1133.
18. Anderson DC. Sex-hormone-binding globulin. Clin Endocrinol (Oxf). 1974; 3:69–96.
19. Andersen RN. Use of gonadotropin and steroid assays in the diagnosis of disorders of female reproduction. In: Givens JR, ed. Gynecologic Endocrinology. Chicago: Year Book Med Publ, 1977:109–126.
20. Andersen RN, Givens JR, Wiser WL, et al. Response of the binding capacity of plasma testosterone-estradiol-binding globulin to norethindrone, 2 mg, and mestranol, 0.1 mg, in polycystic ovarian disease. Am J Obstet Gynecol. 1976; 125:166–169.
21. Anderson DC. The role of sex hormone binding

globulin in health and disease. In: James VHT, Serio M, Guisti G, eds. The Endocrine Function of the Human Ovary. New York: Academic Press, 1976:141–158.

22. Anderson DC, Yen SSC. Effects of estrogens on adrenal 3β-hydroxysteroid dehydrogenase in ovariectomized women. J Clin Endocrinol Metab. 1976; 43:561–570

23. Aono T, Miyake A, Shioji T, et al. Restoration of oestrogen positive feedback effect on LH release by bromocriptine in hyperprolactinaemic patients with galactorrhoea-amenorrhoea. Acta Endocrinol (Kbh). 1979; 91:591–600.

24. Aono T, Miyazaki M, Miyake A, et al. Responses of serum gonadotrophins to LH-releasing hormone and oestrogens in Japanese women with polycystic ovaries. Acta Endocrinol (Kbh). 1977; 85:840–849.

25. Aono T, Miyake A, Shiosi T, et al. Impaired LH release following endogenous estrogen administration in patients with amenorrhea-galactorrhea syndrome. J Clin Endocrinol Metab. 1976; 42:696–702.

26. Apter D, Viinikka L, Vihko R. Hormonal pattern of adolescent menstrual cycles. J Clin Endocrinol Metab. 1978; 47:944–954.

27. Archer DF. Current concepts of prolactin physiology in normal and abnormal conditions. Fertil Steril. 1977; 28:125–134.

28. Archer DF, Josimovich JB. Ovarian response to exogenous gonadotropins in women with elevated serum prolactin. Obstet Gynecol. 1976; 48:155–157.

29. Armstrong DT, Dorrington JH. Estrogen biosynthesis in the ovaries and testes. In: Thomas JA, Singhal RL, eds. Advances in Sex Hormone Research, Vol. 3. Baltimore: University Park Press, 1977:217–258.

30. Armstrong DT, Papkoff H. Stimulation of aromatization of exogenous and endogenous androgens in ovaries of hypophysectomized rats *in vivo* by follicle-stimulating hormone. Endocrinology. 1976; 99:114–1151.

31. Atkinson LE, Hotchkiss J, Fritz GR, et al. Circulating levels of steroids and chorionic gonadotropin during pregnancy in the rhesus monkey, with special attention to the rescue of the corpus luteum in early pregnancy. Biol Reprod. 1975; 12:335–345.

32. Axelrod LR, Goldzieher JW. The polycystic ovary. V. Alternate pathways of steroid aromatization in normal pregnancy and polycystic ovaries. J Clin Endocrinol Metab. 1965; 25:1275–1278.

33. Axelrod LR, Goldzieher JW, Ross SD. Concurrent 3β-hydroxysteroid dehydrogenase deficiency in adrenal and sclerocystic ovary. Acta Endocrinol (Kbh). 1965; 48:392–412.

34. Axelrod LR, Goldzieher JW. Mechanism of biochemical aromatization of steroids. J Clin Endocrinol Metab. 1962; 22:537–542.

35. Axelrod LR, Goldzieher JW. The polycystic ovary. III. Steroid biosynthesis in normal and polycystic ovarian tissue. J Clin Endocrinol Metab. 1962; 22:431–446.

36. Axelrod LR, Goldzieher JW. Enzymic inadequacies of human polycystic ovaries. Arch Biochem Biophys. 1961; 95:547–548.

37. Ayers JWT. Differential response to adrenocorticotropin hormone stimulation in polycystic ovarian disease with high and low dehydroepiandrosterone sulfate levels. Fertil Steril. 1982; 37:645–649.

38. Babaknia A, Calfopoulos P, Jones HW Jr. The Stein-Leventhal syndrome and coincidental ovarian tumors. Obstet Gynecol. 1976; 47:223–224.

39. Baird DT, Corker CS, Davidson DW, et al. Pituitary–ovarian relationships in polycystic ovary syndrome. J Clin Endocrinol Metab. 1977; 45:798–809.

40. Baird DT. Pituitary–ovarian relationships in disorders of menstruation. In: James VHT, Serio M, Giusti G, eds. The Endocrine Function of the Human Ovary. New York: Academic Press, 1976:349–357.

41. Baird DT, Baker TG, McNatty KP, Neal P. Relationship between the secretion of the corpus luteum and the length of the follicular phase of the ovarian cycle. J Repro Fertil. 1975; 45:611–619.

42. Baird DT, Fraser IS. Concentrations of oestrone and oestradiol 17-β in follicular fluid and ovarian venous blood in women. Clin Endocrinol (Oxf). 1975; 4:259–266.

43. Baird DT, Horton R, Longcope C, et al. Steroid dynamics under steady-state conditions. Rec Prog Horm Res. 1969; 25:611–664.

44. Balmaceda JP, Valenzuela GV, Eddy CA, et al. Prostaglandin production by rhesus monkey corpora lutea *in vitro*: effects of estrogen administration. Int J Gynaecol Obstet. 1980; 18:15–18.

45. Balmaceda JP, Asch RH, Fernandez EO, et al. Prostaglandin production by rhesus monkey corpora lutea *in vitro*. Fertil Steril. 1979; 31:214–216.

46. Bar RS, Muggeo M, Kahn CR, et al. Characterization of insulin receptors in patients with the syndromes of insulin resistance and acanthosis nigricans. Diabetologia. 1980; 18:209–216.

47. Bar RS, Muggeo M, Roth J, et al. Insulin resistance, acanthosis nigricans and normal insulin receptors in a young woman: evidence for a postreceptor defect. J Clin Endocrinol Metab. 1978; 47:620–625.

48. Baramki TA, Leddy AL, Woodruff JD. Bilateral

hilus cell tumors of the ovary. Obstet Gynecol. 1983; 62:128–131.

49. Baranowska B, Jeske W, Stopinska U. Prolactin secretion in response to metoclopramide stimulation in polycystic ovary syndrome. Acta Endocrinol, Abstract 54, (Kbh). 1981; 97:S243.

50. Barbieri RL, Makris A, Ryan KJ. Effects of insulin on steroidogenesis in cultured porcine ovarian theca. Fertil Steril. 1983; 40:237–241.

51. Bardin CW, Paulsen CA. The testes. In: Williams RH, ed. Textbook of Endocrinology, 6th Ed. Philadelphia: WB Saunders Co., 1981:293–354.

52. Bardin CW, Hembree WD, Lipsett MB. Suppression of testosterone and androstenedione production rates with dexamethasone in women with idiopathic hirsutism and polycystic ovaries. J Clin Endocrinol Metab. 1968; 28:1300–1306.

53. Bardin CW, Lipsett MB, Edgcomb JH, et al. Studies of testosterone metabolism in a patient with masculinization due to stromal hyperthecosis. New Engl J Med. 1967; 277:399–402.

54. Bardin CW, Lipsett MB. Testosterone and androstenedione blood production rates in normal women and women with idiopathic hirsutism or polycystic ovaries. J Clin Invest. 1967; 46:891–902.

55. Barnes EW, Irvine WJ. Addison's disease, ovarian failure and hypoparathyroidism. Clin Endocrinol Metab. 1975; 4:379–434.

56. Barraclough CA, Wise PM. The role of catecholamines in the regulation of pituitary luteinizing hormone and follicle-stimulating hormone secretion. Endocrinol Rev. 1982; 3:91–119.

57. Barraclough CA. Sex differentiation of cyclic gonadotropin secretion. In: Kaye AM, Kaye M, eds. Advances in the Biosciences, Vol 25, Development of Responsiveness to Steroid Hormones. New York: Pergamon Press, 1979:433–450.

58. Barraclough CA, Gorski RA. Evidence that the hypothalamus is responsible for androgen-induced sterility. Endocrinology. 1961; 68:68–79.

59. Bartuska DG, Bernard AE, Smith EM, et al. Brain damage, hypertrichosis, and polycystic ovaries. Clinical evaluation of 7 cases. Am J Obstet Gynecol. 1967; 99:387–389.

60. Bassi F, Giusti G, Borsi L, et al. Plasma androgens in women with hyperprolactinemic amenorrhoea. Clin Endocrinol (Oxf). 1977; 6:5–10.

61. Bates GW, Whitworth NS. Effect of body weight reduction on plasma androgens in obese, infertile women. Fertil Steril. 1982; 38:406–409.

62. Bayliss RIS, Edwards OM, Starer E. Complications of adrenal venography. Br J Radiol. 1970; 43:531–533.

63. Baxendale PM, Jacobs HS, James VHT. Plasma and salivary androstenedione and dihydrotestos-

terone in women with hyperandrogenism. Clin Endocrinol (Oxf). 1983; 18:447–457.

64. Beck RP, Morcos F, Fawcett D, et al. Adrenocortical function studies during the normal menstrual cycle and in women receiving norethindrone with and without mestranol. Am J Obstet Gynecol. 1972; 112:364–368.

65. Belchetz PE, Plant TM, Nakai Y, et al. Hypophysial responses to continuous and intermittent delivery of hypothalamic gonadotropin-releasing hormone. Science. 1978; 202:631–633.

66. Belisle S, Lehoux JG, Benard B, et al. Ovarian hyperthecosis: in vivo and in vitro correlations of the androgen profile. Obstet Gynecol. 1981; 57:S70–S75.

67. Belisle S, Menard J. Adrenal androgen production in hyperprolactinemic states. Fertil Steril. 1980; 33:396–400.

68. Beloff-Chain AS, Bogdanovic S, Cawthorne MA. Acute regulation of insulin release by the pituitary gland in relation to hyperinsulinemia and obesity. J Endocrinol. 1979; 81:271–279.

69. Ben-David M, Schenker JG. Transient hyperprolactinemia: a correctable cause of idiopathic female infertility. J Clin Endocrinol Metab. 1983; 57:442–444.

70. Ben-David M, Schenker JG. Human ovarian receptors to human prolactin: implication in infertility. Fertil Steril. 1982; 38:182–186.

71. Benedict PH, Cohen RB, Cope O, et al. Ovarian and adrenal morphology in cases of hirsutism or virilism and Stein-Leventhal syndrome. Fertil Steril. 1962; 13:380–395.

72. Benjamin F, Cohen M, Romney SL. Sequential adrenal and ovarian suppression tests in the differential diagnosis of the polycystic ovary syndrome. Fertil Steril. 1970; 21:854–859.

73. Ben-Jonathan N, Peters L. Catecholamines and pituitary prolactin release. J Repro Fertil. 1980; 58:501–502.

74. Berger MJ, Taymor ML, Patton WC. Gonadotropin levels and secretory patterns in patients with typical and atypical polycystic ovarian disease. Fertil Steril. 1975; 26:619–626.

75. Bergh T, Nillius SJ, Wide L. Serum prolactin and gonadotrophin levels before and after luteinizing hormone-releasing hormone in the investigation of amenorrhoea. Br J Obstet Gynaecol. 1978; 85: 945–956.

76. Bergman P, Sjogren B, Hakansson B. Hypertensive form of congenital adrenocortical hyperplasia: analysis of case with coexisting polycystic ovaries. Acta Endocrinol (Kbh). 1962; 40:555–564.

77. Bergstrand H. Luteinisierung der ovarien bei ein falle von basophilem hypophysenadenom mit Cushings symptomenkomplex. Virchow's Arch (Pathol Anat). 1934; 239:413–428.

78. Besser GM. Hyperprolactinaemic-hypogonadism syndromes. Med J Aust. (Suppl) 1978; 2:14–17.

79. Besser GM, Thorner MO, Wass JAH, et al. Absence of uterine neoplasia in patients on bromocriptine. Br Med J. 1977; 2:868.

80. Betson JR Jr, Marshall RA, Chiffelle TL. Scleropolycystic (Stein-Leventhal) ovary with an arrhenoblastoma of the opposite gonad. Am J Obstet Gynecol. 1962; 83:93–100.

81. Biberoglu K, Behrman SJ. Hirsutism: diagnostic approach and stimulation-suppression dynamics of androgens in the female. Int J Fertil. 1982; 27:146–152.

82. Bird CE, Morrow L, Fukumoto Y, et al. Delta⁵-androstenediol: kinetics of metabolism and binding to plasma proteins in normal men and women. J Clin Endocrinol Metab. 1976; 43:1317–1322.

83. Bishun NP, Morton WR. Chromosome mosaicism in Stein-Leventhal syndrome. Br Med J. 1964; 2:1200.

84. Blair AJ, Reuter SR. Adrenal venography in virilized women. JAMA. 1970; 213:1623–1629.

85. Blankstein J, Faiman C, Reyes FI, et al. Adult-onset familial adrenal 21-hydroxylase deficiency. Am J Med. 1980; 68:441–448.

86. Blaustein A. Non-neoplastic cysts of the ovary. In: Blaustein A, ed. Pathology of the Female Genital Tract, 2nd ed. New York: Springer Verlag, 1982:449–463.

87. Blichert-Toft M, Vejlsted H, Hehlet H, et al. Virilizing adrenocortical adenoma responsive to gonadotropin. Acta Endocrinol (Kbh). 1975; 78:77–85.

88. Blum I, Bruhis S, Kaufman H. Clinical evaluation of the effects of combined treatment with bromocriptine and spironolactone in two women with the polycystic ovary syndrome. Fertil Steril. 1981; 35:629–633.

89. Blum I, Kaufman H, Marilus R, et al. Successful treatment of polycystic ovary syndrome with spironolactone or bromocriptine. Obstet Gynecol. 1981; 57:661–665.

90. Bohnet HG, Dahlen HG, Wuttke W, et al. Hyperprolactinemic anovulatory syndrome. J Clin Endocrinol Metab. 1976; 42:132–143.

91. Boisselle A, Tremblay RR. New therapeutic approach to the hirsute patient. Fertil Steril. 1979; 32:276–279.

92. Bongiovanni AM. Acquired adrenal hyperplasia: with special reference to 3β-hydroxysteroid dehydrogenase. Fertil Steril. 1981; 35:599–608.

93. Boyar RM, Katz J, Finkelstein JW, et al. Anorexia nervosa. Immaturity of the 24-hour luteinizing hormone secretory pattern. New Engl J Med. 1974; 291:861–865.

94. Boyar RM, Kapen S, Finkelstein JW, et al. Hypothalamic–pituitary function in diverse hyperprolactinemic studies. J Clin Invest. 1974; 53:1588–1598.

95. Boyar RM, Finkelstein JW, David R, et al. Twenty-four hour patterns of plasma luteinizing hormone and follicle-stimulating hormone in sexual precocity. New Engl J Med. 1973; 289:282–286.

96. Boyar RM, Finkelstein JW, Roffwarg H, et al. Twenty-four-hour luteinizing hormone and follicle-stimulating hormone secretory patterns in gonadal dysgenesis. J Clin Endocrinol Metab. 1973; 37:521–525.

97. Boyar RM, Finkelstein JW, Roffwarg H, et al. Synchronization of augmented luteinizing hormone secretion with sleep during puberty. New Engl J Med. 1972; 287:582–586.

98. Braithwaite SS, Erkman-Balis B, Avila TD. Postmenopausal virilization due to ovarian stromal hyperthecosis. J Clin Endocrinol Metab. 1979; 46:295–300.

99. Brawer JR, van Houten M. Cellular organization of luteinizing hormone-releasing factor delivery systems. In: Naftolin F, Ryan KJ, Davies IJ, eds. Subcellular Mechanisms in Reproductive Neuroendocrinology. Amsterdam: Elsevier Press, 1976:1–31.

100. Brisman K, Efendic S. Pituitary function in the empty sella syndrome. Neuroendocrinol. 1981; 32:70–77.

101. Brooks RV, Jeffcoate SL, London DR, et al. Studies of ovarian androgen secretion. Vermeulen A, Exley D, eds. In: Androgens in Normal and Pathological Conditions, Proceedings of the Second Symposium on Steroid Hormones, Ghent, 1965. Excerpta Medica International Congress Series 1966; 101:108–113.

102. Brooksbank BWL. Endocrinological aspects of hirsutism. Physiol Rev. 1961; 41:623–676.

103. Brown J, Winkelmann RK: Acanthosis nigricans: a study of 90 cases. Medicine. 1968; 47:33–51.

104. Bryner JR, El Gammal T, Acker JD, et al. Intrasellar subarachnoid herniation or empty sella associated with galactorrhea. Obstet Gynecol. 1978; 51:198–203.

105. Bulbrook RD, Hayward JL, Herian M, et al. Effect of steroidal contraceptives on levels of plasma androgen sulphates and cortisol. Lancet. 1973; 1:628–631.

106. Burghen GA, Givens JR, Kitabchi AE. Correlation of hyperandrogenism with hyperinsulinism in polycystic ovarian disease. Fertil Steril. 1980; 50:113–116.

107. Burrow GN, Wortzman G, Newcastle NG, et al. Microadenomas of the pituitary and abnormal sellar tomograms in an unselected autopsy series. New Engl J Med. 1981; 304:156–158.

108. Butler WR, Hotchkiss J, Knobil E. Functional luteolysis in the rhesus monkey: ovarian estrogen and progesterone during the luteal phase of the menstrual cycle. Endocrinology. 1975; 96:1509–1512.

109. Buttram VC Jr, Vaquero C. Post-ovarian wedge resection adhesive disease. Fertil. Steril. 1975; 26:874–876.

110. Buvat J, Siame-Mourot C, Fourlinnie JC, et al. Androgens and prolactin levels in hirsute women with either polycystic ovaries or "borderline ovaries." Fertil Steril. 1982; 38:695–700.

111. Buxton CL, Vande Wiele R. Wedge resection for polycystic ovaries. New Engl J Med. 1954; 251:293–297.

112. Byrd JR, Mahesh VB, Greenblatt RB. Chromosomal studies in the Stein-Leventhal syndrome. J Clin Endocrinol Metab. 1964; 24:939–940.

113. Calne DB, Plotkin C, Williams AC, et al. Long-term treatment of Parkinsonism with bromocriptine. Lancet. 1978; 1:735–738.

114. Camacho AM, Migeon CJ. Isolation, identification and quantitation of testosterone in the urine of normal adults and in patients with endocrine disorders. J Clin Endocrinol Metab. 1963; 23:301–305.

115. Canales ES, Zarate A, Castelazo-Ayala. Primary amenorrhea associated with polycystic ovaries. Endocrine, cytogenetic and therapeutic considerations. Obstet Gynecol. 1971; 37:205–210.

116. Cargille CM, Vaitukaitis JL, Bermudez JA, et al. A differential effect of ethinyl estradiol upon plasma FSH and LH relating to time of administration in the menstrual cycle. J Clin Endocrinol Metab. 1973; 36:87–94.

117. Carmel P, Araki S, Ferin M. Prolonged stalk portal blood collection in rhesus monkeys. Pulsatile release of gonadotropin-releasing hormone (Gn-RH). Endocrinology. 1975; 96:107A.

118. Carmel P, Araki S, Ferin M. Pituitary stalk portal blood collection in rhesus monkeys: evidence for pulsatile release of gonadotropin-releasing hormone (GnRH). Endocrinology. 1976; 99:243–248.

119. Carr BR, Sadler RK, Rochelle DB, et al. Plasma lipoprotein regulation of progesterone biosynthesis by human corpus luteum tissue in organ culture. J Clin Endocrinol Metab. 1981; 52:875–881.

120. Carter JN, Tyson JE, Warne GL, et al. Adrenocortical function in hyperprolactinemic women. J Clin Endocrinol Metab. 1977; 45:973–980.

121. Case Records of the Massachusetts General Hospital (Case 25–1982). New Engl J Med. 1982; 306:1537–1544.

122. Case Records of the Massachusetts General Hospital (Case 6–1976): New Engl J Med. 1976; 294:326–331.

123. Case records of the Massachusetts General Hospital (Case 12–1974). New Engl J Med. 1974; 290:730–736.

124. Case records of the Massachusetts General Hospital (Case 49–1972). New Engl J Med. 1972; 287:1192–1195.

125. Case Records of the Massachussetts General Hospital (Case 8–1965). New Engl J Med. 1965; 272:365–371.

126. Case Records of the Massachusetts General Hospital (Case 89–1961). New Engl J Med. 1961; 265:1210–1214.

127. Case Records of the Massachusetts General Hospital (Case 43481). New Engl J Med. 1957; 257:1086–1091.

128. Case Records of the Massachusetts General Hospital (Case 40072). New Engl J Med. 1954; 250:296–300.

129. Casey JH. Chronic treatment regimens for hirsutism in women: effect on blood production rates of testosterone and on hair growth. Clin Endocrinol (Oxf). 1975; 4:313–325.

130. Casey JH, Nabarro JDH. Plasma testosterone in idiopathic hirsutism, and the changes produced by adrenal and ovarian stimulation and suppression. J Clin Endocrinol Metab. 1967; 27:1431–1435.

131. Castro-Magnana M, Cheruvanky T, Collipp PJ, et al. Transient adrenogenital syndrome due to exposure to danazol *in utero*. Am J Dis Child. 1981; 135:1032–1034.

132. Cathelineau G, Brerault JL, Fiet J, et al. Adrenocortical 11β-hydroxylation defect in adult women with postmenarchial onset of symptoms. J Clin Endocrinol Metab. 1980; 51:287–291.

133. Caufriez A, Sugar J, Quenon M, et al. Serum prolactin (PRL) and dehydroepiandrosterone-sulfate (DHEAS) in patients with hyperprolactinaemia and/or isolated galactorrhoea. Acta Endocrinol (Suppl 212) (Kbh). 1977; 85:140.

134. Cetel NS, Quigley ME, Ropert JF, et al. Synchronized pulsatile release of prolactin and luteinizing hormone in normal cycling and hypogonadal women. 64th Annual Meeting of Endocrine Society, San Francisco, Calif., June 14–16, Abstr 24., 1982.

135. Chamlian DL, Taylor HB. Endometrial hyperplasia in young women. Obstet Gynecol. 1970; 36:659–666.

136. Chang RJ, Nakamura RM, Judd HL, et al. Insulin resistance in nonobese patients with polycystic ovarian disease. J Clin Endocrinol Metab. 1983; 57:356–359.

137. Chang RJ, Laufer LR, Meldrum DR, et al. Ster-

oid secretion in polycystic ovarian disease after ovarian suppression by a long-acting gonadotropin-releasing hormone agonist. J Clin Endocrinol Metab. 1983; 56:897–903.

138. Chang RJ, Mandel FP, Lu JKH, et al. Enhanced disparity of gonadotropin secretion by estrone in women with polycystic ovarian disease. J Clin Endocrinol Metab. 1982; 54:490–494.

139. Chang RJ, Mandel FP, Wolfsen AR, et al. Circulating levels of plasma adrenocorticotropin in polycystic ovary disease. J Clin Endocrinol Metab. 1982; 54:1265–1267.

140. Channing CP, Gagliano P, Hoover DJ, et al. Relationship between human follicular fluid inhibin F activity and steroid content. J Clin Endocrinol Metab. 1981; 52:1193–1198.

141. Channing CP, Schaerf FW, Anderson LD, et al. Ovarian follicular and luteal physiology. In: Greep RO, ed. Reproductive Physiology III, International Review of Physiology, Vol 22, Chap 3. Baltimore: University Park Press, 1980:117–210.

142. Chappel SC, Resko JA, Norman RL, et al. Studies in rhesus monkeys on the site where estrogen inhibits gonadotropins: delivery of 17β-estradiol to the hypothalamus and pituitary gland. J Clin Endocrinol Metab. 1981; 52:1–8.

143. Chappel SC, Holt JA, Spies HG. Inhibin: differences in bioactivity within human follicular fluid in the follicular and luteal stages of the menstrual cycle. Proc Soc Exp Biol Med. 1980; 163.310–314.

144. Charles D, Klein T, Lunn SF, et al. Clinical and endocrinological studies with the isomeric components of clomiphene citrate. J Obstet Gynaecol Br Comm. 1969; 76:1100–1110.

145. Chiocchio SR, Negro-Vilar A, Tramezzani JH: Acute changes in norepinephrine content in the median eminence induced by orchidectomy or testosterone replacement. Endocrinology. 1976; 99:629–634.

146. Christie GA. Comparative potency of ethinyl oestradiol and mestranol. Med J Australia. 1970; 2:202.

147. Christy NP, Warren MP. Disease syndromes of the hypothalamus and anterior pituitary. In: DeGroot LJ, Cahill GF Jr, Odell WD, et al, eds. Endocrinology, Vol 1. New York: Grune & Stratton, 1979:215–252.

148. Chrousos GP, Loriaux DL, Mann DL, et al. Late-onset 21-hydroxylase deficiency mimicking idiopathic hirsutism or polycystic ovarian disease; an allelic variant of congenital virilizing adrenal hyperplasia with a milder enzymatic defect. Ann Int Med. 1982; 96:143–148.

149. Clapp DH, Wiebe RH. The effect of hyperprolactinemia on the diurnal variation of adrenal androgens. Fertil Steril. 1983; 39:749–752.

150. Clayton RN, Catt KJ. Gonadotropin-releasing

151. hormone receptors: characterization, physiological regulation, and relationship to reproductive function. Endocrinol Rev. 1981; 2:186–209.

151. Clayton RN, Catt KJ. Regulation of pituitary gonadotropin-releasing hormone receptors by gonadal hormones. Endocrinology. 1981; 108:887–895.

152. Clayton RN, Harwood JP, Catt KJ. Gonadotropin-releasing hormone binds to luteal cells and inhibits progesterone production. Nature. 1979; 282:90–92.

153. Cohen MB. Surgical management of infertility in the polycystic ovary syndrome. In: Givens JR, ed. The Infertile Female. Chicago: Yearbook Medical Publishers, 1979:273–292.

154. Cohen PN, Givens JR, Wiser WL, et al. Polycystic ovarian disease, maturation arrest of spermiogenesis, and Klinefelter's syndrome in siblings of a family with familial hirsutism. Fertil Steril. 1975; 26:1228–1238.

155. Comite F, Cutler GB Jr, Rivier J, et al. Short-term treatment of idiopathic precocious puberty with a long-acting analogue of luteinizing hormone-releasing hormone. New Engl J Med. 1981; 305:1546–1550.

156. Conn PM, Marian J, McMillan M, et al. Gonadotropin-releasing hormone action in the pituitary: a three step mechanism. Endocrinol Rev. 1981; 2:174–185.

157. Conte FA, Grumbach MM, Kaplan SL, et al. Correlation of luteinizing hormone-releasing factor-induced luteinizing hormone and follicle-stimulating hormone release from infancy to 19 years with the changing pattern of gonadotropin secretion in agonadal patients: relation to the restraint of puberty. J Clin Endocrinol Metab. 1980; 50:163–168.

158. Cooke CW, McEvoy D, Bulaschenko H, et al. Adrenocortical and ovarian function in the hirsute woman. Am J Obstet Gynecol. 1972; 114:65–77.

159. Cooke CW, McEvoy D, Wallach EE. Polycystic ovarian syndrome with unilateral cystic teratoma. Obstet Gynecol. 1972; 39:789–794.

160. Cooper HE, Spellacy WN, Prem KA, et al. Hereditary factors in the Stein-Leventhal syndrome. Am J Obstet Gynecol. 1968; 100:371–387.

161. Copmann TL, Adams WC. Relationship of polycystic ovary induction to prolactin secretion: prevention of cyst formation by bromocryptine in the rat. Endocrinology. 1981; 108:1095–1097.

162. Corbin A, Beattie CW, Rees R, et al. Post-coital contraceptive effects of agonist analogs of luteinizing hormone-releasing hormone. Fertil Steril. 1977; 28:471–475.

163. Corenblum B. Hyperprolactinemic polycystic

ovary syndrome. In: Mahesh VB, Greenblatt RB, eds. Hirsutism and Virilism. Boston: John Wright, PSG Inc., 1983:239–276.

164. Corenblum B, Taylor PJ. The hyperprolactinemic polycystic ovary syndrome may not be a distinct entity. Fertil Steril. 1982; 38:549–552.

165. Corenblum B, Taylor PJ. An investigation of the hyperprolactinemic polycystic ovary (PCOD) syndrome. Fertil Steril (abstr). 1982; 37:292.

166. Corenblum B, LeBlanc FE, Watanabe M: Acromegaly with an adenomatous pharyngeal pituitary. JAMA. 1980; 243:1456–1457.

167. Corenblum B, Taylor PJ. A rationale for the use of bromocriptine in patients with amenorrhea and normoprolactinemia. Fertil Steril. 1980; 34:239–241.

168. Corenblum B, Pairaudeau N, Shewchuk AB. Prolactin hypersecretion and short luteal phase defects. Obstet Gynecol. 1976; 47:486–488.

169. Corral-Gallardo J, Acevedo HA, Perez de Salazar JL, et al. The polycystic ovary: VI. A hilus cell tumor of the ovary associated with polycystic ovarian disease. *In vivo* and *in vitro* studies. Acta Endocrinol (Kbh). 1966; 52:425–442.

170. Correa De Oliveira RF, Novaes LP, Lima MB, et al. A new treatment for hirsutism. Ann Int Med. 1975; 83:817–819.

171. Cortes-Gallegos V, Gallegos AG, Bodolla-Tovar N, et al. Effect of paramethasone acetate on ovarian steroids and gonadotropins. I. Normal menstrual cycle. J Clin Endocrinol Metab. 1975; 41:215–220.

172. Corvol P, Michaud A, Menard J. Antiandrogenic effect of spironolactones: mechanisms of action. Endocrinology. 1975; 97:52–58.

173. Corvol P, Bardin CW. Species distribution of testosterone-binding protein. Biol Reprod. 1973; 8:277–282.

174. Coulam CB, Annegers JF, Kranz JS. Chronic anovulation syndrome and associated neoplasia. Obstet Gynecol. 1983; 61:403–407.

175. Coulam CB, Annegers JF, Kranz JS. The association between pituitary adenoma and chronic anovulation syndrome. Am J Obstet Gynecol. 1982; 143:319–322.

176. Coulam CB, Annegers JF, Abboud CF, et al. Pituitary adenomas and oral contraceptives: a case control study. Fertil Steril. 1979; 31:25–28.

177. Crooke AC, Butt WR, Palmer R, et al. Effect of human pituitary follicular-stimulating and chorionic gonadotrophin in Stein-Leventhal syndrome. Br Med J. 1963; 1:1119–1123.

178. Crosignani PG, Ferrari C, Malinverni A, et al. Effect of central nervous system dopaminergic activation on prolactin secretion in man: evidence for a common central defect in hyperprolactinemic patients with and without radio-

logical signs of pituitary tumors. J Clin Endocrinol Metab. 1980; 51:1068–1073.

179. Crosignani PG, Reschini E, Lembroso GC, et al. Comparison of placebo and bromocriptine in the treatment of patients with normoprolactinaemic amenorrhoea. Br J Obstet Gynecol. 1978; 85:773–775.

180. Cruikshank DP, Chapler FK. Arrhenoblastomas and associated ovarian pathology. Obstet Gynecol. 1974; 43:539–543.

181. Culiner A, Shippel S. Virilism and theca cell hyperplasia of the ovary syndrome. J Obstet Gynecol Br Com. 1949; 56:439–445.

182. Cumming DC, Yang JC, Rebar RW, et al. Treatment of hirsutism with spironolactone. JAMA. 1982; 247:1295–1298.

183. Cumming DC, Quigley ME, Rebar RW, et al. Reduced hypothalamic influences on luteinizing hormone (LH) secretion in polycystic ovarian disease. Fertil Steril (Abstr). 1981; 36:431.

184. Cunningham GR, Goldzieher JW, de la Pena A, et al. The mechanism of ovulation induction by triamcinolone acetonide. J Clin Endocrinol Metab. 1978; 46:8–14.

185. Cutler GB Jr, Loriaux DL. Adrenarche and its relationship to the onset of puberty. Fed Proc. 1980; 39:2384–2390.

186. Daane TA, Dignam WJ, Frankland MV, et al. Daily serum follicle-stimulating hormone, luteinizing hormone, and plasma testosterone and androstenedione in hirsute women with polycystic sclerotic ovaries: effect of diethylstilbestrol and norethindrone acetate. Am J Obstet Gynecol. 1973; 117:392–399.

187. Daniel SAJ, Armstrong DT. Enhancement of follicle-stimulating hormone-induced aromatase activity by androgens in cultured rat granulosa cells. Endocrinology. 1980; 107:1027–1033.

188. D'Armiento M, Reda G, Bisignani G, et al. No linkage between HLA and congenital adrenal hyperplasia due to 17α-hydroxylase deficiency. New Engl J Med. 1983; 308:970–971.

189. Davidson JM, Damassa DA, Smith ER, et al. Feedback control of gonadotropin secretion in the rat. In: Spilman CH, Lobl TJ, Kirton KT, eds. Regulatory Mechanism of Male Reproductive Physiology. Amsterdam: Excerpta Medica, 1976:151–168.

190. Davies IJ, Naftolin F, Ryan KJ, et al. A specific, high affinity, limited-capacity estrogen-binding component in the cytosol of human fetal pituitary and brain tissues. J Clin Endocrinol Metab. 1975; 40:909–912.

191. deGrouchy J, Lamy M, Yaneva H, et al. Further abnormalities of the X chromosome in primary amenorrhea or in severe oligomenorrhea. Lancet. 1961; 2:777–778.

192. deJong FH, Sharpe RM. Evidence for inhibin-

like activity in bovine follicular fluid. Nature. 1976; 263:71–72.

193. deJong FH, Baird DT, van der Molen HJ. Ovarian secretion rates of oestrogens androgens and progesterone in normal women and in women with persistent ovarian follicles. Acta Endocrinol (Kbh). 1974; 77:575–587.

194. Delahunt JW, Clements RV, Ramsay ID, et al. The monocystic ovary syndrome. Br Med J. 1975; 4:621–622.

195. deLange WE, Pratt JJ, Doorenbos H. A gonadotrophin-responsive testosterone-producing adrenocortical adenoma and high gonadotrophin levels in an elderly woman. Clin Endocrinol (Oxf). 1980; 12:21–28.

196. Delforge JP, Thomas K, Roux F, et al. Time relationships between granulosa cell growth and luteinization, and plasma luteinizing hormone discharge in human. I. A morphometric analysis. Fertil Steril. 1972; 23:1–11.

197. del Pozo E, Falaschi P. Prolactin and cyclicity in polycystic ovary syndrome. In: L'Hermire M, Judd SJ, eds. Progress in Reproductive Biology. Basel: S. Karger, 1980:252–259.

198. deMoor P, Heynes W, Bouillon R. Growth hormone and the steroid binding β-globulin of human plasma. J Steroid Biochem. 1972; 3:593–600.

199. Demura R, Ono M, Demura H, et al. Prolactin directly inhibits basal as well as gonadotropin-stimulated secretion of progesterone and 17β-estradiol in the human ovary. J Clin Endocrinol Metab. 1982; 54:1246–1250.

200. deQuijada M, Timmermans HAT, Lamberts SWJ, et al. Tamoxifen enhances the sensitivity of dispersed prolactin-secreting pituitary tumor cells of dopamine and bromocriptine. Endocrinology. 1980; 106:702–706.

201. Desclin L, Flament-Durand J, Gepts W. Transplantation of the ovary to the spleen in rats with persistent estrus resulting from hypothalamic lesions. Endocrinology. 1962; 70:429–436.

202. Deutsch S, Krumholz B, Benjamin I. The utility and selection of laboratory tests in the diagnosis of polycystic ovary syndrome. J Reprod Med. 1978; 20:275–282.

203. deVane GW, Czekala NM, Judd HL, et al. Circulating gonadotropins, estrogens and androgens in polycystic ovarian disease. Am J Obstet Gynecol. 1975; 121:496–500.

204. Dewhurst CJ, Underhill R, Goldmann S, et al. The treatment of hirsutism with cyproterone acetate (an anti-androgen). Br J Obstet Gynaecol. 1977; 84:119–123.

205. Dickerman Z, Prager-Lewin R, Laron Z: Response of plasma LH and FSH to synthetic LH-RH in children at various pubertal stages. Am J Dis Child. 1976; 130:634–638.

206. Dignam WJ, Pion RJ, Lamb FJ, et al. Plasma androgens in women. II. Patients with polycystic ovaries and hirsutism. Acta Endocrinol (Kbh). 1964; 45:254–271.

207. diZerega GS, Goebelsmann U, Nakamura RM. Identification of protein(s) secreted by the preovulatiory ovary which suppresses the follicle response to gonadotropins. J Clin Endocrinol Metab. 1982; 54:1091–1096.

208. diZerega GS, Turner CK, Stouffer RL, et al. Suppression of follicle-stimulating hormone folliculogenesis during the primate ovarian cycle. J Clin Endocrinol Metab. 1981; 52:451–456.

209. diZerega GS, Hodgen GD. Folliculogenesis in the primate ovarian cycle. Endocrinol Rev. 1981; 2:27–49.

210. diZerega GS, Hodgen GD. The primate ovarian cycle. Suppression of human menopausal gonadotropin-induced follicular growth in the presence of the dominant follicle. J Clin Endocrinol Metab. 1980; 50:819–825.

211. Dmowski WP, Rezai P, Auletta FJ, et al. Abnormal follicle-stimulating hormone and luteinizing hormone patterns contrasting with normal estradiol and progesterone secretion in women with longstanding unexplained infertility. J Clin Endocrinol Metab. 1981; 52:1218–1224.

212. Dockerty MB, Mussey I. Malignant lesions of the uterus associated with estrogen-producing ovarian tumors. Am J Obstet Gynecol. 1951; 61:147–153.

213. Domingue JN, Wing D, Wilson CB. Coexisting pituitary adenomas and partially empty sellas. J Neurosurg. 1978; 48:23–28.

214. Dorrington JH, Moon YS, Armstrong DT. Estradiol-17β biosynthesis in cultured granulosa cells from hypophysectomized immature rats; stimulation by follicle-stimulating hormone. Endocrinology. 1975; 97:1328–1331.

215. Drucker WD, David RR. Plasma dehydroepiandrosterone sulfate (DHAS) in normals and patients with hyperprolactinemia. In: Genazzani AR, ed. Adrenal Androgens. New York: Raven Press, 1980:89–94.

216. Drouva SV, Gallo RV. Catecholamine involvement in episodic luteinizing hormone release in adult ovariectomized rats. Endocrinology. 1976; 99:651–658.

217. Ducharme JR, Forest MG, Deperetti E, et al. Plasma adrenal and gonadal steroids in human pubertal development. J Clin Endocrinol Metab. 1976; 42:468–476.

218. Duignan NM. Polycystic ovarian disease. Br J Obstet Gynaecol. 1976; 83:593–602.

219. Duignan NM, Shaw RW, Rudd BT, et al. Sex hormone levels and gonadotrophin release in

the polycystic ovary syndrome. Clin Endocrinol (Oxf). 1975; 4:287–295.

220. Dupon C, Rosenfield RL, Cleary RE. Sequential changes in total and free testosterone and androstenedione in plasma during spontaneous and clomid-induced ovulatory cycles. Am J Obstet Gynecol. 1973; 115:478–483.

221. Dupont B, Pollack MS, Levine LS, et al. Congenital adrenal hyperplasia. In: Terasaki PI, ed. Histocompatibility Testing 1980. Los Angeles: UCLA Tissue Typing Laboratory, 1980:693.

222. DuToit DAH. Polycystic ovaries, menstrual disturbances and hirsutism. In: Stenfert HE, ed. Hyperthecosis. Leiden: Kroese NV, 1951.

223. Easterling WF, Talbert LM, Potter HD. Serum testosterone levels in the polycystic ovary syndrome. Am J Obstet Gynecol. 1974; 120:385–389.

224. Eddy CA, Asch RH, Balmaceda JP. Pelvic adhesions following microsurgical and macrosurgical wedge resection of the ovaries. Fertil Steril. 1980; 33:557–561.

225. Eddy WA. Endometrial carcinoma in Stein-Leventhal syndrome treated with hydroxyprogesterone caproate. Am J Obstet Gynecol. 1978; 131:581–582.

226. Edman CD, Aiman EJ, Porter JC, et al. Identification of the estrogen product of extraglandular aromatization of plasma androstenedione. Am J Obstet Gynecol. 1978; 130:439–447.

227. Edman CD, MacDonald PC. The role of extraglandular estrogen in women in health and disease. In: James VHT, Serio M, Giusti G, eds. The Endocrine Function of the Human Ovary. New York: Academic Press, 1976:135–140.

228. Edwards CRW, Jeffcoate WJ. Bromocriptine and the adrenal cortex. In: Bayliss RIS, Turner P, Maclay WP, eds. Pharmacological and Clinical Aspects of Bromocriptine. Turnbridge Wells: MCS Consultants, 1976:43–49.

229. Elkind-Hirsch K, Ravnikar V, Schiff I, et al. Determinations of endogenous immunoreactive luteinizing hormone-releasing hormone in human plasma. J Clin Endocrinol Metab. 1982; 54:602–607.

230. Erickson GF, Hsueh AJW, Quigley ME, et al. Functional studies of aromatase activity in human granulosa cells from normal and polycystic ovaries. J Clin Endocrinol Metab. 1979; 49:514–519.

231. Erickson GF, Hsueh AJW. Stimulation of aromatase activity by follicle-stimulating homone in rat granulosa cells *in vivo* and *in vitro*. Endocrinology. 1978; 102:1275–1282.

232. Eskey RL, Warberg J, Mical RS, et al. Prostaglandin E_2-induced release of LHRH and hypophysial portal blood. Endocrinology. 1975; 97:816–824.

233. Espey LL. Ovarian proteolytic enzymes and ovulation. Biol Reprod. 1974; 10:216–235.

234. Ettinger B, Golditch IM. Medroxyprogesterone acetate for the evaluation of hypertestosteronism in hirsute women. Fertil Steril. 1977; 28:1285–1288.

235. Ettinger B, Goldfield EB, Burrill KC, et al. Plasma testosterone stimulation-suppression dynamics in hirsute women: correlation with long-term therapy. Am J Med. 1973; 54:195–200.

236. Ettinger B, von Werder K, Thenaers GC, et al. Plasma testosterone stimulation-suppression dynamics in hirsute women. Am J Med. 1971; 51:170–175.

237. Evans TN, Riley GM. Thecoma and polycystic disease of the ovaries. Obstet Gynecol. 1961; 18:52–59.

238. Evans TN, Riley GM. Polycystic ovarian disease. A clinical and experimental study. Am J Obstet Gynecol. 1960; 80:873–888.

239. Evans WS, Schiebinger RJ, Kaiser DL, et al. Serum adrenal androgens in hyperprolactinaemic women prior to, during, and after chronic treatment with bromocriptine. Acta Endocrinol (Kbh). 1982; 101:235–241.

240. Evans WS, Cronin MJ, Thorner MO. Hypogonadism in hyperprolactinemia: proposed mechanisms. In: Ganong WF, Martini L, eds. Frontiers in Neuroendocrinology, Vol 7. New York: Raven Press, 1982:77–122.

241. Evans WS, Rogol A, MacLeod RM, et al. Dopaminergic mechanisms and luteinizing hormone secretion. I. Acute administration of the dopamine agonist bromocriptine does not inhibit luteinizing hormone release in hyperprolactinemic women. J Clin Endocrinol Metab. 1980; 50:103–107.

242. Evron S, Navot D, Laufer N, et al. Induction of ovulation with combined human gonadotropins and dexamethasone in women with polycystic ovarian disease. Fertil Steril. 1983; 40:183–186.

243. Evron S, Shapiro G, Diamant YZ. Induction of ovulation with spironolactone (Aldactone) in anovulatory oligomenorrheic and hyperandrogenic women. Fertil Steril. 1981; 36:468–471.

244. Faglia G, Beck-Peccoz P, Travaglini P, et al. Functional studies in hyperprolactinemic states. In: Crosignani PG, Robyn C, eds. Prolactin and Human Reproduction. New York: Academic Press, 1977:225–238.

245. Faglia G, Travaglini P, Neri V, et al. Occurrence of a virilizing syndrome with 21-hydroxylase deficiency after pregnancy. J Clin Endocrinol Metab. 1969; 29:1325–1329.

246. Falaschi P, del Pozo E, Rocco A, et al. Prolactin

release in polycystic ovary. Obstet Gynecol. 1980; 55:579–582.

247. Falaschi P, Rocco A, Pompei P, et al. High incidence of hyperprolactinemia in polycystic ovary (PCO) syndrome: functional or tumoral origin. 6th International Congress of Endocrinology, (Abstr). 1980:641.

248. Falaschi P, Rocco A, Sciarra F, et al. The effect of short-term bromocryptine administration on PCO syndrome with hyperprolactinemia: a preliminary report. In: Klopper A, Lerner L, Vander Molen HJ, Sciarra F, eds. Research on Steroids, Vol VIII. London: Academic Press, 1979:241–245

249. Falaschi P, Frajese G, Rocco A, et al. High incidence of hyperprolactinemia in PCOD. Clin Endocrinol (Oxf). 1977; 8:427–433.

250. Farber M, Millan VG, Turksoy RN, et al. Diagnostic evaluation of hirsutism in women by selective bilateral adrenal and ovarian venous catheterization. Fertil Steril. 1978; 30:283–288.

251. Farber M, Daoust PR, Rogers J. Hyperthecosis syndrome. Obstet Gynecol. 1974; 44:35–41.

252. Fayez JA, Jonas HS. Assessment of the role of laparoscopic ovarian biopsy. Obstet Gynecol. 1976; 48:397–402.

253. Fayez JA. Selection of patients for clomiphene citrate therapy. Obstet Gynecol. 1976; 47:671–676.

254. Fechner RE, Kaufman RH: Endometrial adenocarcinoma in Stein-Leventhal syndrome. Cancer. 1974; 34:444–452.

255. Feher T, Halmy L. Dehydroepiandrosterone and dehydroepiandrosterone sulfate dynamics in obesity. Can J Biochem. 1975; 53:215–222.

256. Ferin M, Rosenblatt H, Carmel PW, et al. Estrogen-induced gonadotropin surges in female rhesus monkeys after pituitary stalk section. Endocrinology. 1979; 104:50–52.

257. Ferland L, Marchetti B, Seguin C, et al. Dissociated changes of pituitary luteinizing homone-releasing hormone (LH-RH) receptors and responsiveness to the neurohormone induced by 17β-estradiol and LH-RH *in vivo* in the rat. Endocrinology. 1981; 109:87–93.

258. Fern M, Rose DP, Fern EB. Effect of oral contraceptives on plasma androgenic steroids and their precursors. Obstet Gynecol. 1978; 51:541–554.

259. Ferraninni E, Muggeo M, Navalesi R, et al. Impaired insulin degradation in a patient with insulin resistance and acanthosis nigricans. Am J Med. 1982; 73:148–154.

260. Ferriman D, Purdie AW. The inheritance of polycystic ovarian disease and a possible relationship to premature balding. Clin Endocrinol (Oxf). 1979; 11:291–300.

261. Ferriman D, Purdie AW, Tindall WJ. The use

of corticosteroids in infertility associated with hirsuties and oligomenorrhea. Br Med J. 1961; 1:1006–1008.

262. Finkelstein M. Pregnanetriolone, an abnormal urinary steroid. In: Dorfman RI, ed. Methods in Hormone Research, Vol 1. New York: Academic Press, 1971:169–197.

263. Fisher RA, Anderson DC. Simultaneous measurement of unbound testosterone and estradiol fractions in undiluted plasma at 37 degrees C by steady-state gel filtration. Steroids. 1974; 24:809–824.

264. Flier JS, Young JB, Landsberg L. Familial insulin resistance with acanthosis nigricans, acral hypertrophy and muscle cramps. New Engl J Med. 1980; 303:970–973.

265. Flier JS, Kahn CR, Roth J. Receptors, antireceptors antibodies, and mechanism of insulin resistance. New Engl J Med. 1979; 300:413–419.

266. Flier JS, Kahn CR, Roth J, et al. Antibodies that impair insulin receptor binding in an unusual diabetic syndrome with severe insulin resistance. Science. 1975; 190:63–65.

267. Floersheim-Schachar Y, Keller PJ. Treatment of hyperprolactinemia-anovulation syndrome. Fertil Steril. 1977; 28:1158–1163.

268. Forest MG, Bertrand J. Studies of the protein binding of dihydrotestosterone (17β-hydroxy-5α-androstan-3 one) in human plasma in different physiological conditions and effect of medroxyprogesterone (17-hydroxy-6α-methyl-4 pregnene-3,20 dione 17-acetate). Steroids. 1972; 19:197–214.

269. Fortune JE, Armstrong DT. Androgen production by theca and granulosa isolated from proestrus rat follicles. Endocrinology. 1977; 100:1341–1347.

270. Fox H, Langley FA. Andۇoblastoma. In: Tumors of the Ovary. London: William Heinemann Med Books Ltd., 1976:138–163.

271. Fraenkel L. Thecoma and hyperthecosis of the ovary. J Clin Endocrinol Metab. 1943; 3:557–559.

272. France JT, Knox BS. Urinary excretion of testosterone and epitestosterone in hirsutism. Acta Endocrinol (Kbh). 1967; 56:177–187.

273. Franchimont P, Henderson K, Verhoeven G, et al. Inhibin: mechanisms of action and secretion. In: Franchimont P, Channing CP, eds. Intragonadal Regulation of Reproduction. London: Academic Press, 1981:167–191.

274. Franks S, Murray MAF, Jequier AM, et al. Incidence and significance of hyperprolactinaemia in women with amenorrhoea. Clin Endocrinol (Oxf). 1975; 4:597–607.

275. Frantz AG. Prolactin. New Engl J Med. 1978; 298:201–207.

276. Fraser IS, Michie EA, Wide L, et al. Pituitary

gonadotropins and ovarian function in adolescent dysfunctional uterine bleeding. J Clin Endocrinol Metab. 1973; 37:407–414.

277. Frisch RE, McArthur JW. Menstrual cycles: fatness as a determinant of minimum weight for height necessary for their maintenance or onset. Science. 1974; 185:949–951.

278. Frisch RE, Revelle R. Height and weight at menarche and a hypothesis of menarche. Arch Dis Child. 1971; 46:695–701.

279. Frisch RE, Revelle R. Height and weight at menarche and a hypothesis of critical body weights and adolescent events. Science. 1970; 169:397–399.

280. Fritz MA, Speroff L. The endocrinology of the menstrual cycle: the interaction of folliculogenesis and neuroendocrine mechanisms. Fertil Steril. 1982; 38:509–529.

281. Fuller PJ, Pettigrew IG, Pike JW, et al. An adrenal adenoma causing virilization of mother and infant. Clin Endocrinol (Oxf). 1983; 18:143–153.

282. Fulling KH, Mills BK, Swarm RL, et al. Diffuse prolactin cell hyperplasia is the precursor lesion to estrogen-induced and spontaneous adenomatous neoplasia in rats (abstr 563). Presented at the 60th Annual Meeting of the Endocrine Society, Miami, Fla, June 14–16, 1978:356

283. Funder JW, Mercer JE. Cimetidine, a histamine H_2 receptor antagonist, occupies androgen receptors. J Clin Endocrinol Metab. 1979; 48:189–191.

284. Futterweit W. Pituitary tumors and polycystic ovarian disease. Obstet Gynecol. 1983; 62: S74–S79.

285. Futterweit W, Krieger DT, Kase N. Unpublished data, 1984.

286. Futterweit W, Mechanick JI. Unpublished data, 1983.

287. Futterweit W, Scher J, Nunez AE, et al. A case of bilateral dermoid cysts, insulin resistance and polycystic ovarian disease: the association of ovarian tumors with polycystic ovaries with a review of the literature. Mt. Sinai J of Med. 1983; 50:251–255.

288. Futterweit W. Galactorrhea, amenorrhea, hyperprolactinemia and pseudotumor cerebri in a patient with primary empty sella syndrome: case report with review of the literature. Mt Sinai J Med. 1982; 49:514–518.

289. Futterweit W. Endocrine management of transsexual. Hormonal profiles of serum prolactin, testosterone, and estradiol. NY State J Med. 1980; 80:1260–1264.

290. Futterweit W, Krieger DT. Pituitary tumors associated with hyperprolactinemia and polycystic ovarian disease. Fertil Steril. 1979; 31:608–613.

291. Futterweit W, Goodsell CH. Galactorrhea in primary hypothyroidism: report of two cases and review of the literature. Mt. Sinai J Med. 1970; 37:584–589.

292. Futterweit W, Freeman R, Siegel GL, et al. Clinical application of a gas chromatographic method for the combined determination of testosterone and epitestosterone glucuronide in urine. J Clin Endocrinol Metab. 1965; 25:1451–1456.

293. Futterweit W, McNiven NL, Guerra-Garcia R, et al. Testosterone in human urine. Steroids. 1964; 4:137–141.

294. Futterweit W, Margolis SA, Soffer LJ, et al. Effect of urinary gonadotropin inhibitor on the mouse uterine response to various gonadotropins. Endocrinology. 1963; 72:903–907.

295. Fuxe K, Andersson K, Löfström A, et al. Neurotransmitter mechanisms in the control of the secretion of hormones from the anterior pituitary. In: Fuxe K, Hokfelt T, Luft R, eds. Central Regulation of the Endocrine System. New York: Plenum Press, 1979:349–380.

296. Fuxe K, Hökfelt J, Löfström A, et al. On the role of neurotransmitters and hypothalamic hormones and their interactions in hypothalamic and extrahypothalamic control of pituitary function and sexual behavior. In: Naftolin F, Ryan KJ, Davies IJ, eds. Subcellular Mechanisms in Reproductive Neuroendocrinology. Amsterdam: Elsevier Press, 1976:193–246.

297. Gabrilove JL, Seman AT, Sebet R, et al. Virilizing adrenal adenoma with studies on the steroid content of the adrenal venous effluent and a review of the literature. Endocrinol Rev. 1981; 2:462–470.

298. Gabrilove JL, Nicolis GL, Mitty HA. Virilizing adrenocortical adenoma studies by selective adrenal venography. Am J Obstet Gynecol. 1976; 125:180–184.

299. Gabrilove JL, Sharma DC, Dorfman RI. Adrenocortical 11β-hydroxylase deficiency and virilism first manifest in the adult woman. New Engl J Med. 1965; 272:1189–1194.

300. Gallagher TF, Spencer H, Bradlow HL, et al. Steroid production and metabolism in metastatic arrhenoblastoma. J Clin Endocrinol Metab. 1962; 22:970–977.

301. Gambrell RD Jr. Regression of polycystic ovaries by estrogen therapy. Obstet Gynecol. 1976; 47:569–574.

302. Gambrell RD, Greenblatt RB, Mahesh VB. Inappropriate secretion of LH in the Stein-Leventhal syndrome. Obstet Gynecol. 1973; 42:429–440.

303. Gant NF, Hutchinson HT, Siiteri P, et al. Study of the metabolic clearance rate of dehydroisoandrosterone sulfate in pregnancy. Am J Obstet Gynecol. 1971; 111:555–561.

304. Garces LY, Kenny FM, Drash A, et al. Cortisol

secretion rate during fasting of obese adolescent subjects. J Clin Endocrinol Metab. 1968; 28:1843–1847.

305. Garcia JE, Jones GS, Wright GL Jr. Prediction of the time of ovulation. Fertil Steril. 1981; 36:308–315.

306. Garcia JE, Jones GS, Wentz AC. The use of clomiphene citrate. Fertil Steril. 1977; 28:707–717.

307. Gardo S, Papp Z, Smid I, et al. Cytogenetic studies in Stein-Leventhal syndrome Arch Gynäk. 1974; 216:311–315.

308. Gaspard UJ. Role of antiandrogens in the treatment of acne. In: Mahesh VB, Greenblatt RB, eds. Hirsutism and Virilism. Boston: John Wright, PSG Inc., 1983:369–394.

309. Geist SH, Gaines JA. Diffuse luteinization of ovaries associated with masculinization syndrome. Am J Obstet Gynecol. 1942;43:975–983.

310. Geller S, Ayme Y, Lemasson C, et al. Polykystose ovarienne. Sécrétion inappropriée de LH "seule." Micro-adénome hypophysaire à LH? Nouvelle Presse Médicale. 1976; 5:1492.

311. Gemzell CA. Induction of ovulation with human gonadotropins. J Reprod Med. 1977; 18:155–158.

312. Gemzell CA, Diczfalusy E, Tillinger G. Clinical effect of human pituitary follicle-stimulating hormone (FSH). J Clin Endocrinol Metab. 1958; 18:1333–1348.

313. Genazzani AR, Pintor C, Corda R. Plasma levels of gonadotropins, prolactin, thyroxine, and adrenal and gonadal steroids in obese prepubertal girls. J Clin Endocrinol Metab. 1978; 47:974–979.

314. Gibson M, Lackritz R, Schiff I, et al. Abnormal adrenal responses to adrenocorticotropic hormone in hyperandrogenic women. Fertil Steril. 1980; 33:43–48.

315. Ginsburg J, Isaacs AJ, Gore MBR, et al. Use of clomiphene and luteinizing hormone/follicle stimulating hormone-releasing hormone in investigation of ovulatory failure. Br Med J. 1975; 3:130–133.

316. Girard J, Baumann JB, Büchler U, et al. Cyproterone acetate and ACTH adrenal function. J Clin Endocrinol Metab. 1978; 47:581–586.

317. Giusti G, Bassi F, Forti G, et al. Effects of prolactin on androgen secretion by the human adrenal cortex. In: Robyn C, Harter M, eds. Progress in Prolactin Physiology and Pathology. Amsterdam: Elsevier/North-Holland Biomedical Press, 1978:293–303.

318. Giusti G, Bassi F, Borsi L, et al. Effects of prolactin on the human adrenal cortex: plasma dehydroepiandrosterone sulphate in women affected by amenorrhea with hyperprolactinemia. In: Crosignani PG, Robyn C, eds. Prolactin and Human Reproduction. New York: Academic Press, 1977:239–244.

319. Given WP, Gause RW, Douglas RG. Rational therapy for secondary amenorrhea. New Engl J Med. 1950; 243:357–362.

320. Givens JR. Role of oral contraceptives in the treatment of hyperandrogenism of hirsute women. In: Mahesh VB, Greenblatt RB, eds. Hirsutism and Virilism. Boston: John Wright, PSG Inc., 1983:351–367.

321. Givens JR, Wiedemann E, Andersen RN, et al. β-endorphin and β-lipotropin plasma levels in hirsute women: correlation with body weight. J Clin Endocrinol Metab. 1980; 50:975–976.

322. Givens JR. Panel. Endocrine disorders. In: Givens JR, ed. The Infertile Female. Chicago: Year Book Med Publ, 1979:228.

323. Givens JR. Normal and abnormal androgen metabolism. Clin Obstet Gynecol. 1978; 21:115–123.

324. Givens JR. Polycystic ovarian disease In: Givens JR, ed. Gynecologic Endocrinology. Chicago: Year Book Med Publ, 1977:127–142.

325. Givens JR. Hirsutism and hyperandrogenism. In: Stollerman GH, ed. Advances in Internal Medicine, Vol 21. Chicago: Year Book Med Publ, 1976:221–247.

326. Givens JR, Andersen RN, Ragland JB, et al. Effects of norgestrel and metyrapone on pituitary–adrenal–ovarian function. 1976; Obstet Gynecol 48:392–396.

327. Givens, JR, Andersen RN, Umstot ES, et al. Clinical findings and hormonal responses in patients with polycystic ovarian disease with normal versus elevated LH levels. Obstet Gynecol. 1976; 47:388–394.

328. Givens JR, Andersen RN, Wiser WL, et al. The effectiveness of two oral contraceptives in suppressing plasma androstenedione, testosterone, LH, and FSH, and in stimulating plasma testosterone-binding capacity in hirsute women. Am J Obstet Gynecol. 1976; 124:333–339.

329. Givens JR, Andersen RN, Wiser WL, et al. A testosterone-secreting, gonadotropin-responsive pure thecoma and polycystic ovarian disease. J Clin Endocrinol Metab. 1975; 41:845–853.

330. Givens JR, Andersen RN, Ragland JB, et al. Adrenal function in hirsutism. I. Diurnal change and response of plasma androstenedione, testosterone, 17-hydroxyprogesterone, cortisol, LH and FSH to dexamethasone and 1/2 unit of ACTH. J Clin Endocrinol Metab. 1975; 40:988–1000.

331. Givens JR, Wilroy RS, Summitt RL, et al. Features of Turner's syndrome in women with polycystic ovaries. Obstet Gynecol. 1975; 45:619–624.

332. Givens JR, Andersen RN, Wiser WL, et al. Dy-

namics of suppression and recovery of plasma FSH, LH, androstenedione and testosterone in polycystic ovarian disease using an oral contraceptive. J Clin Endocrinol Metab. 1974; 38:727–735.

333. Givens JR, Kerber IJ, Wiser WL, et al. Remission of acanthosis nigricans associated with polycystic ovarian disease and a stromal luteoma. J Clin Endocrinol Metab. 1974; 38:347–355.

334. Givens JR, Andersen RN, Wiser WL, et al. A gonadotropin-responsive adrenocortical adenoma. J Clin Endocrinol Metab. 1974; 38:126–133.

335. Givens JR, Wiser WL, Coleman SA, et al. Familial ovarian hyperthecosis: a study of two families. Am J Obstet Gynecol. 1971; 110:959–972.

336. Glass AR, Dahms WT, Abraham G, et al. Secondary amenorrhea in obesity: etiologic role of weight-related androgen excess. Fertil Steril. 1978; 30:243–244.

337. Glass MR, Shaw RW, Butt WR, et al. An abnormality of oestrogen feedback in amenorrhoea-galactorrhoea. Br Med J. 1975; 3:274–275.

338. Glickman SP, Rosenfield RL, Bergenstal RM, et al. Multiple androgenic abnormalities, including elevated free testosterone, in hyperprolactinemic women. J Clin Endocrinol Metab. 1982; 55:251–257.

339. Goebelsmann U, Kletsky OA, Davajan V. Anovulation and amnorrhea. In: Crosignani PG, Mishell DR, eds. Ovulation in the Human. New York: Academic Press, 1976:167–179.

340. Goldfarb AF, Crawford R. Polycystic ovarian disease, clomiphene, and multiple pregnancies. Obstet Gynecol. 1969; 34:307–309.

341. Goldzieher JW. Polycystic ovarian disease. Fertil Steril. 1981; 35:371–394.

342. Goldzieher JW. Perspectives in polycystic ovarian disease — 1969–77. In: Givens JR, ed. Endocrine Causes of Menstrual Disorders, Chicago: Year Book Med Publ, 1978:307–332.

343. Goldzieher JW. The pill. In: Givens JR, ed. Gynecologic Endocrinology. Chicago: Year Book Med Publ, 1977:193–208.

344. Goldzieher JW, Dozier TS, Smith KD, et al. Improving the diagnostic reliability of rapidly fluctuating plasma hormone levels by optimized multiple-sampling techniques. J Clin Endocrinol Metab. 1976; 43:824–830.

345. Goldzieher JW, Kleber JW, Moses LE, et al. A cross-sectional study of plasma FSH and LH levels in women using sequential, combination or injectable steroid contraceptives over long periods of time. Contraception. 1970; 2:225–245.

346. Goldzieher JW. The interplay of adrenocortical and ovarian function. In: Mack HC, ed. The Ovary, Proceedings of the Second Annual Symposium on the Physiology and Pathology of Human Reproduction. Springfield: Charles C. Thomas, 1968:106–129.

347. Goldzieher JW, Axelrod LR. Clinical and biochemical features of polycystic ovarian disease. Fertil Steril. 1963; 14:631–653.

348. Goldzieher JW, Axelrod LR. The polycystic ovary. II. Urinary steroid exretion. J Clin Endocrinol Metab. 1962; 22:425–430.

349. Goldzieher JW, Green JA. The polycystic ovary. I. Clinical and histologic features. J Clin Endocrinol Metab. 1962; 22:325–338.

350. Gordon GG, Southren AL, Calanog A, et al. The effect of medroxyprogesterone acetate on androgen metabolism in the polycystic ovary syndrome. J Clin Endocrinol Metab. 1972; 35:444–447.

351. Gordon GG, Southren AL, Tochimoto S, et al. Effect of medroxyprogesterone acetate (Provera) on the metabolism and biological activity of testosterone. J Clin Endocrinol. 1970; 30:449–456.

352. Gordon JS, Wu CH, Mikhail G. Daily plasma prolactin in various gynecologic endocrinopathies. Fertil Steril. 1979; 31:385–391.

353. Gourmelen M, Pham-Huu-Trung MT, Bredon MG, et al. 17-hydroxyprogesterone in the cosyntropin test: results in normal and hirsute women and in mild congenital adrenal hyperplasia. Acta Endocrinol (Kbh). 1979; 90:481–489.

354. Granoff AB, Abraham GE. Peripheral and adrenal venous levels of steroids in a patient with virilizing adrenal adenoma. Obstet Gynecol. 1979; 53:111–115.

355. Grant LD, Stumpf WE. Localization of ^{3}H-cstradiol and catecholamines in identical neurons in the hypothalamus. J Histochem Cytochem. 1973; 21:404.

356. Grattarola R. Misdiagnosis of endometrial adenocarcinoma in young women with polycystic ovarian disease. Am J Obstet Gynecol. 1969; 105:498–502.

357. Gray LA, Christopherson WM, Hoover RN. Estrogens and endometrial carcinoma. Obstet Gynecol. 1977; 49:385–389.

358. Green JA, Maqueo M. Histopathology and ultrastructure of an ovarian hilar cell tumor. Am J Obstet Gynecol. 1966; 96:478–485.

359. Green JA, Goldzieher JW. The polycystic ovary. IV. Light and electron microscope studies. Am J Obstet Gynecol. 1965; 91:173–181.

360. Greenblatt RB, Mahesh VB. The androgenic polycystic ovary. Am J Obstet Gynecol. 1976; 125:712–726.

361. Greenblatt RB. In: The Hirsute Female ch. 9. The polycystic ovary syndrome of Stein-Le-

venthal. Springfield, Ill: Charles C. Thomas, 1963:149–178.

362. Greenblatt RB, Barfield WE, Lampros CP. Cortisone in the treatment of infertility. Fertil Steril. 1956; 7:203–212.

363. Groom GV, Griffiths K. Effect of the anti-oestrogen tamoxifen on plasma levels of luteinizing hormone, follicle-stimulating hormone, prolactin, oestradiol and progesterone in normal premenopausal women. J Endocrinol. 1976; 70:421–428.

364. Grosse-Wilde H, Weil J, Albert E, et al. Genetic linkage studies between congenital adrenal hyperplasia and the HLA blood group system. Immunogenetics. 1979; 8:41–48.

365. Grumbach MM, Conte FA. Disorders of sex differentiation. In: Williams RH, ed. Textbook of Endocrinology, Philadelphia: WB Saunders Co., 1981:423–514.

366. Grumbach MM. The neuroendocrinology of puberty. In: Krieger DT, Hughes JC, eds. Neuroendocrinology. Sunderland, Mass: Sinauer Associates, 1980:249–258.

367. Grumbach MM, Roth JC, Kaplan SL, et al. Hypothalamic–pituitary regulation of puberty in man: evidence and concepts derived from clinical research. In: Grumbach MM, Grave DG, Mayer FE, eds. The Control of the Onset of Puberty. New York: John Wiley & Sons, 1974:115–166.

368. Gudelsky GA, Porter JC. Release of dopamine from tuberoinfundibular neurons into pituitary stalk blood after prolactin or haloperidol administration. Endocrinology. 1980; 106:526–529.

369. Gudelsky GA, Porter JC. Morphine and opioid peptide-induced inhibition of the release of dopamine from tuberoinfundibular neurons. Life Sci. 1979; 25:1697–1702.

370. Guillemin R. Beta-lipotropin and endorphins: implications of current knowledge. In: Krieger DT, Hughes JC, eds. Neuroendocrinology. Sunderland, Mass: Sinauer Associates, 1980:67–74.

371. Gulyas BJ, Hodgen GD, Tullner WW, et al. Effects of fetal or maternal hypophysectomy on endocrine organs and body weight in infant rhesus monkeys (Mecaca mulatta) with particular reference to oogenesis. Biol Reprod. 1977; 16:216–227.

372. Gurpide E. Secretion of steroids in normal ovaries. In: Schooler R, ed. Endocrinology of the Ovary. Paris: Editions Sepe, 1978:3–21.

373. Gurpide E. Interpretation of isotopic data from blood-borne compounds. In: Gross F, Labhart A, Lipsett MB et al eds. Tracer Methods in Hormone Research, Monographs on Endocrinology, Vol 8. New York: Springer-Verlag, 1975:105–147.

374. Gustafsson JA, Steinberg A. Influence of prolactin on the metabolism of steroid hormones in rat liver and adrenals. Acta Endocrinol (Kbh). 1975; 78:545–553.

375. Gutai JP, Lee PA, Johnsonbaugh RE, et al. Detection of the heterozygous state in siblings of patients with congenital adrenal hyperplasia due to 21-hydroxylase deficiency. J Pediatr. 1979; 94:770–772.

376. Gutai JP, Kowarski AA, Migeon CJ. Twenty-four hour integrated concentration of progesterone, 17-hydroxyprogesterone and cortisol in normal male subjects. J Clin Endocrinol Metab. 1977; 44:116–120.

377. Gutai JP, Kowarski AA, Migeon CJ. The detection of the heterozygous carrier for congenital virilizing adrenal hyperplasia. J Pediatr. 1977; 90:924–929

378. Gyory G, Kiss C, Feher T, et al. Concentration of unconjugated adrenalgenic hormones and their precursors in normal and polycystic ovaries. Endokrinologie. 1975; 64:181–190.

379. Gysler M, March CM, Mishell DM Jr, et al. A decade's experience with an individualized clomiphene treatment regimen including its effect of the postcoital test. Fertil Steril. 1982; 37:161–167.

380. Gyves MT. The significance of peripheral sclerosis in the Stein-Leventhal syndrome. Fertil Steril. 1970; 21:502–507.

381. Haesslein HC, Lamb EJ. Pituitary tumors in patients with secondary amenorrhea. Am J Obstet Gynecol. 1976; 125:759–767.

382. Hammerstein J, Mickies J, Leo-Rossberg I, et al. Use of cyproterone acetate (CPA) in the treatment of acne, hirsutism, and virilism. J Steroid Biochem. 1975; 6:827–836.

383. Hargrave DC. Chromosome mosaicism in Stein-Leventhal syndrome. Br Med J. 1965; 1:997–998.

384. Harris GW, Naftolin F. The hypothalamus and control of ovulation. Br Med Bull. 1970; 26:3–9.

385. Hatch R, Rosenfield RL, Kim MH, et al. Hirsutism: implications, etiology and management. Am J Obstet Gynecol. 1981; 140:815–830.

386. Haug E, Gautvik KM. Effects of sex steroids on prolactin-secreting rat pituitary cells in culture. Endocrinology. 1976; 99:1482–1489.

387. Healy DL, Pepperell RJ, Stockdale J, et al. Pituitary autonomy in hyperprolactinemic secondary amenorrhea: results of hypothalamic–pituitary testing. J Clin Endocrinol Metab. 1977; 44:809–819.

388. Hillier SG, Reichart LE Jr, van Hall EV. Control of preovulatory follicular estrogen biosynthesis in the human ovary. J Clin Endocrinol Metab. 1981; 52:847–856.

389. Hillier SG, van den Boogaard AMJ, Reichart

LE, et al. Intraovarian sex steroid hormone interactions and the regulation of follicular maturation: aromatization of androgens by human granulosa cells *in vitro.* J Clin Endocrinol Metab. 1980; 50:640–647.

390. Hjortrup A, Kehlet H, Lockwood K, et al. Long-term clinical effects of ovarian wedge resection in polycystic ovarian syndrome. Acta Obstet Gynecol Scand. 1983; 62:55–57.

391. Hochner-Celuikier D, Zylber-Haran E, Shilo S, et al. Increased prolactin response to thyrotropin-releasing hormone in primary ovarian failure. Obstet Gynecol. 1982; 59:280–284.

392. Hopper BR, Yen SSC. Circulatory concentrations of dehydroepiandrosterone and dehydroepiandrosterone sulfate during puberty. J Clin Endocrinol Metab. 1975; 40:458–461.

393. Horton R, Neisler J. Plasma androgens in patients with polycystic ovary syndrome. J Clin Endocrinol Metab. 1968; 28:479–484.

394. Horton R, Frasier SD. Androstenedione and its conversion to plasma testosterone in congenital adrenal hyperplasia. J Clin Invest. 1967; 46:1003–1009.

395. Horton R, Tait JF. *In vivo* conversion of dehydroisoandrosterone to plasma androstenedione and testosterone in man. J Clin Endocrinol Metab. 1967; 27:79–88.

396. Horton R, Romanoff E, Walker J. Androstenedione and testosterone in ovarian venous and peripheral plasma during ovariectomy for breast cancer. J Clin Endocrinol Metab. 1966; 26:1267–1269.

397. Horton R, Tait JF. Androstenedione production and interconversion rates measured in peripheral blood and studies on the possible site of its conversion to testosterone. J Clin Invest. 1966; 45:301–313.

398. Hosseinian AH, Kim MH, Rosenfield RL. Obesity and oligomenorrhea are associated with hyperandrogenism independent of hirsutism. J Clin Endocrinol Metab. 1976; 42:765–769.

399. Hsueh AJW, Jones PBC. Extrapituitary actions of gonadotropin-releasing hormone. Endocrine Rev. 1981; 2:437–461.

400. Hsueh AJW, Wang C, Erickson GF. Direct inhibitory effect of gonadotropin-releasing hormone upon follicle-stimulating hormone induction of luteinizing hormone receptor and aromatase activity in rat granulosa cells. Endocrinology. 1980; 108:1697–1705.

401. Hsueh AJW, Erickson GF. Extrapituitary action of gonadotropin-releasing hormone: direct inhibition of ovarian steroidogenesis. Science. 1979; 204:854–855.

402. Huppert LC. Induction of ovulation with clomiphene citrate. Fertil Steril. 1979; 31:1–8.

403. Huq MS, Pfaff M, Jespersen D, et al. Concurrence of aldosterone, androgen, and cortisol secretion in adrenal venous effluents. J Clin Endocrinol Metab. 1976; 42:230–238.

404. Hutchinson JR, Taylor HB, Zimmerman EA. The Stein-Leventhal syndrome and coincident ovarian neoplasms. Obstet Gynecol. 1966; 28:700–703.

405. Ikkos DG, Dellia-Sifikaki A. Letter: Plasma steroids in hirsutism. Obstet Gynecol. 1975; 46:114–115.

406. Imperato-McGinley J, Peterson RE, Sturla E, et al. Primary amenorrhea associated with hirsutism, acanthosis nigricans, dermoid cysts of the ovaries and a new type of insulin resistance. Am J Med. 1978; 65:389–395.

407. Insler V, Zakut H, Serr DM. Cycle pattern and pregnancy rate following combined clomiphene-estrogen therapy. Obstet Gynecol. Survey 1973; 41:602–607.

408. Ireland K, Woodruff JD. Masculinizing ovarian tumors. Obstet Gynecol Sur. 1976; 31:83–111.

409. Ismail AAA, Davidson DW, Souka AR, et al. The evaluation of the role of androgens in hirsutism and the use of a new anti-androgen "cyproterone acetate" for therapy. J Clin Endocrinol Metab. 1974; 39:81–95.

410. Ito T, Horton R. The source of plasma dihydrotestosterone in man. J Clin Invest. 1971; 50:1621–1627.

411. Jackson RL, Dockerty MD. The Stein-Leventhal syndrome: analysis of 43 cases with special reference to association with endometrial carcinoma. Am J Obstet Gynecol. 1957; 73:161–173.

412. Jacobi J, Lloyd HM, Meares JD. Onset of estrogen-induced prolactin secretion and DNA synthesis by the rat pituitary gland. J Endocrinol. 1977; 72:35–39.

413. Jacobi J, Lloyd HM, Meares JD. Induction of pituitary tumors in male rats by a single dose of estrogen. Horm Metab Res. 1975; 7:228–230.

414. Jafari K, Javaheri G, Ruiz G. Endometrial adenocarcinoma and the Stein-Leventhal syndrome. Obstet Gynecol. 1978; 51:97–100.

415. Jaffe RB. Hyperprolactinemia. In: Givens JR, ed. The Infertile Female. Chicago: Yearbook Med Publ, 1979:439–452.

416. Jaffe RB, Keye WR Jr. Estradiol augmentation of pituitary responsiveness to gonadotropin-releasing hormone in women. J Clin Endocrinol Metab. 1974; 39:850–855.

417. Jaffee W, Russell V, Longcope C, et al. Hyperprolactinemia among women with polycystic ovary syndrome. 60th Annual Meeting of the Endocrine Society. Miami, Florida, June 14–16, Abstr 71., 1978.

418. Janata J, Starka L. Effect of cortisol on the production of ovarian androgens. J Endocrinol. 1964; 29:93–94.

419. Jänne OA, Bardin CW. Mechanism of action of androgens and antiandrogens. In: Mahesh VB, Greenblatt RB, eds. Hirsutism and Virilism. Boston: John Wright, PSG Inc., 1983:283–293.

420. Jayle MF, Weinmann SH, Baulieu EE, et al. Virilisme post-pubertaire discret par deficience de l'hydroxylation en C21. Acta Endocrinol (Kbh). 1958; 29:513–524.

421. Jeffcoate SL. Diagnosis of hyperprolactinaemia. Lancet. 1978; 2:1245–1247.

422. Jeffcoate SL, Brooks RV, London DR, et al. Secretion of C₁₉-steroids and oestrogens in the polycystic ovary syndrome. Ovarian studies *in vivo* and *in vitro* (including studies *in vitro* on a coincidental granulosa cell tumour). J Endocrinol. 1968; 42:229–243.

423. Jeffcoate TNA. The androgenic ovary, with special reference to the Stein-Leventhal syndrome. Am J Obstet Gynecol. 1963; 88:143–156.

424. Jeffcoate WJ, Edwards CRW, Rees LH, et al. Cyproterone acetate (letter). Lancet. 1976; 2:1140.

425. Jones DL, Jacobs HS, James VHT. The relationship between plasma prolactin and dehydroepiandrosterone and dehydroepiandrosterone sulphate levels in patients with hyperprolactinemia. In: Genazzani AR, Thyssen JH, Siiteri PK, eds. Adrenal Androgens. New York: Raven Press, 1980:83–87.

426. Jones GES, Howard JE, Langford H. The use of cortisone in follicular phase disturbances. Fertil Steril. 1953; 4:49–62.

427. Jones PBC, Hsueh AJW. Direct effect of gonadotropin-releasing hormone and its antagonist upon ovarian functions stimulated by FSH, prolactin and LH. Biol Reprod. 1981; 24:747–759.

428. Johnson JE Jr. Outcome of pregnancies following clomiphene citrate therapy. In: Westin B, Wiqvist N, eds. Proceedings of the 5th World Congress on Fertility and Sterility, Stockholm. Amsterdam: Excerpta Medica Foundation, 1967:101.

429. Judd SJ, Rigg LA, Yen SSC. The effects of ovariectomy and estrogen treatment on the dopamine inhibition of gonadotropin and prolactin release. J Clin Endocrinol Metab. 1979; 49:182–184.

430. Judd HL. Endocrinology of polycystic ovarian disease. Clin Obstet Gynecol. 1978; 21:99–144.

431. Judd SJ, Rakoff JS, Yen SSC. Inhibition of gonadotropin and prolactin release by dopamine: effect of endogenous estradiol levels. J Clin Endocrinol Metab. 1978; 47:494–498.

432. Judd HL, McPherson RA, Rakoff JS, et al. Correlation of the effects of dexamethasone administration, urinary 17-ketosteroid and serum androgen levels in patients with hirsutism. Am J Obstet Gynecol. 1977; 128:408–417.

433. Judd HL, Anderson DC, Yen SSC. Delineation of abnormal adrenal function in polycystic ovary syndrome. Gynecol Invest. 1976; 7:76–77.

434. Judd HL, Rigg LA, Anderson DC, et al. The effects of ovarian wedge resection on circulating gonadotropin and ovarian steroid levels in patients with polycystic ovary syndrome. J Clin Endocrinol Metab. 1976; 43:347–355.

435. Judd HL, Scully RE, Herbst AL, et al. Familial hyperthecosis: comparison of endocrinologic and histologic findings with polycystic ovarian disease. Am J Obstet Gynecol. 1973; 117:976–982.

436. Judd HL, Yen SSC. Serum androstenedione and testosterone levels during the menstrual cycle. J Clin Endocrinol Metab. 1973; 36:475–481.

437. Judd HL, Scully RE, Atkins L, et al. Pure gonadal dysgenesis with progressive hirsutism. New Engl J Med. 1970; 282:881–889.

438. Kable WT, Yussman MA. Testosterone-secreting adrenal adenoma. Fertil Steril. 1979; 32:610–611.

439. Kahn CR, Podskalny JM. Demonstration of a primary (? genetic) defect in insulin receptors in fibroblasts from a patient with the syndrome of insulin resistance and acanthosis nigricans type A. J Clin Endocrinol Metab. 1980; 50:1139–1141.

440. Kahn CR, Flier JS, Bar RS, et al. The syndromes of insulin resistance and acanthosis nigricans. Insulin-receptor disorders in man. New Engl J Med. 1976; 294:739–745.

441. Kamrava MM, Seibel MM, Berger MJ, et al. Reversal of persistent anovulation in polycystic ovarian disease by administration of chronic low-dose follicle-stimulating hormone. Fertil Steril. 1982; 37:520–523.

442. Kandeel FR, London DR, Butt WR, et al. Adrenal function in subgroups of the PCO syndrome assessed by a long ACTH test. Clin Endocrinol (Oxf). 1980; 13:601–612.

443. Kandeel FR, Butt WR, London DR, et al. Oestrogen amplification of LH-RH response in the polycystic ovary syndrome and response to clomiphene. Clin Endocrinol (Oxf). 1978; 9:429–441.

444. Kandeel FR, Rudd BT, Butt WR, et al. Androgen and cortisol responses to ACTH stimulation in women with hyperprolactineamia. Clin Endocrinol (Oxf). 1978; 9:123–130.

445. Kandeel F, Butt WR, London DR. Regulation of serum prolactin levels by oestrone and oes-

trone sulphate in normally menstruating women. Acta Endocrinol (Kbh) (Suppl). 1977; 212:42.

446. Karam K, Hajj S. Hyperthecosis syndrome. Acta Obstet Gynecol Scand. 1979; 58:73–79.

447. Karsch JF, Krey LC, Weick RF, et al. Functional luteolysis in the rhesus monkey: the role of estrogen. Endocrinology. 1973; 92:1148–1152.

448. Kase N. Steroid synthesis in abnormal ovaries. III. Polycystic ovaries. Am J Obstet Gynecol. 1964; 90:1268–1273.

449. Kater CE, Biglieri EG. Distinctive plasma aldosterone, 18-hydroxycorticosterone, and 18-hydroxydeoxycorticosterone profile in the 21-, 17α-, and 11β-hydroxylase deficiency types of congenital adrenal hyperplasia. Am J Med. 1983; 75:43–48.

450. Katz M, Carr PJ, Cohen BM, et al. Hormonal effects of wedge resection of polycystic ovaries. Obstet Gynecol. 1978; 51:437–444.

451. Katz M, Carr PJ. Abnormal luteinizing hormone response patterns to synthetic gonadotropin-releasing hormone in patients with polycystic ovarian syndrome. J Endocrinol. 1976; 70:163–171.

452. Keettel WC, Bradbury JT, Stoddard FJ. Observations on the PCO syndrome. Am J Obstet Gynecol. 1957; 73:954–965.

453. Kemmann E, Jones JR. Sequential clomiphene citrate-menotropin therapy for induction or enhancement of ovulation. Fertil Steril. 1983; 39:772–779.

454. Kemmann E, Tavakoli F, Shelden RM, et al. Induction of ovulation with menotropins in women with polycystic ovary sydrome. Am J Obstet Gynecol. 1981; 141:58–64.

455. Kendall JW, Sloop PR. Dexamethasone-suppressible adrenocortical tumor. New Engl J Med. 1968; 279:532–535.

456. Keye WR, Jaffe RB. Modulation of pituitary gonadotropin response to gonadotropin-releasing hormone by estradiol. J Clin Endocrinol Metab. 1974; 38:805–810.

457. Kim MH, Rosenfield RL, Hosseinian AH, et al. Ovarian hyperandrogenism with normal and abnormal histologic findings of the ovaries. Am J Obstet Gynecol. 1979; 134:445–452.

458. Kim MH, Rosenfield RL, Dupon C. The effects of dexamethasone on plasma free androgens during the normal menstrual cycle. Am J Obstet Gynecol. 1976; 126:982–986.

459. Kim MH, Hosseinian AH, Dupon C. Plasma levels of estrogens, androgens, and progesterone during normal and dexamethasone-treated cycles. J Clin Endocrinol Metab. 1974; 39:706–712.

460. Kirschner MA. Adrenal and gonadal venous catheterization studies in hirsute women. In: Mahesh VB, Greenblatt RB, eds. Hirsutism and Virilism. Boston: John Wright, PSG Inc., 1983:309–332.

461. Kirschner MA. Polycystic and sclerocystic ovaries. In: Krieger DT, Bardin CW, eds. Current Therapy of Infertility. St. Louis: C.V. Mosby Co., 1983:404–409.

462. Kirschner MA, Zucker IR, Jespersen DL. Ovarian and adrenal vein catheterization studies in women with idiopathic hirsutism. In: James VHT, Serio M, Giusti G, eds. The Endocrine Function of the Ovary. New York: Academic Press, 1976:443–456.

463. Kirschner MA, Zucker IR, Jespersen D. Idiopathic hirsutism—an ovarian abnormality. New Engl J Med. 1976; 294:637–640.

464. Kirschner MA, Sinhamahaptra S, Zucker IR, et al. The production, origin, and role of dehydroepiandrosterone and delta⁵-androstenediol as androgen prehormones in hirsute women. J Clin Endocrinol Metab. 1973; 37:1183–1189.

465. Kirschner MA, Bardin WC. Androgen production and metabolism in normal and virilized women. Metabolism. 1972; 21:667–688.

466. Kirschner MA, Jacobs JB. Combined ovarian and adrenal vein catheterization to determine the site of androgen overproduction in hirsute women. J Clin Endocrinol Metab. 1971; 33:199–209.

467. Kirschner MA, Bardin CW, Hembree WC, et al. Effect of estrogen administration on androgen production and plasma luteinizing hormone in hirsute women. J Clin Endocrinol Metab. 1970; 30:727–732.

468. Kirschner MA, Lipsett MB, Collins DR. Plasma ketosteroids and testosterone in man: a study of the pituitary–testicular axis. J Clin Invest. 1965; 44:657–665.

469. Kistner RW. Sequential use of clomiphene citrate and human menopausal gonadotropin in ovulation induction. Fertil Steril. 1976; 27:72–82.

470. Kistner RW. Peri-tubal and peri-ovarian adhesions subsequent to wedge resection of the ovaries. Fertil Steril. 1969; 20:35–42.

471. Kleinberg DL, Noel GL, Frantz AG. Galactorrhea: a study of 235 cases, including 48 with pituitary tumors. New Engl J Med. 1977; 296:589–600.

472. Kletzky OA, Davajan V, Mishell DR Jr. The effect of gonadotropin-releasing hormone on ovarian estradiol secretion. Am J Obstet Gynecol. 1982; 142:427–431.

473. Kletzky OA, Davajan V, Nakumura RM, et al. Classification of secondary amenorrhea based on distinct hormonal patterns. J Clin Endocrinol Metab. 1975; 41:660–668.

474. Kley HK, Bartmann E, Krüskemper HL. A simple and rapid method to measure non-protein-bound fractions of cortisol, testosterone and oestradiol by equilibrium dialysis: comparison with centrifugal filtration. Acta Endocrinol (Kbh). 1977; 85:209–219.

475. Klibanski A, Beitins IZ, Zervas NT, et al. α-subunit and gonadotropin responses to luteinizing hormone-releasing hormone in hyperprolactinemic women before and after bromocriptine. J Clin Endocrinol Metab. 1983; 56:774–780.

476. Klingensmith GJ, Wentz AC, Meyer WJ III, et al. Gonadotropin output in congenital adrenal hyperplasia before and after adrenal suppression. J Clin Endocrinol Metab. 1976; 43:933–936.

477. Klopper A, Hall M. New synthetic agent for the induction of ovulation: preliminary trials in women. Br Med J. 1971; 1:152–154.

478. Knobil E. The neuroendocrine control of the menstrual cycle. Rec Prog Horm Res. 1980; 36:53–88.

479. Knobil E, Plant TM, Wildt L, et al. Control of the rhesus monkey menstrual cycle: permissive role of hypothalamic gonadotropin-releasing hormone. Science. 1980; 207:1371–1373.

480. Knobil E, Plant TM. The hypothalamic regulation of LH and FSH secretion in the rhesus monkey. In: Reichlin S, Baldessarini RJ, Martin JB, eds. The Hypothalamus. New York: Raven Press, 1978:359–372.

481. Knobil E. On the control of gonadotropin secretion in the rhesus monkey. Rec Prog Horm Res. 1974; 30:1–46.

482. Koike K, Aono T, Miyake A, et al. Induction of ovulation in patients with normoprolactinemic amenorrhea by combined therapy with bromocriptine and clomiphene. Fertil Steril. 1981; 35:138–141.

483. Kopelman PG, Pilkington TRE, White N, et al. Abnormal sex steroid secretion and binding in massively obese women. Clin Endocrinol (Oxf). 1980; 12:363–369.

484. Korenman SG, Sherman BM. Further studies of gonadotropin and estradiol secretion during the preovulatory phase of the human menstrual cycle. J Clin Endocrinol Metab. 1973; 36:1205–1209.

485. Korenman SG, Kirschner MA, Lipsett MB. Testosterone production in normal virilized women and in women with the Stein-Leventhal syndrome or idiopathic hirsutism. J Clin Endocrinol Metab. 1965; 25:798–803.

486. Korth-Schutz S, Levin LS, New MI. Dehydroepiandrosterone sulfate (DS) levels, a rapid test for abnormal adrenal androgen secretion. J Clin Endocrinol Metab. 1976; 42:1005–1013.

487. Korth-Schutz S, Levine LS, Merkatz IR, et al. An unusual case of Cushing's syndrome, hilus cell tumor and polycystic ovaries. J Clin Endocrinol Metab. 1974; 38:794–800.

488. Kovacs K, Ilse G, Ryan N, et al. Pituitary prolactin cell hyperplasia. Horm Res. 1980; 12:87–95.

489. Kovacs K, Ryan N, Horvath E, et al. Prolactin cell adenomas of the human pituitary. Pathologic features of prolactin cells in the nontumorous portions of the anterior lobe. Horm Metab Res. 1978; 10:409–412.

490. Kraus FT, Neubecker RD. Luteinization of the ovarian theca in infants and children. Am J Clin Path. 1962; 37:389–397.

491. Kraus FT. Gynecologic Pathology. St. Louis: C.V. Mosby Co., 1957:320–326.

492. Krensky AM, Bongiovanni AM, Marino J, et al. Identification of heterozygote carriers of congenital adrenal hyperplasia by radioimmunoassay of serum 17-OH progesterone. J Pediatr. 1977; 90:930–933.

493. Krieger DT. Cushing's syndrome. Gross F, Grumbach MM, Labhart A et al eds. In: Monographs on Endocrinology, Vol 22. New York: Springer-Verlag, 1982:73–118.

494. Krieger DT. The hypothalamus and neuroendocrine pathology. In: Krieger DT, Hughes JC, eds. Neuroendocrinology. Sunderland, Mass: Sinauer Associates, 1980:13–22.

495. Krieger DT. The hypothalamus and neuroendocrinology. In: Krieger DT, Hughes JC, eds. Neuroendocrinology. Sunderland, Mass: Sinauer Associates, 1980:3–12.

496. Kurachi K, Aono T, Minagawa J, et al. Congenital malformations of newborn infants after clomiphene-induced ovulation. Fertil Steril. 1983; 40:187–189.

497. Kurisaka M, Tindall SC, Takei Y. Cystic prolactinoma of the pituitary following surgery for polycystic ovaries. Neurol Med Chir (Tokyo). 1983; 23:55–60.

498. Kuttenn F, Rigaud C, Wright F, et al. Treatment of hirsutism by oral cyproterone acetate and percutaneous oestradiol. J Clin Endocrinol Metab. 1980; 51:1107–1111.

499. Kuttenn F, Mowszowicz I, Schaison G, et al. Androgen production and skin metabolism in hirsutism. J Endocrinol. 1977; 75:83–91.

500. Laatikainen TJ, Apter DL, Paavonen JA, et al. Steroids in ovarian and peripheral venous blood in polycystic ovarian disease. Clin Endocrinol (Oxf). 1980; 13:125–134.

501. Lachelin GCL, Judd HL, Swanson SC, et al. Long-term effects of nightly dexamethasone administration in patients with polycystic ovarian disease. J Clin Endocrinol Metab. 1982; 55:768–773.

502. Lachelin GCL, Barnett M, Hopper BR, et al. Adrenal function in normal women and women with the polycystic ovary syndrome. J Clin Endocrinol Metab. 1979; 49:892–898.

503. Lachelin GCL, Abu-Fadil S, Yen SSC. Functional aberration of hyperprolactinemia-amenorrhea. J Clin Endocrinol Metab. 1977; 44:1163–1174.

504. Lamotte M, Houdart R, Pasteels J, et al. Adénome hypophysaire prolactinique. Presse Médicale. 1966; 74:1025–1030.

505. Laron Z, Pollack MS, Zamir R, et al. Late onset 21-hydroxylase deficiency and HLA in the Ashkenazi population: a new allele at the 21-hydroxylase locus. Hum Immunol. 1980; 1:55–66.

506. Larson BA, Vanderlaan WP, Judd HL, et al. A testosterone-producing adrenal cortical adenoma in an elderly woman. J Clin Endocrinol Metab. 1976; 42:882–887.

507. Larsson-Cohn U, Johansson EDB, Wide L, et al. Effects of continuous daily administration of 0.5 mg of norethindrone on the plasma levels of progesterone and the urinary excretion of luteinizing hormone, pregnanediol, and total oestrogens. Acta Endocrinol (Kbh). 1970; 63:216–224.

508. Lasley BL, Wang CW, Yen SSC. The effects of estrogen and progesterone on the functional capacity of the gonadotrophs. J Clin Endocrinol Metab. 1975; 41:820–826.

509. Lavric MV. Galactorrhea and amenorrhea with polycystic ovaries. Am J Obstet Gynecol. 1969; 104:814–817.

510. Lawrence DM, McGarrigle HHG, Radwanska E, et al. Plasma testosterone and androstenedione levels during monitored induction of ovulation in infertile women with "simple" amenorrhoea and with polycystic ovary syndrome. Clin Endocrinol (Oxf). 1976; 5:609–618.

511. Leblanc H, Lachelin GCL, Abu-Fadil S, et al. Effects of dopamine infusion on pituitary hormone secretion in humans. J Clin Endocrinol Metab. 1976; 43:668–674.

512. Lee PA, Xenakis T, Winer J, et al. Puberty in girls: correlation of serum levels of gonadotropins, prolactin, androgens, estrogens, and progestins with physical changes. J Clin Endocrinol Metab. 1976; 43:775–784.

513. Lee PA, Gareis FJ. Evidence for partial 21-hydroxylase deficiency among heterozygote carriers of congenital adrenal hyperplasia. J Clin Endocrinol Metab. 1975; 41:415–418.

514. Lee PA, Kowarski A, Gigeon CJ, et al. Lack of correlation between gonadotropin and adrenal androgen levels in agonadal children. J Clin Endocrinol Metab. 1975; 40:664–669.

515. Leichter SB, Jacobs LS. Normal gestation and diminished androgen responsiveness in an untreated patient with 21-hydroxylase deficiency. J Clin Endocrinol Metab. 1976; 42:575–581.

517. Lemarchand-Beraud T, Zufferey MM, Reymond M, et al. Maturation of the hypothalamo-pituitary-ovarian axis in adolescent girls. J Clin Endocrinol Metab. 1982; 54:241–246.

517. Leme CE, Wajchenberg BL, Lerario AC, et al. Acanthosis nigricans, hirsutism, insulin resistance and insulin receptor defect. Clin Endocrinol (Oxf). 1982; 17:43–49.

518. Lenton EA, Sobowale OS, Cooke ID. Prolactin concentrations in ovulatory but infertile women: treatment with bromocriptine. Br Med J. 1977; 2:1179–1181.

519. Leon N, Becak W, Becak ML, et al. On the etiology of the Stein-Leventhal syndrome. Acta Genet (Basel). 1963; 13:252–262.

520. Leong DA, Frawley LS, Neill JD. Neuroendocrine control of prolactin secretion. Ann Rev Physiol. 1983; 45:109–127.

521. Leventhal ML. Amenorrhea and sterility caused by bilateral polycystic ovaries. Am J Obstet Gynecol. 1941; 41:516–517.

522. Levine LS, Dumont B, Lorenzen F, et al. Cryptic 21-hydroxylase deficiency in families of patients with classical congenital adrenal hyperplasia. J Clin Endocrinol Metab. 1980; 51:1316–1324.

523. Levine LS, Zachmann M, New MI, et al. Genetic mapping of the 21-hydroxylase deficiency gene within the HLA linkage group. New Engl J Med. 1978; 299:911–915.

524. Lieberman ME, Maurer RA, Gorski J. Estrogen control of prolactin synthesis in vitro. Proc Natl Acad Sci USA. 1978; 75:5946–5949.

525. Lim NY, Dingman JF. Measurement of testosterone excretion and production rate by glass paper chromatography. J Clin Endocrinol Metab. 1965; 25:563–570.

526. Lindner HR, Tsafriri A, Lieberman ME, et al. Gonadotropic action on cultured graafian follicles: induction of maturation division of the mammalian oocyte and differentiation of the luteal cell. Rec Prog Horm Res. 1974; 30:79–138.

527. Lloyd CW, Lobotsky J, Segre EJ, et al. Plasma testosterone and urinary 17-ketosteroids in women with hirsutism and polycystic ovaries. J Clin Endocrinol Metab. 1966; 26:314–324.

528. Lloyd CW, Moses AM, Lobotsky J, et al. Studies of adrenocortical function of women with idiopathic hirsutism: response to 25 units of ACTH. J Clin Endocrinol Metab. 1963; 23:413–418.

529. Lobo RA, Goebelsmann U, Horton R. Evidence for the importance of peripheral tissue

events in the development of hirsutism in polycystic ovary syndrome. J Clin Endocrinol Metab. 1983; 57:393–397.

530. Lobo RA, Granger LR, Paul WL, et al. Psychological stress and increases in urinary norepinephrine metabolites, platelet serotonin, and adrenal androgens in women with polycystic ovary syndrome. Am J Obstet Gynecol. 1983; 145:456–503.

531. Lobo RA, Kletzky OA, Campeau JD, et al. Elevated bioactive luteinizing hormone in women with the polycystic ovary syndrome. Fertil Steril. 1983; 39:674–678.

532. Lobo RA, Goebelsmann U. Effect of androgen excess on inappropriate gonadotropin secretion as found in the polycystic ovary syndrome. Am J Obstet Gynecol. 1982; 142:394–401

533. Lobo RA, Goebelsmann U, Horton R. Hirsutism in polycystic ovary syndrome (PCO). Abstract. Thirtieth Annual Meeting of the Pacific Coast Fertility Society, Oct 13–17. Fertil Steril. 1982; 38:278.

534. Lobo RA, Kletzky OA, diZerega GS. Elevated serum bioactive luteinizing hormone (LH) concentrations in women with polycystic ovary syndrome (PCO). Fertil Steril (Suppl). 1982; 37:301–302.

535. Lobo RA, Gysler M, March CM, et al. Clinical and laboratory predictors of clomiphene response. Fertil Steril. 1982; 37:168–174.

536. Lobo RA, Kletzky OA. Normalization of androgen and sex hormone-binding globulin levels after treatment of hyperprolactinemia. J Clin Endocrinol Metab. 1982; 56:562–566.

537. Lobo RA, Paul W, March CW, et al. Clomiphene and dexamethasone in women unresponsive to clomiphene alone. Obstet Gynecol. 1982; 60:497–502.

538. Lobo RA, Goebelsmann U. Evidence for reduced 3β-ol-hydroxysteroid dehydrogenase activity in some hirsute women thought to have polycystic ovary syndrome. J Clin Endocrinol Metab. 1981; 53:394–400.

539. Lobo RA, Granger L, Goebelsmann U, et al. Elevations in unbound serum estradiol as a possible mechanism for inappropriate gonadotropin secretion in women with PCO. J Clin Endocrinol Metab. 1981; 52:156–158.

540. Lobo RA, Paul WL, Goebelsmann U. Serum levels of DHEAS in gynecologic endocrinopathy and infertility. Obstet Gynecol. 1981; 57:607–612.

541. Lobo RA, Goebelsmann U. Adult manifestation of congenital adrenal hyperplasia due to incomplete 21-hydroxylase deficiency mimicking polycystic ovarian disease. Am J Obstet Gynecol. 1980; 138:720–726.

542. Lobo RA, Kletzky OA, Kaptein EM, et al. Prolactin modulation of dehydroepiandrosterone sulfate secretion. Am J Obstet Gynecol. 1980; 138:632–636.

543. Lobo RA, Goebelsmann U. Incomplete 21-hydroxylase and 3β-ol-dehydrogenase deficiences in hirsute women. In: Proceedings of the 62nd Annual Meeting of the Endocrine Society, (abstr 456), Washington DC: 1980:188.

544. Lobo RA, Paul WL, Goebelsmann U. Dehydroepiandrosterone sulfate as an indicator of adrenal androgen function. Obstet Gynecol. 1980; 57:69–73.

545. Longcope C, Layne DS, Tait JF. Metabolic clearance rate and interconversion of estrone and 17β-estradiol in normal males and females. J Clin Invest. 1968; 47:93–106.

546. Longcope C, Williams KIH. The metabolism of estrogens in normal women after pulse injections of ³H-estradiol and ³H-estrone. J Clin Endocrinol Metab. 1974; 38:602–607.

547. Lorber DL, McKenna TJ, Rabinowitz D. Plasma pregnenolone and 17-OH-pregnenolone in hirsute amenorrhoeic patients. Acta Endocrinol (Kbh). 1978; 87:566–576.

548. Lorenzen F, Pang S, New M, et al. Studies of the C-21 and C-19 steroids and HLA genotyping in siblings and parents of patients with congenital adrenal hyperplasia due to 21-hydroxylase deficiency. J Clin Endocrinol Metab. 1980; 50:572–577.

549. Loriaux DL, Menard R, Taylor A, et al. Spironolactone and endocrine dysfunction. Ann Int Med. 1976; 85:630–636.

550. Loriaux DL, Malmak LR, Noall MW. Contribution of plasma dehydroepiandrosterone sulfate to testosterone in a virilized patient with an arrhenoblastoma. J Clin Endocrinol Metab. 1970; 31:702–704.

551. Louvet JP, Harman SM, Schreiber JR, et al. Evidence for a role of androgens in follicular maturation. Endocrinology. 1975; 97:366–372.

552. Lucis OJ, Hollenberg CH, MacDonald SA, et al. Polycystic ovaries associated with congenital adrenal hyperplasia. Can Med Assoc J. 1966; 94:1–7.

553. Lunde O. Hyperprolactinaemia in polycystic ovary syndrome. Ann Chir Gynaecol. 1981; 70:197–201.

554. Lundy LE, Lee SG, Levy W, et al. The ovulatory cycle. A histologic, thermal, steroid, and gonadotropin correlation. Obstet Gynecol. 1974; 44:14–25.

555. Lyon MF. X-chromosome inactivation and developmental patterns in mammals. Biol Rev. 1972; 47:1–35.

556. MacDonald PC, Edman CD, Homsell DL, et al. Effect of obesity on conversion of plasma an-

drostenedione to estrone in postmenopausal women with and without endometrial cancer. Am J Obstet Gynecol. 1978; 130:448–455.

557. MacDonald PC, Siiteri PK. The relationship between the extraglandular production of estrone and the occurrence of endometrial neoplasia. Gynecol Oncol. 1974; 2:259–263.

558. MacGregor AH, Johnson JE, Bunde CA. Further clinical experience with clomiphene citrate. Fertil Steril. 1968; 19:616–620.

559. MacLeod RM, Kimura H, Login I. Inhibition of prolactin secretion by dopamine and piribedil (ET-495). In: Pecile A, Muller EE, eds. Growth Hormone and Related Peptides. Amsterdam: Excerpta Medica, 1976:443–453.

560. Macourt DC. A new synthetic agent for the induction of ovulation. Med J Aust. 1974; 1:631–632.

561. Madden JD, Milewich L, Parker CR, et al. The effect of oral contraceptive treatment on the serum concentration of dehydroepiandrosterone sulfate. Am J Obstet Gynecol. 1978; 132:380–384.

562. Madden JD, Milewich L, Gomez-Sanchez C, et al. The effect of oral contraceptive treatment on the serum concentration of dehydroepiandrosterone sulfate and ACTH. Gynecol Invest. 1977; 8:16.

563. Magendantz HG, Jones DED, Schomber DW. Virilization during pregnancy associated with polycystic ovary disease. Obstet Gynecol. 1972; 40:156–162.

564. Magoffin DA, Reynolds DS, Erickson GF. Direct inhibitory effect of GnRH on androgen secretion by ovarian interstitial cells. Endocrinology. 1981; 109:661–663.

565. Magrini G, Pellaton M, Felber JP. Prolactin-induced modifications of testosterone metabolism in man. Acta Endocrinol (Kbh) (Suppl 212). 1977; 85:143.

566. Magrini G, Ebiner JR, Burckhardt P, et al. Study on the relationship between plasma prolactin levels and androgen metabolism in man. J Clin Endocrinol Metab. 1976; 43:944–947.

567. Mahajan DK, Billiar RB, Jassani M, et al. Ethinyl estradiol administration and plasma steroid concentrations in ovariectomized women. Am J Obstet Gynecol. 1978; 130:398–402.

568. Mahesh VB, Toldeo SPA, Mattar E. Hormone levels following wedge resection in polycystic ovary syndrome. Obstet Gynecol. 1978; 51:S64–S69.

569. Mahesh VB, Greenblatt RB. Steroid secretions in the normal and polycystic ovary. Rec Prog Horm Res. 1964; 20:341–394.

570. Mahesh VB, Greenblatt RB, Aydar CK, et al. Urinary steroid exretion patterns in hirsutism. I. Use of adrenal and ovarian suppression tests in the study of hirsutism. J Clin Endocrinol Metab. 1964; 24:1283–1292.

571. Mahesh VB, Greenblatt RB. Isolation of dehydroepiandrosterone and 17α-hydroxy-delta⁵-pregnenolone from the polycystic ovaries of the Stein-Leventhal syndrome. J Clin Endocrinol Metab. 1962; 22:441–448.

572. Malarkey WB. Nonpuerperal lactation and normal prolactin regulation. J Clin Endocrinol Metab. 1975; 40:198–204.

573. Mandel FP, Chang RJ, Dupont B, et al. HLA genotyping in family members and patients with familial polycystic ovarian disease. J Clin Endocrinol Metab. 1983; 56:862–867.

574. Mandel FP, Voet RL, Weiland AJ, et al. Steroid secretion by masculinizing and "feminizing" hilus cell tumors. J Clin Endocrinol Metab. 1981; 52:779–784.

575. Mansell H, Hertig AT. Granulosa-theca cell tumors and endometrial carcinoma: a study of their relationship and a survey of 80 cases. Obstet Gynecol. 1955; 6:385–394.

576. March CM, Goebelsmann U, Nakamura RM, et al. Roles of estradiol and progesterone in eliciting the midcycle luteinizing hormone and of follicle-stimulating hormone surges. J Clin Endocrinol Metab. 1979; 49:507–513.

577. Marder ML, Channing CP, Schwartz NB. Suppression of serum follicle-stimulating hormone in intact and acutely ovariectomized rats by porcine follicular fluid. Endocrinology. 1977; 101:1639–1642.

578. Marik J, Hulka J. Luteinized unruptured follicle syndrome: a subtle cause of infertility. Fertil Steril. 1978; 29:270–274.

579. Maroulis GB. Evaluation of hirsutism and hyperandrogenemia. Fertil Steril. 1981; 36:273–305.

580. Maroulis GB. Unpublished data, 1981.

581. Maroulis GB. Comparison of ovarian morphology with the source of hyperandrogenism in hirsute patients. Fertil Steril (abstract). 1980; 33:239.

582. Maroulis GB, Manlimos FS, Abraham GE. Comparison between urinary 17-ketosteroids and serum androgens in hirsute patients. Obstet Gynecol. 1977; 49:454–458.

583. Maroulis GB, Manlimos FS, Garza R, et al. Serum cortisol and 11-deoxy cortisol levels in hirsute premenopausal women. Obstet Gynecol. 1976; 48:388–391.

584. Maroulis GB, Abraham GE. Ovarian and adrenal contributions to peripheral steroid levels in postmenopausal women. Obstet Gynecol. 1976; 48:150–154.

585. Marshall JR. Induction of ovulation. In: Givens JR, ed. The Infertile Female. Chicago: Year Book Med Publ, 1979:261–272.

586. Marshall WA. Postnatal growth. In: Falkner F, Tanner JM, eds. Human Growth, Vol II. New York: Plenum Press, 1978;141–181.

587. Martin JB, Reichlin S, Brown GM. Neuropharmacology of anterior pituitary control. In: Clinical Neuroendocrinology. Philadelphia: F.A. Davis Co., 1977:45–59.

588. Martin WH, Rogol AD, Kaiser DL, et al. Dopaminergic mechanisms and luteinizing hormone (LH) secretion. II. Differential effects of dopamine and bromocriptine on LH release in normal women. J Clin Endocrinol Metab. 1981; 52:650–656.

589. Marut EL, Williams RF, Cowan BD, et al. Pulsatile pituitary gonadotropin secretion during maturation of the dominant follicle in monkeys: estrogen positive feedback enhances the biological activity of LH. Endocrinology. 1981; 109:2270–2272.

590. Marynick SP, Chakmakjian ZH, McCaffree DL, et al. Androgen excess in cystic acne. New Engl J Med. 1983; 308:981–986.

591. Maschler I, Salzberger M, Finkelstein M. Ovarian enzymatic divergence in patients with polycystic ovary syndrome excreting urinary pregnanetriolone. Acta Endocrinol (Kbh). 1976; 82:366–379.

592. Maschler I, Salzberger M, Finkelstein M. 11β-hydroxylase with affinity to C-21-deoxysteroids from ovaries of patients with polycystic ovary syndrome. J Clin Endocrinol Metab. 1975; 41:999–1002.

593. Mathur RS, Moody LO, Landrebe SC, et al. Sex-hormone-binding globulin in clinically hyperandrogenic women: association of plasma concentrations with body weight. Fertil Steril. 1982; 38:207–211.

594. Mauseth RS, Hansen JA, Smith EK, et al. Detection of heterozygotes for congenital adrenal hyperplasia: 21-hydroxylase deficiency—a comparison of HLA typing and 17-OH progesterone response to ACTH infusion. J Pediatr 1980; 97:749–753.

595. Mauvais-Jarvis P, Kuttenn F, Mowszowicz I. Hirsutism of ovarian origin. Gross F, Grumbach MM, Labhart A et al. eds. In: Hirsutism. Monographs on Endocrinology, Vol 19. New York: Springer-Verlag, 1981:74–82.

596. Mauvais-Jarvis P, Kuttenn F, Mowszowicz I. Hirsutism of ovarian origin. Gross F, Grumbach MM, Labhart A et al. eds. In: Hirsutism. Monographs on Endocrinology, Vol. 19. New York: Springer-Verlag, 1981:60–73.

597. Mauvais-Jarvis P, Kuttenn F, Mowszowicz I. Hirsutism of ovarian origin. Gross F, Grumbach MM, Labhart A et al. eds. In: Monographs on Endocrinology, Vol 19. New York: Springer-Verlag, 1981:18–30.

598. Mauvais-Jarvis P, Kuttenn F, Gauthier-Wright F. Testosterone 5α-reduction in human skin as an index of androgenicity. In: James VHT, Serio M, Giusti G, eds. The Endocrine Function of the Human Ovary. New York: Academic Press, 1976:481–494.

599. Mayar MQ, Tarnovsky GK, Reeves JJ. Ovarian growth and uptake of iodinated D-Leu, des-Gly, NH_2-LHRH ethylamide in hCG-treated rats. Proc Soc Exp Biol Med. 1979; 161:216–219.

600. McArthur JW, Ingersoll FM, Worcester J. The urinary excretion of interstitial-cell and follicle-stimulating hormone activity by women with diseases of the reproductive system. J Clin Endocrinol Metab. 1958; 18:1202–1215.

601. McBride RA, Sturgis SH, Crigler JF. Gynandroblastoma. Report of a case with hormonal studies. Obstet Gynecol. 1962; 19:914–925.

602. McCann SM, Krulich L, Ojeda SR, et al. Neurotransmitters in the control of anterior pituitary function. In: Fuxe K, Hökfelt T, Luft R, eds. Central Regulation of the Endocrine System. New York: Plenum Press, 1979:329–347.

603. McCann SM. Luteinizing-hormone-releasing-hormone. New Engl J Med. 1977; 296:797–802.

604. McCann SM. Regulation of the secretion of follicle-stimulating hormone (FSH) and luteinizing hormone (LH). In: Knobil ET, Sawyer WH, eds. Handbook of Physiology, Vol IV. Baltimore: Williams and Wilkins, 1974:489–517,

605. McConway MG, England P, Black WP, et al. Ovarian morphology and hormone profiles in women with primary oligomenorrhea. In: Klopper A, Lerner L, Vander Molen HJ, eds. Research on Steroids, Vol VIII. London: Academic Press, 1979:247–248.

606. McCormack JT, Plant TM, Hess DL, et al. The effect of luteinizing hormone-releasing hormone (LHRH) antiserum administration on gonadotropin secretion in the rhesus monkey. Endocrinology. 1977; 100:663–667.

607. McDonald TW, Malkasian GD, Gaffey TA. Endometrial cancer associated with feminizing ovarian tumors and polycystic ovarian disease. Obstet Gynecol. 1977; 49:654–658.

608. McDonough PG. Amenorrhea–etiologic approach to diagnosis. Fertil Steril. 1978; 30:1–15.

609. McDonough PG, Mahesh VB, Ellegood JO: Steroid, follicle-stimulating hormone, and luteinizing hormone profiles in identical twins with polycystic ovaries. Am J Obstet Gynecol. 1972; 113:1072–1078.

610. McKeel DW Jr, Fowler M, Jacobs LS. The high prevalence of prolactin cell hyperplasia in the

human adenohypophysis. 60th Annual Meeting of the Endocrine Society, Miami, Fla, June 14–16, Abstract 557, 1978.

611. McKeel DW Jr, Jacobs LS. Nonadenomatous pituitary prolactin cell hyperplasia in patients with pathologic hyperprolactinemia. 59th Annual Meeting of Endocrine Society, Chicago. Illinois, Abstract 136, 1977.

612. McKenna TJ. The adrenal cortex and menstrual disorders. In: Givens JR, ed. Endocrine Causes of Menstrual Disorders. Chicago: Year Book Med Publ, 1978:371–407.

613. McKenna TJ, Miller RB, Liddle GW. Plasma pregnenolone and 17α-OH-pregnenolone in patients with adrenal tumors, ACTH excess, or idiopathic hirsutism. J Clin Endocrinol Metab. 1977; 44:231–236.

614. McKenna TJ, Jennings AS, Liddle GW, et al. Pregnenolone, 17-OH-pregnenolone and testosterone in plasma of patients with congenital adrenal hyperplasia. J Clin Endocrinol Metab. 1976; 42:918–925.

615. McNatty KP, Makris A, Osathanondh R, et al. Effects of luteinizing hormone on steroidogenesis by thecal tissue from human ovarian follicles in vitro. Steroids. 1980; 36:53–63.

616. McNatty KP, Smith DM, Makris A, et al. The intraovarian sites of androgen and estrogen formation in women with normal and hyperandrogenic ovaries as judged by in vitro experiments. J Clin Endocrinol Metab. 1980; 50:755–763.

617. McNatty KP: Relationship between plasma prolactin and the endocrine microenvironment of the developing human antral follicle. Fertil Steril. 1979; 32:433–438.

618. McNatty KP, Smith DM, Makris A, et al. The microenvironment of the human antral follicle: interrelationships among the steroid levels in antral fluid, the population of granulosa cells, and the status of the oocyte in vivo and in vitro. J Clin Endocrinol Metab. 1979; 49:851–860.

619. McNatty KP, Makris A, DeGrazia C, et al. The production of progesterone, androgens, and estrogens by granulosa cells, thecal tissue, and stromal tissue from human ovaries in vitro. J Clin Endocrinol Metab. 1979; 49:687–699.

620. McNatty KP, Makris A, Reinhold VN, et al. Metabolism of androstenedione by human ovarian tissue in vitro with particular reference to reductase and aromatase activity. Steroids. 1979; 34:429–443.

621. McNatty KP. Cyclic changes in antral fluid hormone concentrations in humans. Clin Endocrinol Metab. 1978; 7:577–600.

622. McNatty KP, Baird DT, Bolton A, et al. Concentration of oestrogens and androgens in human ovarian venous plasma and follicular fluid throughout the menstrual cycle. J Endocrinol. 1976; 71:77–85.

623. McNatty KP, Henderson KM, Sawers RS. Effects of prostaglandin $F_{2\alpha}$ and E_2 on the production of progesterone by human granulosa cells in tissue culture. J Endocrinol. 1975; 67:231–240.

624. McNatty KP, Hunter WM, McNeilly AS, et al. Changes in the concentration of pituitary and steroid hormones in the follicular fluid of human graafian follicles throughout the menstrual cycle. J Endocrinol. 1975; 64:555–571.

625. McNatty KP, Sawers RS. Relationship between the endocrine environment within the graafian follicle and the subsequent rate of progesterone secretion by human granulosa cells in vitro. J Endocrinol. 1975; 66:391–400.

626. McNatty KP, Sawers R, McNeilly AS. A possible role for prolactin in control of steroid secretion by the human graafian follicle. Nature. 1974; 240:653–655.

627. McNeill TH, Sladek JR Jr. Fluorescence-immunocytochemistry: simultaneous localization of catecholamines and gonadotropin-releasing hormone. Science. 1978; 200:72–74.

628. McNeilly AS, Sharpe RM, Davidson DW, et al. Inhibition of gonadotropin secretion by induced hyperprolactinemia in the male rat. J Endocrinol. 1978; 79:59–68.

629. Mechanick JI, Futterweit W. Hypothesis: aberrant puberty and polycystic ovarian disease. Int J Fertil. 1984; In press.

630. Meikle AW, Stringham JD, Wilson DE, et al. Plasma 5α-reduced androgens in men and hirsute women: role of adrenals and gonads. J Clin Endocrinol Metab. 1979; 48:969–975.

631. Meites J, Bruni JF, van Vugt DA, et al. Relation of endogenous opioid peptides and morphine to neuroendocrine functions. Life Sci. 1979; 24:1325–1336.

632. Meldrum DR, Chang RJ, Lu J, et al. "Medical oophorectomy" using a long-acting GnRH agonist—a possible new approach to the treatment of endometriosis. J Clin Endocrinol Metab. 1982; 54:1081–1083.

633. Meldrum DR, Frumar AM, Shamonki IM, et al. Ovarian and adrenal steroidogenesis in a virilized patient with gonadotropin-resistant ovaries and hilus cell hyperplasia. Obstet Gynecol. 1980; 56:216–221.

634. Meldrum DR, Abraham GE. Peripheral ovarian venous concentrations of various steroid hormones in virilizing ovarian tumors. Obstet Gynecol. 1979; 53:36–43.

635. Menard RH, Guenther TM, Kon H. Studies on the destruction of adrenal and testicular cytochrome P-450 by spironolactone. J Biol Chem. 1979; 254:1726–1733.

636. Menard RH, Loriaux DL, Bartter FC, et al. The effect of the administration of spironolactone on the concentration of plasma testosterone, estradiol and cortisol in male dogs. Steroids. 1978; 31:771–782.

637. Merker E, Futterweit W. Postpartum amenorrhea, diabetes insipidus and galactorrhea. Report of a case and review of the literature. Am J Med. 1974; 56:554–558.

638. Metcalf MG, Espiner EA, Donald RA. Lack of effect of prolactin suppression on plasma dehydroepiandrosterone sulphate. Clin Endocrinol (Oxf). 1979; 10:539–544.

639. Migeon CJ, Rosenwaks Z, Lee PA, et al. The attenuated form of congenital adrenal hyperplasia as an allelic form of 21-hydroxylase deficiency. J Clin Endocrinol Metab. 1980; 51:647–649.

640. Milewicz A, Silber D, Kirschner MA. Therapeutic effects of spironolactone in polycystic ovary syndrome. Obstet Gynecol. 1983; 61:429–432.

641. Minaker K, Rowe J, Pallotta J, et al. Reduced insulin clearance in patients with cellular insulin resistance (abstr). Diabetes (suppl 1). 1981; 30:36.

642. Mishell DR Jr, March CM. Induction of ovulation. In: Mishell DR Jr, Davajan V, eds. Reproductive Endocrinology, Infertility and Contraception. Philadelphia: F.A. Davis Co., 1979:317–337.

643. Molitch ME, Goodman RH, Post KD, et al. Surgical cure of prolactinoma reverses abnormal prolactin response to carbidopa/L-dopa. J Clin Endocrinol Metab. 1982; 55:1118–1123.

644. Molitch ME, Reichlin S. Hyperprolactinemic disorders. Disease-A-Month, (June). Chicago: YearBook Med Publ, 1982. 1–58.

645. Moll GW Jr, Rosenfield RL. Plasma free testosterone in the diagnosis of adolescent polycystic ovary syndrome. J Pediatr. 1983; 102:461–464.

646. Moll GW Jr, Rosenfield RL. Testosterone binding and free plasma androgen concentrations under physiological conditions: characterization by flow dialysis technique. J Clin Endocrinol Metab. 1979; 49:730–736.

647. Moltz L, Rommler A, Schwartz U, Peripheral steroid–gonadotropin interactions and diagnostic significance of double-stimulation tests with luteinizing hormone-releasing hormone in polycystic ovarian disease. Am J Obstet Gynecol. 1979; 134:813–818.

648. Monroe SE, Levine L, Chang RJ, et al. Prolactin-secreting pituitary adenomas. V. Increased gonadotroph responsivity in hyperprolactinemic women with pituitary adenomas. J Clin Endocrinol Metab. 1981; 52:1171–1178.

649. Moon RM. Sites of steroid production in ovine graafian follicles in culture. J Endocrinol. 1977; 73:143–150.

650. Moon YS, Tsang BK, Simpson C, et al. 17β-estradiol biosynthesis in cultured granulosa and thecal cells of human ovarian follicles: stimulation by follicle-stimulating hormone. J Clin Endocrinol Metab. 1978; 47:263–267.

651. Moon YS, Dorrington JH, Armstrong DT. Stimulatory action of follicle-stimulating hormone on estradiol 17-β secretion by hypophysectomized rat ovaries in organ culture. Endocrinology. 1975; 97:244–247.

652. Moore A, Magee F, Cunningham S, et al. Adrenal abnormalities in idiopathic hirsutism. Clin Endocrinol (Oxf). 1983; 18:391–399.

653. Moore RY. Central neural control of circadian rhythms. In: Ganong WF, Martini L, eds. Frontiers in Neuroendocrinology. New York: Raven Press, 1978:185–206.

654. Moore JG, Schifrin BS, Erez S. Ovarian tumors in infancy, childhood, and adolescence. Am J Obstet Gynecol. 1967; 99:913–922.

655. Mori T, Fujita Y, Nihnobu K, et al. Significance of atretic follicles as the site of androgen production in polycystic ovaries. J Endocrinol Invest. 1982; 5:209–215.

656. Morimoto I, Edmiston A, Hawks D, et al. Studies on the origin of androstanediol and androstanediol glucuronide in young and elderly men. J Clin Endocrinol Metab. 1981; 52:772–778.

657. Morrow LB, Burrow GN, Murrow PJ. Inhibition of adrenal protein synthesis by steroids in vitro. Endocrinology. 1967; 80:883–888.

658. Mortimer RH, Lev-Gur M, Freeman R, et al. Pituitary response to bolus and continuous intravenous infusion of luteinizing hormone-releasing factor in normal women and women with polycystic ovarian syndrome. Am J Obstet Gynecol. 1978; 130:630–634.

659. Mortimer CH, Besser GM, Hook J, et al. Intravenous, intramuscular, subcutaneous and intranasal administration of LH/FSH-RH: the duration of effect and occurrence of asynchronous pulsatile release of LH and FSH. Clin Endocrinol (Oxf). 1974; 3:19–26.

660. Moult PJA, Rees LH, Besser GM. Pulsatile gonadotrophin secretion in hyperprolactinaemic amenorrhoea and the response to bromocriptine therapy. Clin Endocrinol (Oxf). 1982; 16:153–162.

661. Moult PJA, Grossman A, Evans JM, et al. The effect of naloxone on pulsatile gonadotrophin release in normal subjects. Clin Endocrinol (Oxf). 1981; 14:321–324.

662. Motohashi T, Wu CH, Abdel-Rahman HA, et al. Estrogen/androgen balance in health and

disease. Am J Obstet Gynecol. 1979; 135:89–95.

663. Mowszowicz I, Melanitou E, Doukani A, et al. Androgen binding capacity and 5α-reductase activity in pubic skin fibroblasts from hirsute patients. J Clin Endocrinol Metab. 1983; 56:1209–1213.

664. Mowszowicz I, Melanitou E, Kirchhoffer MO, et al. Dihydrotestosterone stimulates 5α-reductase activity in pubic skin fibroblasts. J Clin Endocrinol Metab. 1983; 56:320–325.

665. Mroueh AM, Siler-Khodr TM. Ovarian refractoriness to gonadotropins in cases of inappropriate lactation: restoration of ovarian function with bromocryptine. J Clin Endocrinol Metab. 1976; 43:1398–1401.

666. Muhr C, Bergstrom K, Grimelius L. A parallel study of the roentgen anatomy of the sella turcica and the histopathology of the pituitary gland in 205 autopsy specimens. Neuroradiology. 1981; 21:55–65

667. Nabarro JDN. Pituitary prolactinomas. Clin Endocrinol (Oxf). 1982; 17:129–155.

668. Naftolin F, Tolis G. Neuroendocrine regulation of the menstrual cycle. Clin Obstet Gynecol. 1978; 21:17–29.

669. Naftolin F, Ryan KJ, Petro Z. Aromatization of androstenedione by the anterior hypothalamus of adult male and female rats. Endocrinology. 1972; 90:295–298.

670. Nagamani M, Lingold JC, Gomez LG, et al. Clinical and hormonal studies in hyperthecosis of the ovaries. Fertil Steril. 1981; 36:326–332.

671. Nakai Y, Plant TM, Heiss DL, et al. On the sites of the negative and positive feedback actions of estradiol in the control of gonadotropin secretion in the rhesus monkey. Endocrinology. 1978; 102:1008–1014.

672. Nakano R, Yamoto M, Iwasaki M. Effects of oestrogen and prostaglandin $F_{2\alpha}$ on luteinizing hormone receptors in human corpora lutea. J Endocrinol. 1981; 88:401–408.

673. Nebel L, Safriel OJ, Salzberger M, et al. Coelomic mesothelium-like cells in the ovarian stroma of patients with the polycystic ovary syndrome (Stein-Leventhal syndrome). Am J Obstet Gynecol. 1971; 111:766–772.

674. Neill JD. Neuroendocrine control of prolactin secretion. In: Martini L, Ganong WF, eds. Frontiers in Neuroendocrinology. New York: Raven Press, 1980:129–155.

675. Neill JD, Patton JM, Dailey RA, et al. Luteinizing hormone-releasing hormone (LHRH) in pituitary stalk blood of rhesus monkeys: relationship to level of LH release. Endocrinology. 1977; 101:430–434.

676. Neill JD, Dailey RA, Tsou RC, et al. Immunoreactive LH-like substances in serum of hypophysectomized and prepubertal monkeys: inactive in an *in vitro* LH bioassay. Endocrinology. 1977; 100:856–861.

677. Netter A, Bloch-Michel H, Salomon Y, et al. Study of karotypes in Stein-Leventhal syndrome. Ann Endocrinol (Paris). 1961; 22:841–849.

678. New MI, Dupont B, Pang S, et al. An update of congenital adrenal hyperplasia. Recent Prog Horm Res. 1981; 37:105–181.

679. New MI, Lorenzen F, Pang S, et al. "Acquired" adrenal hyperplasia with 21-hydroxylase deficiency is not the same genetic disorder as congenital adrenal hyperplasia. J Clin Endocrinol Metab. 1979; 48:356–359.

680. Neuwirth RS. A method of bilateral ovarian biopsy at laparoscopy in infertility and chronic anovulation. Fertil Steril. 1972; 23:361–366.

681. Newmark S, Dluhy RG, Williams GH, et al. Partial 11- and 21-hydroxylase deficiencies in hirsute women. Am J Obstet Gynecol. 1977; 127:594–598.

682. Nicolis GL, Babich AM, Mitty HA, et al. Observations in the cortisol content of human adrenal venous blood. J Clin Endocrinol Metab. 1974; 38:638–645.

683. Nicolis GL, Gabrilove JL. Studies on the efficiency of adrenocortical 11β-hydroxylation in the human subject. J Clin Endocrinol Metab. 1969; 29:831–836.

684. Nieschlag E, Loriaux DL, Ruger HJ, et al. The secretion of dehydroepiandrostenone and dehydroepiandrosterone sulphate in man. J Endocrinol. 1973; 57:123–134.

685. Nillius S, Wide L. Effects of oestrogen on serum levels of LH and FSH. Acta Endocrinol (Kbh). 1970; 65:583–594.

686. Nilsson L, Hillensjo T, Ekholm C. Pre-ovulatory changes in rat follicular cyclic AMP and sensitivity to gonadotropins. Acta Endocrinol (Kbh). 1977; 86:384–393.

687. Nimrod A, Erickson GF, Ryan KJ. A specific FSH receptor in rat granulosa cells: properties of binding *in vitro*. Endocrinology. 1976; 98:56–64.

688. Nimrod A, Ryan KJ. Aromatization of androgens by human abnormal and breast fat tissue. J Clin Endocrinol Metab. 1975; 40:367–372.

689. Nisula BC, Dunn JF. Measurement of the testosterone binding parameters for both testosterone–estradiol binding globulin and albumin in individual serum samples. Steroids. 1979; 34:771–791.

690. Nolin JM. Intracellular prolactin in rat corpus luteum and adrenal cortex. Endocrinology. 1978; 102:402–406.

691. Norman RL, Lindstrom SA, Gliessman P, et al. Reinitiation of ovulatory cycles in pituitary

stalk-sectioned (SS) rhesus monkeys: observations on the use of Silastic membranes as barriers. 64th Annual Meeting of the Endocrine Society, June 16–18, San Francisco, California. Abstract 815, 1982.

692. Norman RL, Lindstrom SA, Gliessman P. Gonadotropin secretion in the stalk-sectioned rhesus macaque: observations after gonadotropin-releasing hormone (GnRH) treatment. Presented at the Fourteenth Annual Meeting of the Society for the Study of Reproduction, August 10–13, Corvallis, Oregon. Abstract 170, 1981.

693. Novak DJ, Lauchlan SC, McCawley JC, et al. Virilization during pregnancy. Am J Med. 1970; 49:281–290.

694. Ober KP, Hennessy JF. Spironolactone therapy for hirsutism in a hyperandrogenic woman. Ann Int Med. 1978; 89:643–644.

695. O'Dea JPK, Wieland RG, Hallberg MC, et al. Effect of dietary weight loss on sex steroid binding, sex steroids, and gonadotropins in obese postmenopausal women. J Lab Clin Med. 1979; 93:1004–1008.

696. Oelsner G, Serr DM, Mashiach S, et al. The study of induction of ovulation with menotropins: analysis of results of 1897 treatment cycles. Fertil Steril. 1978; 30:538–544.

697. O'Herlihy C, Pepperell RJ, Robinson HP. Ultrasound timing of human chorionic gonadotropin administration in clomiphene-stimulated cycles. Obstet Gynecol. 1982; 59:40–45.

698. O'Herlihy C, Pepperell RJ, Evans JH. The significance of FSH elevation in young women with disorders of ovulation. Br Med J. 1980; 281:1447–1450.

699. Ory SJ. Clinical uses of luteinizing hormone-releasing hormone. Fertil Steril. 1983; 39:577–591.

700. Osborn RH, Yannone ME. Plasma androgens in the normal and androgenic female: a review. Obstet Gynecol Surv. 1971; 26:195–228.

701. Pal SB. Urinary excretion of testosterone and epitestosterone in men, women and children, in health and disease. Clin Chim Acta 1971; 33:215–227.

702. Pang S, Levine LS, Stoner E, et al. Nonsalt-losing congenital adrenal hyperplasia due to 3β-hydroxysteroid dehydrogenase deficiency with normal glomerulosa function. J Clin Endocrinol Metab. 1983; 56:808–818.

703. Pang S, Levine LS, Lorenzen F, et al. Hormonal studies in obligate heterozygotes and siblings of patients with 11β-hydroxylase deficiency congenital adrenal hyperplasia. J Clin Endocrinol Metab. 1980; 50:586–589.

704. Parisi L, Tramonti M, Casciano S, et al. The role of ultrasound in the study of polycystic ovarian disease. J Clin Ultrasound. 1982; 10:167–172.

705. Parker CR Jr, Bruneteau DW, Greenblatt RB, et al. Peripheral ovarian and adrenal vein steroids in hirsute women: acute effects of human chorionic gonadotropin and adrenocorticotrophic hormone. Fertil Steril. 1975; 26:877–888.

706. Parker LN, Chang S, Odell WD. Adrenal androgens in patients with chronic marked elevation of prolactin. Clin Endocrinol (Oxf). 1978; 8:1–5.

707. Parker LN, Sack J, Fisher DA, et al. The adrenarche: prolactin, gonadotropins, adrenal androgens, and cortisol. J Clin Endocrinol Metab. 1978; 46:396–401.

708. Parker R, Ming PML, Rajan R, et al. Clinical and cytogenetic studies of patients with polycystic ovary disease. Am J Obstet Gynecol. 1980; 137:656–659.

709. Parkes D. Bromocriptine. New Engl J Med. 1979; 301:873–878.

710. Pasquali R, Venturoli S, Paradis F, et al. Insulin and C-peptide levels in obese patients with polycystic ovaries. Horm Metab Res. 1982; 14:284–287.

711. Patton WC, Berger MJ, Thompson IE, et al. Pituitary gonadotropin responses to synthetic luteinizing hormone-releasing hormone in patients with typical and atypical polycystic ovary disease. Am J Obstet Gynecol. 1975; 121:382–386.

712. Pauerstein CJ, Eddy CA, Croxatto HD, et al. Temporal relationships of estrogen, progesterone, and luteinizing hormone levels to ovulation in women and infrahuman primates. Am J Obstet Gynecol. 1978; 130:876–886.

713. Paulson JD, Keller DW, Wiest WG, et al. Free testosterone concentration in serum: elevation is the hallmark of hirsutism. Am J Obstet Gynecol. 1977; 128:851–857.

714. Pearl GS, Takei Y, Kurisaka M, et al. Cystic prolactinoma. A variant of "transitional cell tumor" of the pituitary. Am J Surg Pathol. 1981; 5:85–90.

715. Pehrson J, Vaitukaitis JL. Altered dopaminergic control of gonadotropin and prolactin secretion in polycystic ovary syndrome. San Francisco: 64th Annual Meeting of Endocrine Society, June 16–18, Abstr 294, 1982.

716. Perel E, Killinger DW. The interconversion and aromatization of androgens by human adipose tissue. J Steroid Biochem. 1979; 10:623–627.

717. Perloff WH, Smith KD, Steinberger E. Effect of prednisone on female infertility. Int J Fertil. 1965; 10:31–40.

718. Peters H, McNatty KP. Ovulation. Peters H,

McNatty KP (eds) In: The Ovary. London: Elek Science, 1980:75–84.

719. Peters H, McNatty KP. Morphology of the ovary. Peters H, McNatty KP (eds) In: The Ovary. London: Elek Science, 1980:12–35.

720. Peterson EP, Behrman SJ. Laparoscopy of the infertile patient. Obstet Gynecol. 1970; 36:363–367.

721. Pfaff DW. Luteinizing hormone-releasing factor potentiates lordosis behavior in hypophysectomized ovariectomized female rats. Science. 1973; 182:1148–1149.

722. Photopulos GJ, McCartney WH, Walton LA, et al. Computerized tomography applied to gynecologic oncology. Am J Obstet Gynecol. 1979; 135:381–383.

723. Pittaway DE, Andersen RN, Coleman SA Jr, et al. Human ovarian 17β-hydroxysteroid oxidoreductase activity: a comparison of normal and polycystic ovarian tissues. J Clin Endocrinol Metab. 1983; 56:715–719.

724. Pituitary Adenoma Study Group. Pituitary adenomas and oral contraceptives: a multicenter case-control study. Fertil Steril. 1983; 39:753–760.

725. Plant TM, Nakai Y, Belchetz P, et al. Sites of action of estradiol and phentolamine in the inhibition of the pulsatile, circhoral discharges of LH in the rhesus monkey (Macaca mulatta). Endocrinology. 1978; 102:1015–1018.

726. Plunkett ER, Moon YS, Zamecnik J, Armstrong DT. Preliminary evidence of a role for prostaglandin F in human follicular function. Am J Obstet Gynecol. 1975; 123:391–397.

727. Plymate SR, Fariss BL, Bassett ML, et al. Obesity and its role in polycystic ovary syndrome. J Clin Endocrinol Metab. 1981; 52:1246–1248.

728. Poindexter AN, Buttram VC Jr, Besch PK, et al. Prolactin receptors in the ovary. Fertil Steril. 1979; 31:273–277.

729. Pollack MS, Levine LS, O'Neill GJ, et al. HLA linkage and B14, DR1, BfS haplotype association with the genes for late onset and cryptic 21-hydroxylase deficiency. Am J Hum Genet. 1981; 33:540–550.

730. Posner BI, Kelly PA, Shiu RPC, et al. Studies of insulin growth hormone and prolactin binding: tissue distribution, species variation and characterization. Endocrinology. 1974; 96:521–531.

731. Prunty FG. Hirsutism, virilism, and apparent virilism, and their gonadal relationships. J Endocrinol. 1967; 38:203–227.

732. Prunty FG, Brooks RV, Mattingly D. Development of hirsutism after puberty. Br Med J. 1958; 2:1554–1557.

733. Quigley ME, Rakoff JS, Yen SSC. Increased luteinizing hormone sensitivity to dopamine inhibition in polycystic ovary syndrome. J Clin Endocrinol Metab. 1981; 52:231–234.

734. Quigley ME, Yen SSC. The role of endogenous opiates on LH secretion during the menstrual cycle. J Clin Endocrinol Metab. 1980; 51:179–181.

735. Quigley ME, Sheehan KL, Casper RF, et al. Evidence for increased dopaminergic and opioid activity in patients with hypothalamic hypogonadotropic amenorrhea. J Clin Endocrinol Metab. 1980; 50:949–954.

736. Raj SG, Thompson IE, Berger MJ, et al. Diagnostic value of androgen measurements in polycystic ovary syndrome. Obstet Gynecol. 1978; 52:169–171.

737. Raj SG, Thompson IE, Berger MJ, et al. Clinical aspects of the polycystic ovary syndrome. Obstet Gynecol. 1977; 49:552–556.

738. Raj SG, Berger MJ, Grimes EM, et al. The use of gonadotropins for the induction of ovulation in women with polycystic ovarian disease. Fertil Steril. 1977; 28:1280–1284.

739. Rajaniemi HJ, Ronnberg L, Kauppila A, et al. Luteinizing hormone receptors in ovarian follicles of patients with polycystic ovarian disease. J Clin Endocrinol Metab. 1980; 52:1054–1057.

740. Raymond V, Beaulieu M, Labrie F, et al. Potent antidopaminergic activity of estradiol at the pituitary level on prolactin release. Science. 1978; 200:1173–1175.

741. Rebar RW, Yen SSC. Endocrine rhythms in gonadotropins and ovarian steroids with reference to reproductive processes. In: Krieger DT, ed. Endocrine Rhythms. New York: Raven Press, 1979:259–298.

742. Rebar R, Judd HL, Yen SSC, et al. Characterization of the inappropriate gonadotropin secretion in polycystic ovary syndrome. J Clin Invest. 1976; 57:1320–1329.

743. Rebar R, Perlman D, Naftolin F, et al. The estimation of pituitary luteinizing hormone secretion. J Clin Endocrinol Metab. 1973; 37:917–927.

744. Reichlin S. Neuroendocrinology. In: Williams RH, ed. Textbook of Endocrinology, Philadelphia: WB Saunders Co., 1981:589–645.

745. Reichlin S. The prolactinoma problem. New Engl J Med. 1979; 300:313–315.

746. Reid RL, Hoff JD, Yen SSC, et al. Effects of exogenous β-endorphin on pituitary hormone secretion and its disappearance rate in normal human subjects. J Clin Endocrinol Metab. 1981; 52:1179–1184.

747. Reuter SR, Blair AJ, Schteingart DF, et al. Adrenal venography. Radiology 1967; 89:805–814.

748. Reyes FI, Broditsky RS, Winter JSD, et al. Studies on human sexual development. II. Fetal and

maternal serum gonadotropin and sex steroid concentrations. J Clin Endocrinol Metab. 1974; 38:612–617.

749. Richards JS. Hormonal control of ovarian follicular development: a 1978 perspective. Rec Prog Horm Res. 1979; 35:343–373.

750. Richards JS, Midgley AR Jr. Protein hormone action: a key to understanding ovarian follicular and luteal cell development. Biol Reprod. 1976; 14:82–94.

751. Richards JS, Williams JJ: Luteal cell receptor content for prolactin (PRL) and luteinizing hormone (LH): regulation by LH and PRL. Endocrinology 1976; 99:1571–1581.

752. Riddick DH, Hammond CG. Adrenal virilism due to 21-hydroxylase deficiency in the postmenarchial female. Obstet Gynecol. 1975; 45:21–24.

753. Rivarola MA, Saez JM, Jones HW Jr, et al. The secretion of androgens by the normal, polycystic and neoplastic ovaries. Johns Hopkins Hosp Bull. 1967; 121:82–90.

754. Rivarola MA, Saez JM, Migeon CJ. Studies of androgens in patients with congenital adrenal hyperplasia. J Clin Endocrinol Metab. 1967; 27:624–630.

755. Rizkallah TH, Tovell HMM, Kelly WG. Production of estrone and fractional conversion of circulating androstenedione to estrone in women with endometrial carcinoma. J Clin Endocrinol Metab. 1975; 40:1045–1056.

756. Roberts DW, Haines M. Is there a Stein-Leventhal syndrome? Br Med J. 1960; 1:1709–1711.

757. Roberts JS, McCracken JA. Prostaglandin $F_{2\alpha}$ production by the brain during estrogen-induced secretion of luteinizing hormone. Science. 1975; 190:894–896.

758. Robyn C, Tukumbane M. Hyperprolactinemia and hirsutism. In: Mahesh VB, Greenblatt RB, eds. Hirsutism and Virilism. Boston: John Wright, PSG Inc., 1983:189–204.

759. Rocco A, Falaschi P, Pompei P, et al. Chronic anovulation in polycystic ovary syndrome: role of hyperprolactinemia and its suppression with bromocryptine. In: Zichella L, Pancheri P, eds. Psychoneuroendocrinology in Reproduction. Elsevier, North-Holland Biomedical Press, New York. 1979:387–394.

760. Rodriguez-Rigau LJ, Smith KD, Tcholakian RK, et al. Effect of prednisone on plasma testosterone levels and on duration of phases of the menstrual cycle in hyperandrogenic women. Fertil Steril. 1979; 32:408–413.

761. Rodriguez-Sierra JF, Blake CA. Catecholestrogens and release of anterior pituitary gland hormones. II. Prolactin. Endocrinology. 1982; 110:325–329.

762. Rodriguez-Sierra JF, Blake CA. Catecholestro-

gens and release of anterior pituitary gland hormones. I. LH. Endocrinology. 1982; 110:318–324.

763. Rogers J, Mitchell GW Jr. The relation of obesity to menstrual disturbances. New Engl J Med. 1952; 247:53–55.

764. Rolland R, Lequin RM, Schellekens LA, et al. The role of prolactin in the restoration of ovarian function during the early post-partum period in the human female. I. A study during physiological lactation. Clin Endocrinol (Oxf). 1975; 4:15–25.

765. Roncari DAK, Van RLR. Promotion of human adipocyte precursor replication by 17β-estradiol in culture. J Clin Invest. 1977; 62:503–508.

766. Ropert JC, Quigley ME, Yen SSC. Endogenous opiates modulate pulsatile luteinizing hormone release in humans. J Clin Endocrinol Metab. 1981; 52:583–585.

767. Rose LI, Underwood RH, Newmark SH, et al. Pathophysiology of spironolactone-induced gynecomastia. Ann Intern Med. 1977; 87:398–403.

768. Rosenfeld RS, Hellman L, Gallagher TF. Metabolism and interconversion of dehydroisoandrosterone and dehydroisoandrosterone sulfate. J Clin Endocrinol Metab. 1972; 35:187–193.

769. Rosenfield RL, Miller WL. Congenital adrenal hyperplasia. In: Mahesh VB, Greenblatt RB, eds. Hirsutism and Virilism. Boston: John Wright, PSG Inc., 1983:87–119.

770. Rosenfield RL, Bickel S, Razdan AK. Amenorrhea related to progestin excess in congenital adrenal hyperplasia. Obstet Gynecol. 1980; 56:208–215.

771. Rosenfield RL, Rich BH, Wolfsdorf JI, et al. Pubertal presentation of congenital delta⁵-3β-hydroxysteroid dehydrogenase deficiency. J Clin Endocrinol Metab. 1980; 51:345–353.

772. Rosenfield RL. Letter to the editor. New Engl J Med. 1976; 295:232.

773. Rosenfield RL. Studies of the relation of plasma androgen levels to androgen action in women. J Ster Biochem. 1975; 6:695–702.

774. Rosenfield RL, Ehrlich EN, Cleary RE. Adrenal and ovarian contributions to the elevated free plasma androgen levels in hirsute women. J Clin Endocrinol Metab. 1972; 34:92–98.

775. Rosenfield RL. Plasma testosterone binding glubulin and indexes of the concentration of unbound plasma androgens in normal and hirsute subjects. J Clin Endocrinol Metab. 1971; 32:717–728.

776. Rosenwaks Z, Lee PA, Jones GS, et al. An attenuated form of congenital adrenal hyperplasia. J Clin Endocrinol Metab. 1979; 49:335–339.

777. Rosenwaks Z, Wentz AC, Jones GS, et al. Endo-

metrial pathology and estrogens. Obstet Gynecol. 1979; 53:403–410.

778. Ross CT, Vande Wiele RL, Frantz AG. The ovaries and the breasts. In: Williams RH, ed. Textbook of Endocrinology. Philadelphia: WB Saunders Co., 1981:355–411.

779. Rossier J. Functions of β-endorphin and enkephalins in the pituitary. In: Ganong WF, Martini L, eds. Frontiers in Neuroendocrinology, Vol 7. New York: Raven Press, 1982:191–209.

780. Roth JC, Kelch RP, Kaplan SL, et al. FSH and LH response to luteinizing hormone-releasing factor in prepubertal and pubertal children, adult males and patients with hypogonadotropic and hypergonadotropic hypogonadism. J Clin Endocrinol Metab. 1972; 35:926–930.

781. Roy S, Mahesh VB, Greenblatt RB. Effect of dehydroepiandrosterone and delta^4-androstenedione on the reproductive organs of female rats: production of cystic changes in the ovary. Nature. 1962; 196:42–43.

782. Rubens B, Vermeulen A. Investigation of hirsutism. In: Genazzani A, Thijssen JHH, Siiteri P, et al., eds. Adrenal Androgens. New York: Raven Press, 1980:283–287.

783. Ruiz-Velasco V, Rosas-Arceo J, Matute MM. Chemical inducers of ovulation: comparative results. Int J Fertil. 1979; 24:61–64.

784. Rust LA, Israel R, Mishell DR Jr. An individualized graduated therapeutic regimen for clomiphene citrate. Am J Obstet Gynecol. 1974; 120:785–790.

785. Ryan KJ, Petro A, Kaiser J. Steroid formation by isolated and recombined ovarian granulosa and thecal cells. J Clin Endocrinol Metab. 1968; 28:355–358.

786. Saez JM, Forest MG, Morera AM, et al. Metabolic clearance rate and blood production rate of testosterone and dihydrotestosterone in normal subjects, during pregnancy and in hyperthyroidism. J Clin Invest. 1972; 51:1226–1234.

787. Sakakura M, Takebe K, Nakagawa S. Inhibition of luteinizing hormone secretion induced by synthetic LRH by long-term treatment with glucocorticoids in human subjects. J Clin Endocrinol Metab. 1975; 40:774–779.

788. Santen RJ, Ruby EB. Enhanced frequency and magnitude of episodic luteinizing hormone-releasing hormone discharge as a hypothalamic mechanism for increased luteinizing hormone secretion. J Clin Endocrinol Metab. 1979; 48:315–319.

789. Santen RJ, Bardin CW. Episodic luteinizing secretion in man. Pulse analysis. Clinical interpretation, physiological mechanism. J Clin Invest. 1973; 52:2617–2628.

790. Sarker DK, Gottschall PE, Meites J. Damage to hypothalamic dopaminergic neurons is associated with development of prolactin-secreting pituitary tumors. Science. 1982; 218:684–686.

791. Sarker DK, Miki N, Xie QW, et al. Estrogen can inhibit "short loop feedback" action of prolactin on prolactin release. 64th Annual Meeting of the Endocrine Society, June 16–18, San Francisco, Calif., Abstr 864, 1982.

792. Sarris S, Swyer GIM, Ward RHT, et al. The treatment of mild adrenal hyperplasia and associated infertility with prednisone. Br J Obstet Gynaecol. 1978; 85:251–253.

793. Sassin JF, Frantz AG, Kapen S, et al. The nocturnal rise of human prolactin is dependent on sleep. J Clin Endocrinol Metab. 1973; 37:436–440.

794. Saunders DB, Hunter JC, Haase HR, et al. Treatment of luteal phase inadequacy with bromocriptine. Obstet Gynecol. 1979; 53:287–289.

795. Schally AV, Arimura A, Baba Y, et al. Isolation and properties of the FSH and LH-releasing hormone. Biochem Biophys Res Commun. 1971; 43:393–399.

796. Schindler AE, Ebert A, Friedrich E. Conversion of androstenedione to estrone by human fat tissue. J Clin Endocrinol Metab. 1972; 35:627–630,

797. Schlechte J, Sherman B, Halmi N, et al. Prolactin-secreting pituitary tumors in amenorrheic women: a comprehensive study. Endocrinol Rev. 1980; 1:295–308.

798. Schneider APG, Bohnet HG, Mühlenstedt D. Prolactin in female infertility. Acta Endocrinol (Kbh) (Suppl 212). 1977; 85:17.

799. Schneider G, Genel M, Bongiovanni AM, et al. Persistent testicular delta^5-isomerase-3β-hydroxysteroid dehydrogenase (delta^5-3β-HSD) deficiency in the delta^5-3β-HSD form of congenital adrenal hyperplasia. J Clin Invest. 1975; 55:681–690.

800. Schoemaker J, Wentz AC, Jones GS, et al. Stimulation of follicular growth with "pure" FSH in patients with anovulation and elevated LH levels. Obstet Gynecol. 1978; 51:270–277.

801. Schreiber JR, Ross GT. Further characterization of a rat ovarian testosterone receptor with evidence for nuclear translocation. Endocrinology. 1976; 99:590–596.

802. Schteingart DE, Woodbury MC, Tsao HS, et al. Virilizing syndrome associated with an adrenal cortical adenoma secreting predominantly testosterone. Am J Med. 1979; 67:140–146.

803. Schultz KD, Geiger W, del Pozo E, et al. Pattern of sexual steroids, prolactin and gonadotropin hormones during prolactin inhibition in normally cycling women. Am J Obstet Gynecol. 1978; 132:561–566.

804. Schwartz M, Jewelewicz R. The use of gonado-

tropins for induction of ovulation. Fertil Steril. 1981; 35:3–12.

805. Sciarra F, Toscano V, Concolino G, et al. Simultaneous estimation of four plasma androgens before and after dynamic tests in women with hirsutism: correlation with long-term therapy. Horm Res. 1976; 7:16–27.

806. Scoggins BA, Oddie DJ, Hare WSC, et al. Preoperative lateralisation of aldosterone-producing tumours in primary aldosteronism. Ann Intern Med. 1972; 76:891–897.

807. Scott RB, Wharton LR. The effect of testosterone on experimental endometriosis in Rhesus monkeys. Am J Obstet Gynecol. 1959; 78:1020–1027.

808. Scully RE, Cohen RB. Oxidative-enzyme activity in normal and pathologic human ovaries. Obstet Gynecol. 1964; 24:667–681.

809. Scully RE. Androgenic lesions of the ovary. In: Grady HG, Smith DE, eds. The Ovary. Baltimore: Williams & Wilkins, 1963:143–174.

810. Scully RE, Richardson GS. Luteinization of the stroma of metastatic cancer involving the ovary and its endocrine significance. Cancer. 1961; 14:827–840.

811. Seibel MM, Kamrava M, McArdle C, et al. Ovulation induction and conception using subcutaneous pulsatile luteinizing hormone-releasing hormone. Obstet Gynecol. 1983; 61:292–298.

812. Seltzer CC. Some re-evaluations of the build and blood pressure study, 1959, as related to ponderal index, somatotype and mortality. New Eng J Med. 1966; 274:254–259.

813. Senior BE, Cawood ML, Oakey RE, et al. A comparison of the effects of clomiphene and tamoxifen treatment on the concentrations of oestradiol and progesterone in the peripheral plasma of infertile women. Clin Endocrinol (Oxf). 1978; 8:382–389.

814. Seppälä M, Hirvonen E, Ranta T. Bromocriptine treatment of secondary amenorrhea. Lancet. 1976; 1:1154–1156.

815. Seppälä M, Hirvonen E, Ranta T. Hyperprolactinaemia and luteal insufficiency. Lancet. 1976; 1:229–230.

816. Seppälä M, Unnerus HA, Hirvonen E, et al. Bromocriptine increases plasma estradiol-17β concentration in amenorrhea patients with normal serum prolactin. J Clin Endocrinol Metab. 1976; 43:474–477.

817. Seppälä M, Hirvonen E, Unnerus HA, Ranta T, et al. Prolactin and testosterone: independent circulating levels in hyperprolactinemic and normoprolactinemic amenorrhea. The effect of prolactin suppression by bromocriptine. J Clin Endocrinol Metab. 1976; 43:198–200.

818. Seppälä M, Hirvonen E. Raised serum prolactin levels associated with hirsutism and amenorrhoea. Br Med J. 1975; 4:144–145.

819. Seppälä M, Hirvonen E, Ranta T, et al. Raised serum prolactin levels in amenorrhoea. Br Med J. 1975; 2:305–306.

820. Serio M, Dell'Acqua S, Calabresi E, et al. Androgen secretion by the human ovary: measurement of androgens in the ovarian venous blood. In: James VHT, Serio M, Giusti G, eds. The Endocrine Function of the Human Ovary. New York: Academic Press, 1976:471–479.

821. Sfikakis AP, Ikkas DG, Diamandopoulos KN. Urinary estrogen secretion after metyrapone administration to patients with polycystic ovary syndrome. J Endocrinol. 1967; 39:61–69.

822. Shapiro AG. Pituitary adenoma, menstrual disturbance, hirsutism and abnormal glucose tolerance. Fertil Steril. 1981; 35:226–229.

823. Shapiro G, Evron S. A novel use of spironolactone: treatment of hirsutism. J Clin Endocrinol Metab. 1980; 51:429–432.

824. Shapiro S, Kaufman DW, Slone D, et al. Recent and past use of conjugated estrogens in relation to adenocarcinoma of the endometrium. New Engl J Med. 1980; 303:485–489.

825. Sharma DC, Forchielli E, Dorfman RI. Inhibition of enzymatic steroid 11β-hydroxylation by androgens. J Biol Chem. 1963; 238:572–575.

826. Sharpe RM, Fraser HM. HCG stimulation of testicular LHRH-like activity. Nature. 1980; 287:642–643.

827. Shaw RW. Neuroendocrinology of the menstrual cycle in humans. J Clin Endocrinol Metab. 1978; 7:531–559.

828. Shaw RW, Duignan NM, Butt WR, et al. Modification by sex steroids of LHRH response in the polycystic ovary syndrome. Clin Endocrinol (Kbh). 1976; 5:495–502.

829. Shaw RW, Butt WR, London DR. Effect of oestrogen pretreatment on subsequent response to luteinizing hormone-releasing hormone (LH-RH) in normal women. Clin Endocrinol (Oxf). 1975; 4:297–304.

830. Shaw RW, Duignan NM, Butt WR, et al. Hypothalamic–pituitary relationships in the polycystic ovary syndrome: serum gonadotrophin levels following injection of oestradiol benzoate. Br J Obstet Gynaecol. 1975; 82:952–957.

831. Shaw RW, Butt WR, London DR. Pathological mechanism to explain some cases of amenorrhoea without organic disease. Br J Obstet Gynaecol. 1975; 82:337–340.

832. Shaw RW, Butt WR, London DR, et al. Variation in response to synthetic luteinizing hormone-releasing hormone (LH-RH) at different phases of the same menstrual cycle in normal

women. J Obstet Gynaecol Br Com. 1974; 81:632–639.

833. Shearman RP, Fraser IS. Impact of new diagnostic methods on the differential diagnosis and treatment of secondary amenorrhoea. Lancet. 1977; 1:1195–1197.

834. Shearman RP, Cox RI. Clinical and chemical correlations in the Stein-Leventhal syndrome. Am J Obstet Gynecol. 1965; 92:747–754.

835. Shepard MK, Balmaceda JP, Leija CG. Relationship of weight to successful induction of ovulation with clomiphene citrate. Fertil Steril. 1979; 32:641–645.

836. Sherman BM, Chapler FK, Crickard K, et al. Endocrine consequences of continuous antiestrogen therapy with tamoxifen in premenopausal women. J Clin Invest. 1979; 64:398–404.

837. Sherman BM, Harris CE, Schlechte J, et al. Pathogenesis of prolactin-secreting pituitary adenomas. Lancet. 1978; 2:1019–1021.

838. Shippel S. The ovarian theca cell: Part IV. The hyperthecosis syndrome. J Obstet Gynaecol Br Emp. 1955; 62:321–353.

839. Shippel S. The ovarian theca cell: Part II. Variable endometrial responses to ovarian thecal activity. J Obstet Gynaecol Br Com. 1950; 57:372–387.

840. Shiu RPC, Friesen HG. Properties of a prolactin receptor from the rabbit mammary gland. Biochem J. 1974; 140:301–311.

841. Short RV: Further observations on the defective synthesis of ovarian steroids in the Stein-Leventhal syndrome. J Endocrinol. 1962; 24:359–365.

842. Short RV, London DR. Defective biosynthesis of ovarian steroids in the Stein-Leventhal syndrome. Br Med J. 1961; 1:1724–1727.

843. Siiteri PK, Schwarz BE, MacDonald PC. Estrogen receptors and the estrone hypothesis in relation to endometrial and breast cancer. Gynecol Oncol. 1974; 2:228–238.

844. Siiteri PK, MacDonald PC. Role of extraglandular estrogen in human endocrinology. In: Greep RO, Astwood EB, eds. Handbook of Physiology: Endocrinology, Vol II, Section 7. Washington DC: American Physiological Society, 1973:615–629.

845. Siler TM, Yen SSC. Augmented response to synthetic LRF in hypogonadal state. J Clin Endocrinol Metab. 1973; 37:491–494.

846. Silverman AJ, Antunes JL, Ferin M, et al. The distribution of luteinizing hormone releasing hormone (LHRH) in the hypothalamus of the rhesus monkey: light microscopic studies using immunoperoxidase technique. Endocrinology. 1977; 101:134–142.

847. Sizonenko PC, Paunier I. Hormonal changes in puberty. III. Correlation of plasma dehydro-epiandrosterone, testosterone, FSH, and LH with stages of puberty and bone age in normal boys and girls and in patients with Addison's disease or hypogonadism or premature or late adrenarche. J Clin Endocrinol Metab. 1975; 41:894–904.

848. Smith DC, Prentice RL, Bauermeister DE. Endometrial carcinoma: histopathology, survival, and exogenous estrogens. Gynecol Obstet Invest. 1981; 12:169–179.

849. Smith DC, Prentice R, Thompson DL, et al. Association of exogenous estrogen and endometrial carcinoma. New Engl J Med. 1975; 293:1164–1167.

850. Smith HC, Posen S, Clifton-Bligh P, et al. A testosterone-secreting adrenal cortical adenoma. Aust N Z J Med. 1978; 8:171–175.

851. Smith KD, Rodriguez-Rigau LJ, Tcholakian RK, et al. The relation between plasma testosterone levels and the lengths of phases of the menstrual cycle. Fertil Steril. 1979; 32:403–407.

852. Smith KD, Steinberger E, Perloff WH: Polycystic ovarian disease. A report of 301 patients. Am J Obstet Gynecol. 1965; 93:994–1001.

853. Smythe GA, Brandstater JF: Oestrogen-induced hyperprolactinaemia in the rat: reduced concentrations of hypothalamic dopamine and the effects of bromocriptine. Aust J Biol Sci. 1980; 33:329–339.

854. Sobrinho LG, Kase NG, Grunt JA. Changes in adrenocortical function of patients with gonadal dysgenesis after treatment with estrogen. J Clin Endocrinol Metab. 1971; 33:110–114.

855. Soffer LJ, Fogel M. Urinary concentration of gonadotrophin (ICSH)-inhibiting sustance in Stein-Leventhal syndrome. J Clin Endocrinol Metab. 1964; 24:656–659.

856. Sohval AR, Churg J, Cobin RH, et al. Histopathology and ultrastructure of ovarian hilus cell tumors. Gynecol Oncol. 1979; 7:79–101.

857. Sohval AR. The syndrome of pure gonadal dysgenesis. Am J Med. 1965; 38:615–625.

858. Sohval AR. Diseases of the Ovary. In: Soffer LJ, ed. Diseases of the Endocrine Glands, 2nd ed. Philadelphia: Lea & Febiger, 1956:664–741.

859. Sommers SC, Wadman PJ. Pathogenesis of polycystic ovaries. Am J Obstet Gynecol. 1956; 72:160–169.

860. Sommers SC, Hertig AT, Bengloff H. Genesis of endometrial carcinoma. II. Cases 19 to 35 years old. Cancer. 1949; 2:957–963.

861. Southren AL, Gordon GG, Tochimoto S, et al. Testosterone and androstenedione metabolism in the polycystic ovary syndrome; studies of the percentage binding of testosterone in plasma. J Clin Endocrinol Metab. 1969; 29:1356–1363.

862. Sowers JR, Fayez J. Effect of dexamethasone on

gonadotropin responsiveness to luteinizing hormone-releasing hormone and clomiphene in women with secondary amenorrhea. Am J Obstet Gynecol. 1979; 134:325–328.

863. Spaeth DG, Osawa Y: Estrogen biosynthesis. III. Stereo-specificity of aromatization by normal and diseased human ovaries. J Clin Endocrinol Metab. 1974; 38:783–786.

864. Spasov SA, Dokumov SI. Dermatoglyphic investigations of patients with Stein-Leventhal syndrome. Obstet Gynecol. 1973; 42:877–880.

865. Spaulding SW, Masuda T, Osawa Y. Increased 17β-hydroxysteroid dehydrogenase activity in a masculinizing adrenal adenoma in a patient with isolated testosterone overproduction. J Clin Endocrinol Metab. 1980; 50:537–540.

866. Speert H. Carcinoma of the endometrium in young women. Surg Gynecol Obstet. 1949; 88:332–336.

867. Spellacy WN, Cantor B, Kalra PS, et al. The effect of varying prolactin levels on pituitary luteinizing hormone and follicle-stimulating hormone response to gonadotropin-releasing hormone. Am J Obstet Gynecol. 1978; 132:157–164.

868. Speroff L. Getting high on running. Fertil Steril. 1981; 36:149–151.

869. Speroff L, Glass RH, Kase NG. Induction of ovulation. In: Clinical Gynecologic Endocrinology and Infertility, 2nd ed, Baltimore: Williams & Wilkins Co., 1978:375–391.

870. Speroff L, Glass RH, Kase NG. Steroid contraception. In: Clinical Gynecologic Endocrinology, 2nd Ed. Baltimore: Williams and Wilkins, 1978:283–310.

871. Speroff L. The adrenogenital syndrome and its obstetrical aspects. A review of the literature and case report. Obstet Gynecol Surv. 1965; 20:185–214.

872. Stahl NL, Teeslink GR, Greenblatt R. Ovarian, adrenal and peripheral testosterone levels in the polycystic ovary syndrome. Am J Obstet Gynecol. 1973; 117:194–200.

873. Starer F. Percutaneous suprarenal venography. Br J Radiol. 1965; 38:675–681.

874. Stein IF. Duration of fertility following ovarian wedge resection—Stein-Leventhal syndrome. West J Surg. 1964; 72:237–242.

875. Stein IF. Multiple pregnancy following wedge resection in the Stein-Leventhal syndrome. Int J Fertil. 1964; 9:343–350.

876. Stein IF. The management of bilateral polycystic ovaries. Fertil Steril. 1955; 6:189–205.

877. Stein IF, Cohen MR, Elson R. Results of bilateral ovarian wedge resection in 47 cases of sterility. Am J Obstet Gynecol. 1949; 58:267–274.

878. Stein IF. Bilateral polycystic ovaries. Am J Obstet Gynecol. 1945; 50:385–396.

879. Stein IF, Cohen MR. Surgical treatment of bilateral polycystic ovaries—amenorrhea and sterility. Am J Obstet Gynecol. 1939; 38:465–480.

880. Stein IF, Leventhal ML. Amenorrhea associated with bilateral polycystic ovaries. Am J Obstet Gynecol. 1935; 29:181–191.

881. Steinberg WH. The morphology, androgenic function, hyperplasia and tumors of the ovarian hilus cells. Am J Path. 1949; 25:493–521.

882. Steinberger E, Rodriguez-Rigau LJ, Smith KD. The prognostic value of acute adrenal suppression and stimulation tests in hyperandrogenic women. Fertil Steril. 1982; 37:187–192.

883. Steinberger E, Smith KD, Rodriguez-Rigau LJ. Hyperandrogenism and female infertility. In: Crosignani PG, Rubin BL, eds. Endocrinology of Human Infertility: New aspects. London: Academic Press, 1981:327–342.

884. Steinberger E, Smith KD, Tcholakian RK, et al. Testosterone levels in female partners of infertile couples. Am J Obstet Gynecol. 1979; 133:133–138.

885. Stenchever MA, MacIntyre MN, Jarvis JA, et al. Cytogenetic evaluation of 41 patients with Stein-Leventhal syndrome. Obstet Gynecol. 1968; 32:794–801.

886. Stewart ME, Pochi PE. Antiandrogens in the skin. Int J Dermatol. 1978; 17:167–179.

887. Stoffer SS, McKeel DW Jr, Randall RV, et al. Pituitary prolactin cell hyperplasia with autonomous prolactin secretion and primary hypothyroidism. Fertil Steril. 1981; 36:682–685.

888. Stouffer RL, Nixon WE, Gulyas BJ, et al. Gonadotropin-sensitive progesterone production by rhesus monkey luteal cells in vitro: a function of age of the corpus luteum during the menstrual cycle. Endocrinology. 1977; 100:506–512.

889. Stripp B, Taylor AA, Bartter FC, et al. Effect of spironolactone on sex hormones in man. J Clin Endocrinol Metab. 1975; 41:777–781.

890. Sutton C. The limitations of laparoscopic ovarian biopsy. J Obstet Gynaecol Br Comm. 1974; 81:317–320.

891. Swanson M, Sauerbrei EE, Cooperberg PL. Medical implications of ultrasonically detected polycystic ovaries. J Clin Ultrasound. 1981; 9:219–222.

892. Swanson IA, McNatty KP, Baird DT. Concentration of prostaglandin F$_2$ and steroids in the human corpus. J Endocrinol. 1977; 73:115–122.

893. Swolin K. Laparoscopy as an operating tool in female sterility. J Reprod Med. 1977; 19:167–170.

894. Sykes DW, Ginsburg J. The use of laparoscopic

ovarian biopsy to assess gonadal function. Am J Obstet Gynecol. 1972; 112:408–413.

895. Tacchi D. Ovarian dysfunction. In: Ovarian Gynaecology, London: WB Saunders Co, 1976:102–117.

896. Tagatz GE, Gurpide E. Hormone secretion by the human ovary. In: Greep RO, Astwood ED, eds. Handbook of Physiology, Section 7: Endocrinology, Vol II, Pt 1. Baltimore: Williams & Wilkins, American Physiological Society. 1973:603–613.

897. Tajima C, Fukushima T. Endocrine profiles in tamoxifen-induced ovulatory cycles. Fertil Steril. 1983; 40:23–30.

898. Talbert LM. Clomiphene citrate induction of ovulation. Fertil Steril. 1983; 39:742–743.

899. Talbert LM, Sloan C. The effect of low-dose oral contraceptive on serum testosterone levels in polycystic ovary disease. Obstet Gynecol. 1979; 53:694–679.

900. Tanabe K, Gagliano P, Channing CP, et al. Levels of inhibin-F activity and steroids in human follicular fluid from normal women and women with polycystic ovarian disease. J Clin Endocrinol Metab. 1983; 57:24–31.

901. Tang VW, Faiman C. Premature ovarian failure: a search for circulating factors against gonadotropin receptors. Am J Obstet Gynecol. 1983; 146:816–821.

902. Taw RL, Jones EG. Polycystic ovaries and menstrual irregularities. Am J Obstet Gynecol. 1963; 86:626–639.

903. Taylor SI, Dons RF, Hernandez E, et al. Insulin resistance associated with androgen excess in women with autoantibodies to the insulin receptor. Ann Int Med. 1982; 97:851–855.

904. Taymor ML, Seibel MM, Smith D, et al. Ovulation timing by luteinizing hormone assay and follicle puncture. Obstet Gynecol. 1983; 62:191–195.

905. Taymor ML, Clark BJ, Sturgis SH: The polycystic ovary. A clinical and laboratory study. Am J Obstet Gynecol. 1963; 86:188–196.

906. Teperman L, Futterweit W, Zappula R, et al. Oral contraceptive history as a risk indicator in patients with pituitary tumors and hyperprolactinemia: a case comparison study of twenty patients. Neurosurgery. 1980; 7:571–573.

907. Thomas PK, Ferriman DG. Variations in facial and pubic hair growth in white women. Am J Phys Anthropol. 1957; 15:171–180.

908. Thompson CR, Hanson LM. Pergonal (menotropins): a summary of clinical experience in the induction of ovulation and pregnancy. Fertil Steril. 1970; 21:844–853.

909. Thompson IE, Taymor ML. Clinical and evolutive aspects of the polycystic ovary. In: Tozzini RI, Reeves G, Pineda RL, eds. Endocrine Phy-siopathology of the Ovary. Amsterdam: Elsevier Press, 1980:295–306.

910. Thorner MO, Schran HF, Evans WS, et al. A broad spectrum of prolactin suppression by bromocriptine in hyperprolactinemic women: a study of serum prolactin and bromocriptine levels after acute and chronic administration of bromocriptine. J Clin Endocrinol Metab. 1980; 50:1026–1033.

911. Thorner MO. Prolactin: clinical physiology and the significance and management of hyperprolactinemia. In: Martini L, Besser GM, eds. Clinical Neuroendocrinology. New York: Academic Press, 1977:319–361.

912. Thorner MO, Besser GM. Hyperprolactinaemia and gonadal function: results of bromocriptine treatment. In: Crosignani PG, Robyn C, eds. Prolactin and Human Reproduction. New York: Academic Press, 1977:285–301.

913. Thorner MO, Besser GM, Jones A, et al. Bromocriptine treatment of female infertility: report of 13 pregnancies. Br Med J. 1975; 4:694–697.

914. Thorner MO, McNeilly AS, Hagan C, et al. Long-term treatment of galactorrhoea and hypogonadism with bromocriptine. Br Med J. 1974; 2:419–422.

915. Toaff R, Toaff ME, Gould S, et al. Role of androgenic hyperactivity in anovulation. Fertil Steril. 1978; 29:407–413.

916. Toaff R, Toaff ME, Peyser MR. Infertility following wedge resection of the ovaries. Am J Obstet Gynecol. 1976; 124:92–96.

917. Toaff ME, Toaff R, Chayen R. Congenital adrenal hyperplasia caused by 11β-hydroxylase deficiency with onset of symptoms after one spontaneous pregnancy. Am J Obstet Gynecol. 1975; 121:202–204.

918. Toledo SPA, Pena EP, Assis LM, et al. Sindrome dos ovarios policisticos familiar (tipo Stein-Leventhal). Rev Ass Med Brasil. 1977; 23:79–82.

919. Tolis G. Prolactin: Physiology and pathology. In: Krieger DT, Hughes JC, eds. Neuroendocrinology. Sunderland, Mass: Sinauer Associates, 1980:321–328.

920. Tolis G, Franks S. Physiology and pathology of prolactin secretion. In: Tolis G, Labrie F, Martin JB, Naftolin F, eds. Clinical Neuroendocrinology. New York: Raven Press, 1979:291–317.

921. Tolis G, Naftolin F: Induction of menstruation with bromocryptine in patients with euprolactinaemic amenorrhoea. Am J Obstet Gynecol. 1976; 126:426–429.

922. Trace RJ, Keaty EC, McCall ML. An investigation of ovarian tissue and urinary 17-ketoster-

oids in patients with bilateral polycystic ovaries. Am J Obstet Gynecol. 1960; 79:310–315.

923. Travaglini P, Faglia G. Pregnanetriolone excretion in Stein-Leventhal syndrome. Acta Endocrinol (Kbh). 1971; 68:826–832.

924. Tremblay RR, Kowarski A, Park IJ, et al. Blood production rate of dihydrotestosterone in the syndrome of male pseudohermaphroditism. J Clin Endocrinol Metab. 1972; 35:101–107.

925. Tsai CC, Yen SSC. The effect of ethinyl estradiol administration during early follicular phase of the cycle on the other gonadotropin levels and ovarian function. J Clin Endocrinol Metab. 1971; 33:917–923.

926. Tsai CC, Yen SSC. Acute effects of intravenous infusion of 17β-estradiol on gonadotropin release in pre- and post-menopausal women. J Clin Endocrinol Metab. 1971; 32:766–771.

927. Tsang BK, Moon YS, Simpson CW, et al. Androgen biosynthesis in human ovarian follicles: cellular source, gonadotropic control, and adenosine 3'5'-monophosphate mediation. J Clin Endocrinol Metab. 1979; 48:153–158.

928. Tsapoulis AD, Zourlas PA, Comninos AC. Observations on 320 infertile patients with human gonadotropins (human menopausal gonadotropin/human chorionic gonadotropin). Fertil Steril. 1978; 29:492–495.

929. Tucci JR, Zäh W, Kalderon AE. Endocrine studies in an arrhenoblastoma responsive to dexamethasone, ACTH, and human chorionic gonadotropin. Am J Med. 1973; 55:687–694.

930. Tucker HSG, Lankford HV, Gardner DF, et al. Persistent defect in regulation of prolactin secretion after successful pituitary tumor removal in women with the galactorrhea–amenorrhea syndrome. J Clin Endocrinol Metab. 1980; 51:968–971.

931. Tulchinsky D, Chopra IJ. Estrogen androgen unbalance in patients with hirsutism and amenorrhea. J Clin Endocrinol Metab. 1974; 39:164–169.

932. Turkalj I, Braun P, Krupp P. Surveillance of bromocriptine in pregnancy. JAMA. 1982; 247:1589–1591.

933. Turski PH, Newton TH, Horten BH. Sella contour: anatomic polytomographic correlation. Am J Neuroradiol. 1981; 137:213–216.

934. Tzingounis VA, Aksu MF, Natrajan PK, et al. The significance of adrenal and ovarian catheterization in patients with polycystic ovary syndrome. Int J Gynaecol Obstet. 1979; 17:78–82.

935. Tzingounis VA, Alperin H, Natrajan PK. Radiographic abnormalities in patients with Stein-Leventhal syndrome. Int J Gynaecol Obstet. 1978; 16:167–169.

936. Vale W, Spiess J, Rivier C, et al. Characterization of a 41-residue ovine hypothalamic peptide that stimulates secretion of corticotropin and β-endorphin. Science. 1981; 213:1394–1397.

937. Valenta LJ, Sostrin RD, Eisenberg H, et al. Diagnosis of pituitary tumors by hormone assays and computerized tomography. Am J Med. 1982; 72:861–873.

938. Valkov IM, Dokumov SI. Effect of ovarian wedge resection for the Stein-Leventhal syndrome on plasma FSH, LH, oestradiol and testosterone levels and on the responses of the pituitary to intravenous LHRH. Br J Obstet Gynaecol. 1977; 84:539–542.

939. van Campenhout J, Simmer H, Dignam W, et al. Polycystic sclerotic ovaries. Lancet. 1963; 2:1380–1381.

940. Vandenberg G, DeVane G, Yen SSC. Effects of exogenous estrogen and progestin on pituitary responsiveness to synthetic luteinizing hormone-releasing factor. J Clin Invest. 1974; 53:1750–1754.

941. van der Steeg HJ, Coelingh Bennink HJT. Bromocriptine for induction of ovulation in normoprolactinaemic post-pill anovulation. Lancet. 1977; 1:502–504.

942. vande Wiele RL. Anorexia nervosa and the hypothalamus. In: Krieger DT, Hughes JC, eds. Neuroendocrinology. Sunderland, Mass: Sinauer Associates, 1980:205–211.

943. van Hall EV, Mastboom JL. Luteal phase insufficiency in patients treated with clomiphene. Am J Obstet Gynecol. 1969; 103:165–171.

944. Vara P, Niemineva K: Small cystic degeneration of ovaries as incidental finding in gynecological laparotomies. Acta Obstet Gynecol Scand. 1951; 31:94–107.

945. Vejlsted H, Albrachtsen R. Biochemical and clinical effect of ovarian wedge resection in the polycystic ovary syndrome. Obstet Gynecol. 1976; 47:575–580.

946. Vekemans M, Delvoye P, L'Hermite M, et al. Serum prolactin levels during the menstrual cycle. J Clin Endocrinol Metab. 1977; 44:989–993.

947. Vemer HM, Rolland R. The influence of exogenous oestradiol benzoate on the pituitary responsiveness to LHRH during the puerperium in women. Clin Endocrinol (Oxf). 1982; 16:251–258.

948. Vermeulen A. Androgen secretion by adrenals and gonads. In: Mahesh VB, Greenblatt RB, eds. Hirsutism and Virilism. Boston: John Wright, PSG Inc., 1983:17–34.

949. Vermeulen A, Ando S, Verdonck L. Prolactinomas, testosterone-binding globulin, and androgen metabolism. J Clin Endocrinol. 1982; 54:409–412.

950. Vermeulen A, Deslypere JP, Schelfhout W, et

al. Adrenocortical function in old age; response to acute adrenocorticotropin stimulation. J Clin Endocrinol Metab. 1982; 54:187–191.

951. Vermeulen A, Ando S. Prolactin and adrenal androgen secretion. Clin Endocrinol (Oxf). 1978; 8:295–303.

952. Vermeulen A, Suy E, Rubens R. Effect of prolactin on plasma DHEA(S) levels. J Clin Endocrinol Metab. 1977; 44:1222–1225.

953. Vermeulen A, Verdonck L. Plasma androgen levels during the menstrual cycle. Am J Obstet Gynecol. 1976; 125:491–494.

954. Vermeulen A, Stoica T, Verdonck L. The apparent free testosterone concentration, an index of androgenicity. J Clin Endocrinol Metab. 1971; 33:759–767.

955. Vermeulen A, Verdonck L, Vandersiraften M, Orif N: Capacity of the testosterone-binding globulin in human plasma and influence of specific binding of testosterone on its metabolic clearance rate. J Clin Endocrinol Metab. 1969; 29:1470–1480.

956. Vician L, Shupnick MA, Gorski J. Effects of estrogen on primary ovine pituitary cell cultures: stimulation of prolactin secretion, synthesis, and prolactin messenger ribonucleic acid activity. Endocrinology. 1979; 104:736–743.

957. Vigersky RA, Mehlman I, Glass AR, et al. Treatment of hirsute women with cimetidine: a preliminary report. New Engl J Med. 1980; 303:1042–1044.

958. Virutamasen P, Wright KH, Wallach EE. Effects of prostaglandin E_2 and $F_{2\alpha}$ on ovarian contractility in the rabbit. Fertil Steril. 1972; 23:675–682.

959. von Werder K, Eversmann T, Rjosk HK, et al. Treatment of hyperprolactinemia. In: Ganong WF, Martini L, eds. Frontiers in Neuorendocrinology, Vol 7. New York: Raven Press, 1982:123–159.

960. Wallach EE. Induction of ovulation. In: Garcia CR, Mastroianni L Jr, Amelar RD, et al. eds. Current Therapy of Infertility. St. Louis: CV Mosby Co, 1982:157–160.

961. Wang CF, Gemzell C. The use of human gonadotropins for the induction of ovulation in women with polycystic ovarian disease. Fertil Steril. 1980; 33:479–486.

962. Wang CF, Hsueh AJW, Erickson GF. Induction of functional prolactin receptors by follicle-stimulating hormone in rat granulosa cells *in vivo* and *in vitro*. J Biol Chem. 1979; 254:11330–11336.

963. Wang CF, Lasley BL, Lein A, et al. The functional changes of the pituitary gonadotrophs during the menstrual cycle. J Clin Endocrinol Metab. 1976; 42:718–728.

964. Wang CF, Yen SSC. Direct evidence of estro-

gen modulation of pituitary sensitivity to luteinizing hormone-releasing factor during the menstrual cycle. J Clin Invest. 1975; 55:201–204.

965. Warren JC, Salhanick HA. Steroid biosynthesis in the human ovary. J Clin Endocrinol Metab. 1961; 21:1218–1230.

966. Weinheimer B, Oertel GW, Leppla W, et al. Plasma steroid concentrations of adrenal venous blood from women with and without hirsutism. Vermeulen A, Exley D (eds) In: Androgens in Normal and Pathological Conditions. Excerpta Medica Foundation Int Cong Series, Ghent 1966; 101:36–41.

967. Weiner RI, Ganong WF. Role of brain monoamines and histamine in regulation of anterior pituitary secretion. Physiol Rev. 1978; 58:905–976.

968. Weinstein D, Polishuk WZ. The role of wedge resection of the ovary as a cause for mechanical sterility. Surg Gynecol Obstet. 1975; 141:417–418.

969. Weiss NS, Szekley DR, Austin DF. Increasing incidence of endometrial cancer in the United States. New Engl J Med. 1976; 294:1259–1262.

970. Wentz AC, White RI Jr, Migeon CJ, et al. Differential ovarian and adrenal vein catheterization. Am J Obstet Gynecol. 1976; 125:1000–1007.

971. Wentz AC, Gutai JP, Jones GS, et al. Ovarian hyperthecosis in the adolescent patient. J Pediatr 1976; 88:488–493.

972. Wentz AC, Jones GS, Sapp KC. Effect of clomiphene on gonadotropin responses to LRH administration in secondary amenorrhea and oligomenorrhea. Obstet Gynecol. 1976; 47:677–683.

973. Wentz AC, Jones GS, Sapp KC: Pulsatile gonadotropin output in menstrual dysfunction. Obstet Gynecol. 1976; 47:309–318.

974. Werk EE Jr, Sholiton LJ, Kalejs L. Testosterone-secreting adrenal adenoma under gonadotropin control. New Engl J Med. 1973; 289:767–770.

975. Westfahl PK, Kling OR. Relationship of estradiol to luteal function in the cycling baboon. Endocrinology. 1982; 110:64–69.

976. White MC, Ginsburg J. The hirsute female. In: Crosignani PG, Rubin BL, eds. Endocrinology of Human Infertility: New Aspects. London: Academic Press, 1981:397–325.

977. White SS, Ojeda SR. Changes in ovarian LHRH receptor content during the onset of puberty in the female rat. Endocrinology. 1981; 108:347–349.

978. Wiebe RH, Morris CV. Testosterone/androstenedione ratio in the evaluation of women with

ovarian androgen excess. Obstet Gynecol. 1983; 61:279–284.

979. Wild RA, Umstot ES, Andersen RN, et al. Adrenal function in hirsutism. II. Effect of an oral contraceptive. J Clin Endocrinol Metab. 1982; 54:676–681.

980. Wildt L, Hutchinson JS, Marshall G, et al. On the site of action of progesterone in the blockade of the estradiol-induced gonadotropin discharge in the rhesus monkey. Endocrinology. 1981; 109:1293–1294.

981. Wildt L, Hausler A, Marshall G, et al. Frequency and amplitude of gonadotropin-releasing hormone stimulation and gonadotropin secretion in the rhesus monkey. Endocrinology. 1981; 109:376–385.

982. Wildt L, Marshall G, Knobil E. Experimental induction of puberty in the infantile female rhesus monkey. Science. 1980; 207:1373–1375.

983. Williams GH, Rose LI, Jagger PI, et al. A Turner's syndrome variant with polycystic ovaries and idiopathic myocardial hypertrophy. Ann Int Med. 1969; 70:571–576.

984. Williamson JG, Ellis JD. The induction of ovulation by tamoxifen. J Obstet Gynaecol Br Comm. 1973; 80:844–847.

985. Wilroy RS, Givens JR, Wiser WL, et al. Hyperthecosis: An inheritable form of polycystic ovarian disease. Birth Defects. 1975; 11:81–85.

986. Wilson EA, Erickson GF, Zarutski P, et al. Endocrine studies of normal and polycystic ovarian tissues in vitro. Am J Obstet Gynecol. 1979; 134:56–63.

987. Wilson EA. Diagnostic and therapeutic uses of sex steroids. In: Givens JR, ed. Endocrine Causes of Menstrual Disorders. Chicago: Year Book Med Publ, 1978:333–361.

988. Wilson SJ, Young BK, Katz M, et al. A gonadotropin-responsive virilizing granulosa tumor. Diag Gynecol Obstet. 1980; 2:275–281

989. Wingrave SJ, Kay CR, Vessey MP. Oral contraception and pituitary adenomas. Br Med J. 1980; 1:685–686.

990. Winter JSD, Faiman C, Reyes FI. Normal and abnormal pubertal development. Clin Obstet Gynecol. 1978; 21:67–86.

991. Winter JSD, Faiman C, Hobson WC, et al. Pituitary–gonadal relations in infancy. I. Patterns of serum gonadotropin concentrations from birth to four years of age in man and chimpanzee. J Clin Endocrinol Metab. 1975; 40:545–551.

992. Witorsch RJ, Kitay JI. Pituitary hormones affecting adrenal 5α-reductase activity: ACTH, growth hormone and prolactin. Endocrinology. 1972; 91:764–769.

993. Wood GP, Boronow RC. Endometrial adenocarcinoma and the polycystic ovary syndrome. Am J Obstet Gynecol. 1976; 124:140–142.

994. Woodard TL, Burghen GA, Kitabchi AE, et al. Glucose intolerance and insulin resistance in aplastic anemia treated with oxymetholone. J Clin Endocrinol Metab. 1981; 53:905–908.

995. Woodruff JD, Parmley TH. Virilizing ovarian tumors. In: Mahesh VB, Greenblatt RB, eds. Hirsutism and Virilism. Boston: John Wright, PSG Inc., 1983:129–158.

996. Wortsman J, Soler NG. Abnormalities of fuel metabolism in the polycystic ovary syndrome. Obstet Gynecol. 1982; 60:342–345.

997. Wortsman J, Singh KB, Murphy J. Evidence for the hypothalamic origin of the polycystic ovary syndrome. Obstet Gynecol. 1981; 58:137–141.

998. Wortsman J, Hirschowitz JS. Galactorrhea and hyperprolactinemia during treatment of polycystic ovary syndrome. Obstet Gynecol. 1980; 55:460–463.

999. Wright CS, Steele SJ, Jacobs HS. Value of bromocriptine in unexplained primary infertility: a double blind controlled study. Br Med J. 1979; 1:1037–1039.

1000. Wright F, Giacomini M. Reduction of dihydrotestosterone to androstanediols by human female skin in vitro. J Ster Biochem. 1980; 13:639–643.

1001. Wright F, Mowszowicz I, Mauvais-Jarvis P. Urinary 5α-androstane-3a, 17β-diol radioimmunoassay: a new clinical evaluation. J Clin Endocrinol Metab. 1978; 47:850–854.

1002. Wu CH. Estrogen–androgen balance in hirsutism. Fertil Steril. 1979; 32:269–275.

1003. Wu CH. Plasma hormones in clomiphene citrate therapy. Obstet Gynecol. 1977; 49:443–448.

1004. Wu RL, Shearman RP, Fraser IA. Is diagnostic gonadotrophin stimulation useful? Aust NZ J Obstet Gynaecol. 1980; 20:47–52.

1005. Wynder EL, Escher GC, Mantel N. An epidemiological investigation of cancer of the endometrium. Cancer. 1966; 19:489–520.

1006. Yamaji T, Ibayashi H: Plasma DHEA-S in normal and pathological conditions. J Clin Endocrinol Metab. 1969; 29:273–278.

1007. Yanaihara T, Troen P. Studies of the human testis. III. Effect of estrogen on testosterone formation in human testis in vitro. J Clin Endocrinol Metab. 1972; 34:968–973.

1008. Yarkoni S, Polishuk WZ, Spitz IM, et al. Inhibitory effect of hyperprolactinemia on induction of ovulation by gonadotropins. Fertil Steril. 1977; 28:772–774.

1009. Yates J, Deshpande N. Kinetic studies on the enzyme catalysing the conversion of 17α-hydroxyprogesterone and dehydroepiandros-terone in the human adrenal gland *in vitro.* J Endocrinol. 1974; 60:27–35.

1010. Yen SSC. Neuroendocrine regulation of the menstrual cycle. In: Krieger DT, Hughes JC, eds. Neuroendocrinology. Sunderland, Mass: Sinauer Associates, 1980:259–272.

1011. Yen SSC. The polycystic ovary syndrome. Clin Endocrinol (Oxf). 1980; 12:177–207.

1012. Yen SSC. Studies of the role of dopamine in the control of prolactin and gonadotropin secretion in humans. In: Fuxe K, Hokfelt T, Luft R, eds. Central Regulation of the Endocrine System. New York: Plenum Press, 1979:387–416.

1013. Yen SSC. Chronic anovulation due to inappropriate feedback system. In: Yen SSC, Jaffe R, eds. Reproductive Endocrinology. Philadelphia: WB Saunders Co., 1978:297–323.

1014. Yen SSC. The adenohypophysis; functional behavior of the gonadotrophs as target cells. In: Naftolin F, Ryan KJ, Davies IJ, eds. Subcellular Mechanisms in Reproductive Endocrinology. Amsterdam: Elsevier Press, 1976: 453–469.

1015. Yen SSC, Chaney C, Judd HL. Functional aberrations of the hypothalamic–pituitary system in polycystic ovary syndrome: a consideration of the pathogenesis. In: James VHT, Serio M, Giusti G, eds. The Endocrine Function of the Human Ovary. New York: Academic Press, 1976:373–385.

1016. Yen SSC, Lasley BL, Wang CF, et al. Recent advances in the neuroendocrine regulation of gonadotropin secretion In: James VHT, Serio M, Giusti G, eds. The Endocrine Function of the Human Ovary. New York: Academic Press, 1976:333–347.

1017. Yen SSC, Lasley BL, Wang CF, et al. The operating characteristics of the hypothalamic–pituitary system during the menstrual cycle and observations of biological action of somatostatin. Recent Prog Horm Res. 1975; 31:321–363.

1018. Yen SSC, Vandenberg G, Siler TM. Modulation of pituitary responsiveness to LRF by estrogen. J Clin Endocrinol Metab. 1974; 39:170–177.

1019. Yen SSC, Vandenberg G, Tsai CC, et al. Causal relationship between the hormonal variables in the menstrual cycle. In: Ferin M, Halberg F, Richart RM, Vande Wiele RL, eds. Biorhythms and Human Reproduction. New York: John Wiley & Sons, 1974:219–238.

1020. Yen SSC, Rebar R, Vandenberg G, et al. Clinical studies with synthetic LRF. In: Gual C, Rosenberg E, eds. Hypothalamic Hypophysiotropic Hormones: Physiological and Clinical Studies. Amsterdam: Excerpta Medica, 1973:217–229.

1021. Yen SSC, Rebar R, Vandenberg G, et al. Pituitary gonadotrophin responsiveness to synthetic LRF in subjects with normal and abnormal hypothalamic–pituitary–gonadal axis. J Reprod Fertil (Suppl). 1973; 20:137–161.

1022. Yen SSC, Vandenberg G, Rebar R, et al. Variation of pituitary responsiveness to synthetic LRF during different phases of the menstrual cycle. J Clin Endocrinol Metab. 1972; 35:931–934.

1023. Yen SSC, Tsai CC, Vandenberg G, et al. Gonadotropin dynamics in patients with gonadal dysgenesis. A model for the study of gonadotropin regulation. J Clin Endocrinol Metab. 1972; 35:897–904.

1024. Yen SSC, Tsai CC, Naftolin F, et al. Pulsatile patterns of gonadotropin release in subjects with and without ovarian function. J Clin Endocrinol Metab. 1972; 34:671–675.

1025. Yen SSC, Tsai CC. Acute gonadotropin release induced by exogenous estradiol during the mid-follicular phase of the menstrual cycle. J Clin Endocrinol Metab. 1972; 34:298–305.

1026. Yen SSC, Tsai CC. The effect of ovariectomy on gonadotropin release. J Clin Invest. 1971; 50:1149–1153.

1027. Yen SSC, Tsai CC. The biphasic pattern in the feedback action of ethinyl estradiol on the release of pituitary FSH and LH. J Clin Endocrinol Metab. 1971; 33:882–887.

1028. Yen SSC, Vela P, Ryan KJ. Effect of clomiphene citrate in polycystic ovarian syndrome relationship between serum gonadotropin and corpus luteum function. J Clin Endocrinol Metab. 1970; 31:7–13.

1029. Yen SSC, Vela P, Rankin J. Inappropriate secretion of follicle-stimulating hormone and luteinizing hormone in polycystic ovarian disease. J Clin Endocrinol Metab. 1970; 30:435–442.

1030. Ying SY, Ling N, Bohlen P, et al. Gonadocrinins: peptides in ovarian follicular fluid stimulating the secretion of pituitary gonadotropins. Endocrinology. 1981; 108:1206–1215.

1031. Young JR, Jaffe RB. Strength-duration characteristics of estrogen effects on gonadotropin response to gonadotropin-releasing hormone in women. II. Effects of varying concentrations of estradiol. J Clin Endocrinol Metab. 1976; 42:432–442.

1032. Yuzpe AA, Rioux JE. The value of laparoscopic ovarian biopsy. J Reprod Med. 1975; 15:57–59.

1033. Zarate A, Canales ES, de la Cruz A, et al. Pituitary response to synthetic LH-RH in Stein-Leventhal syndrome and functional amenorrhea. Obstet Gynecol. 1973; 41:803–808.

1034. Zarate A, Canales ES, Soria J, et al. Ovarian refractoriness during lactation in women: effect of gonadotropin stimulation. Am J Obstet Gynecol. 1972; 112:1130–1132.

1035. Zarate A, Hernandez-Ayup S, Rios-Montiel A. Treatment of anovulation in the Stein-Leventhal syndrome. Analysis of 90 cases. Fertil Steril. 1971; 22:188–193.

1036. Zeleznik AJ. Premature elevation of systemic estradiol reduces serum levels of follicle-stimulating hormone and lengthens the follicular phase of the menstrual cycle in rhesus monkeys. Endocrinology. 1981; 109:352–355.

1037. Zeleznik AJ, Midgley AR, Reichert LE. Granulosa cell maturation in the rat: increased binding of human chorionic gonadotropin following treatment with follicle-stimulating hormone *in vivo*. Endocrinology. 1974; 95:818–825.

1038. Ziel HK, Finkle WD. Increased risk of endometrial carcinoma among users of conjugated estrogens. New Engl J Med. 1975; 293:1167–1170.

1039. Zimmerman EA. Evaluation of the patient with an asymptomatic enlarged sella turcica. In: Tindal GT, Collins WF, eds. Clinical Management of Pituitary Disorders. New York: Raven Press, 1979:171–178.

1040. Zorn EM, Wieland RG, Hallberg MC. 17β-ol androgens and free index in hirsute and hirsute obese women. Fertil Steril. 1976; 27:916–920.

1041. Zourlas PA, Jones HW Jr. Stein-Leventhal syndrome with masculinizing ovarian tumors. Report of 3 cases. Obstet Gynecol. 1969; 34:861–866.

Index